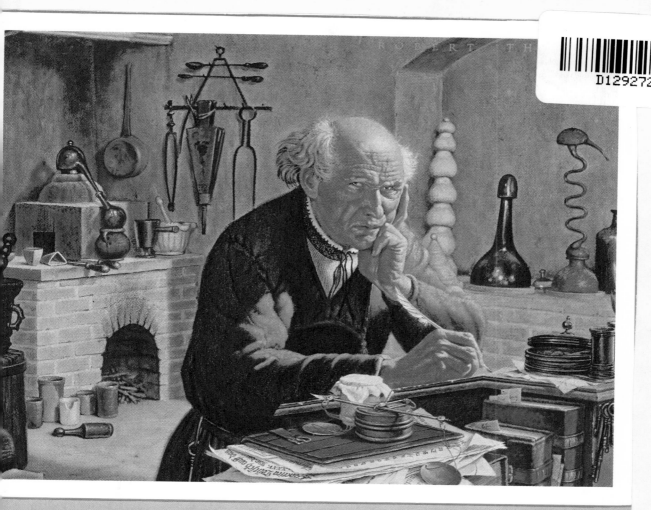

e field of medical history is a most fascinating and ructive one, and nobody who has approached it escaped its charm.

here have been several illustrated histories of icine; yet this attempt to present the history of icine in text accompanied by specially commis- ed original oil paintings, is unique. This technique several definite advantages, not the least of which at it allows a systematic coverage independent of t pictorial material has been left by the accidents story. Inclusion or exclusion of the one or the other rical personality or episode may forever be debat- ; yet no competent or objective critic will deny the plan of *Great Moments In Medicine* as a whole ally gives a complete and fair image of the evolu- of medicine.

picture—especially if it is lively and colorful, eys many facets of history more easily, more eably, and more strikingly than the written word e could do. On the other hand, the reader will find

most excellently presented those ramifications and bits of comparative information which pictures alone can- not give, and guidance and inspiration for further study.

Unique, too, has been the sponsorship of this monu- mental undertaking by a pharmaceutical house. While entailing a large investment both in time and money, this project has been carried on in such good taste that only commendation can accrue to its sponsors.

Ten years of intensive study and over a quarter million miles of travel were devoted by the author- artist team to research for this series of stories and paintings. Where possible, actual sites where events had taken place were visited; and expert advisors in many fields of history and science were consulted.

This book has been produced with a fine sense of responsibility and as much accuracy as available historical evidence permitted. It can therefore be recommended for enjoyment as well as for educational and reference purposes.

Great Moments
in Medicine

Great Moments
in Medicine

The stories and paintings in the series

A History of Medicine
in Pictures

By

PARKE, DAVIS & COMPANY

Stories By

GEORGE A. BENDER

Paintings By

ROBERT A. THOM

DETROIT
NORTHWOOD INSTITUTE PRESS
1966

CONTENTS

PREFACE

MEDICINE, the profession of the art and science of prevention, cure, or relief of disease, has a history inextricably interwoven with the history of the human race. When recorded history came into being, the practice of medicine was old.

The profession has a proud heritage of more than fifty centuries of service to humanity, built upon a foundation of concern for the welfare of fellow men and women.

It was to immortalize the high lights of service of these countless generations of medical men in a new and different way that Parke-Davis undertook development of *A History of Medicine in Pictures*. These original paintings, supplementing stories of outstanding persons and events whose contributions have moved Medicine forward, provide a new and different approach to a concept all too little appreciated by those of us who are beneficiaries of longer lives and better health brought about by better medicines and better medical practitioners.

Among all who have contributed to make *Great Moments in Medicine* possible, special thanks must go to Artist Robert A. Thom for his sincere interest and cooperation, his indefatigable research, and his enlightened pictorial interpretations; to Dr. Erwin H. Ackerknecht for his expert advice and guidance, and his good-humored but firm counsel to the author-artist team; and to Parke-Davis executives whose breadth of vision made this project possible.

If, from these combined efforts, there results a better understanding of the contribution of medicine to world health, then this project will have fulfilled the aims of those who have given to it long hours of planning, of conference, of labor, of search, and of research.

GEORGE A. BENDER

Detroit, Michigan

MEDICINE IN ANCIENT EGYPT

ROOTS of the profession of medicine are buried far back before the dawn of history. Nearly as old as mankind itself, practice of medical procedures in some form has paralleled man's development. In not a few instances, the quality or lack of quality of medical service has profoundly influenced the course of civilizations. Throughout the dawning millennia and much of their recorded history, medicine was intimately associated with the magico-religious practices of various peoples groping for the light of knowledge and a better way of life.

The most ancient records presently known indicate the existence of two centers of civilizations having nearly equal development in two of the world's great river systems: in Mesopotamia, between the Tigris and the Euphrates; and in the Nile valley of northeastern Africa. Organized peoples, enjoying the natural habitational advantages of these areas, were flourishing 6,000 years ago.

Methods of recording events began some ten centuries later, about 3000 B.C., and from that point on, history has for its base a series of factual foundations. However, when recorded history dawned, medicine was already a well-developed profession, and its practitioners had a heritage of experience, knowledge and beliefs handed down from a long line of predecessors by precept and word-of-mouth through countless centuries.

Egypt first became an organized nation about 3000 B.C. Medical interest centers upon a period in the Third Dynasty (2980-2900 B.C.) when Egypt had an ambitious Pharaoh named Zoser; and Zoser, in turn, had for his chief counselor and minister a brilliant noble named Imhotep (whose name means "he who cometh in peace"). Imhotep is said to have constructed the famous step pyramid of Sakkarah, near Memphis, for Pharaoh Zoser. A versatile man, Imhotep seems to have been a priest, a magician, and a poet. But in the Egyptian writings of the Greco-Roman period (third century, B.C.) Imhotep is represented as a physician, and is assigned the role of god of medicine in Egypt. The Greeks identified him with their Asklepios, to whom was attributed

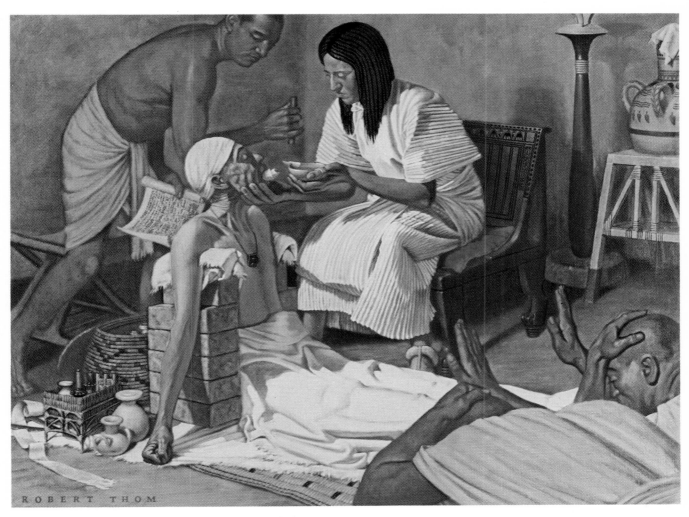

MEDICINE IN ANCIENT EGYPT

An Egyptian physician of the Eighteenth Dynasty (1500-1400 B.C.), clothed in clean white linen and a wig, as became the dignity of his status, is confronted with a patient having symptoms of lockjaw (described in an ancient scroll now known as the Edwin Smith papyrus). With sure, sympathetic hands, the physician treats the patient, who is supported by a "brick chair." Directions for treatment appear on the scroll held by his assistant. Specially trained priests observe prescribed magico-religious rites. Egyptian medicine occupied a dominant position in the world of the ancients for 2500 years.

a similar regard. In this later period, temples were erected to Imhotep in which patients looked for and supposedly found relief in their sleep.

There is a close association in Egyptian medicine between religion and magic. Egyptian physicians used many drugs, but thought their effects primarily magical. The papyri (so called because they were written on sheets prepared from the papyrus plant) dealing exclusively with medicine abound with magic formulas and prayers. "In some cases in which human help seemed to be impossible," observes Hermann Ranke, "a last attempt was made to get help from a supernatural source . . ." a practice not incompatible with that of the religious-minded physician of today who through prayer seeks aid and guidance. The gods of the Egyptians were no less real to them than is our deity to us.

Medicine as practiced by the ancient Egyptians was not primitive, however. Just as they had transcended primitive levels in statecraft, agriculture, technology, and especially architecture and art, so did the Egyptians also reach higher levels in medicine. Some medical papyri are predominantly religious, but others are predominantly empirico-rational. Strangely enough, those recording the more rational observations stem from the earliest periods (1600-1500 B.C.). Among these are the Edwin Smith papyrus and the Ebers papyrus. The first was intended primarily for the use of a surgeon; the latter is a collection of recipes for the physician. Each of these documents, though ancient in its own right, appears by language and explanations to reflect traditions much older. Says Ranke of the Smith papyrus: "That the bulk of the main text goes back to the Old Kingdom (about 2500 B.C.) is shown by a great number of glosses [explanatory notes] added to the text of some of the cases, which explains words that in the course of time had become obsolete." Breasted dates the Smith papyrus in the seventeenth century B.C., but states that it is a copy of a document at least one thousand years older.

Dealing primarily with wounds, the Edwin Smith papyrus is admired for the diagnostic acumen exhibited in the case histories detailed, where symptoms such as feeble pulse (2500 years before reference to the pulse appears in Greek medical treatises), palsy, and deafness are all recorded and referred to as due to one common cause—a head wound. In addition to many surgical conditions, a great number of recognizable internal afflictions are reported in the papyri, such as worms, eye diseases, diabetes, rheumatism and schistosomiasis. The ancient existence of some of these conditions is confirmed by palaeo-pathology (the examination of bones and tissues of mummies for evidence of disease); and, unfortunately, those afflictions are still prevalent in Egypt.

The papyri prescribe many rational methods of treatment, such as diet, physiotherapy, and drugs. Many of the drugs named undoubtedly were worthless, but some, such as tannic acid, turpentine, gentian, senna, and lead, and copper salts, are still used in medical practice. Castor oil, used externally and internally, was a great favorite with the doctors of Egypt. The style used in prescription writing today is much the same as when these papyri were written.

The cases of the Edwin Smith papyrus are not only systematically constructed, each within itself, but their arrangement throughout is a systematic one. First comes a superscription, which briefly gives the name of the illness. This is followed by a careful description, which always begins with the words, "If you examine a man who . . ." has this or that illness. Then comes a diagnosis that always begins with the words, "You should say" he suffered from this or that ailment. This diagnosis always ends with the words: "An ailment which . . ." and then one of three possibilities follows. The surgeon may say: "An ailment which I shall treat," or, "An ailment which I shall combat," or, "An ailment which I will not treat." (The latter discrimination was practiced by some physicians in almost all periods and was regarded as ethical up to the eighteenth century.) Except in entirely hopeless cases, there followed a method of treatment, beginning with the words, "You must do . . ." this or that. Then the healing substances are given.

Of the 48 surgical dissertations in the Smith papyrus, Case 7 is of particular interest. According to Breasted's translation, it reads, in part:

"[If thou examinest a man having a gaping wound in his head, penetrating to the bone, (and) perforating the sutures of his skull], thou should palpate his wound, (although) he shudders exceedingly. Thou shouldst cause him to lift his face; if it is painful for him to open his mouth, (and) his heart beats feebly; if thou observe his spittle hanging at his two lips and not falling off, while he discharges blood from *both his nostrils (and) from both his ears; he suffers with stiffness in his neck, (and) is unable to look at his two shoulders and his breast, thou shouldst say regarding him: [here the findings are restated]. An ailment with which I will contend."*

Directions for treatment follow:

"Now as soon as thou findest that the cord of that man's mandible, his jaw, is contracted, thou shouldst have made for him something hot, until he is comfortable, so that his mouth opens. Thou shouldst bind it with grease, honey, (and) lint, until thou knowst that he has reached a decisive point."

Two other possible examinations are outlined—the second, in which:

"The flesh of that man has developed fever . . . his countenance is clammy with sweat, the ligaments of his neck are tense, his face is ruddy, (and) . . . the odor of the chest of his head [crown] is like the urine of sheep, his mouth is bound, (and) both his eyebrows are drawn, while his face is as if he wept . . ." This, the ancient author admonishes, is *"An ailment not to be treated."*

The ancient observer offers a third possible finding:

"If, however, thou findest that that man has become pale and has already shown exhaustion . . . Thou shouldst have made for him a wooden brace padded with linen and put into his mouth. Thou shouldst have made for him a draught of the w'h fruit [probably a nutritious fruit or grain]. His treatment is sitting, placed between two supports of brick, until thou knowest he has reached a decisive point."

This early physician evidently recognized that if tetanus had invaded the wound, there was little he could do; but until he was certain, he would try to improve the patient's condition.

Egyptian physicians were highly respected all over the ancient world for thousands of years. Homer regarded them as the best in his time. Egyptian physicians were called to the courts of Persian emperors and other Eastern potentates; and only in the sixth century B.C. were they replaced by Greek physicians. Beyond the psychotherapeutic values of magic and religion, Egyptian medical men made solid advances in observation and rational treatment. Their contributions are worthy of a place beside other accomplishments of this great ancient civilization. The dominant position occupied by Egyptian medicine for 2,500 years seems fully justified.

WORLD EVENTS AND MEDICAL HISTORY

The history of Medicine and lives of persons who contributed to its advance were influenced by shifting populations, political changes, and social developments.

Dates, persons, and events of significance to the evolution of Medicine include:

B. C.

550,000	End of Pliocene Age. First known race of man — *Pithecanthropus erectus*.
110,000	Second race—*Eoanthropus*.
50,000	Third race—*Neanderthal*.
35,000	Beginning of Late Palaeolithic Age. Fourth race—*Cro-Magnon*.
7000-2000	Neolithic Age in Europe.
5000-4500	Dawn of Sumerian, Egyptian, and Minoan cultures.
3400-2500	Old Kingdom: Egypt.
2980	Imhotep.
2900-2625	Age of the pyramid builders.
2500	Surgical operations depicted upon tomb of Pharaohs at Saqquarah.
2445-1731	Middle Kingdom: Egypt.
2000	Code of Hammurabi (Babylon).
2000-1000	Bronze Age in Europe.
1500	Edwin Smith Papyrus. Ebers Papyrus.
1237	Death of Asclepius.
1000-500	Earlier Iron Age in Europe.
950	Homer.
800	Period of Brahminic medicine. Building of Carthage.
753	Founding of Rome.
600	Massage and acupuncture practiced by the Japanese.
580-489	Pythagoras.
550	Buddha, Confucius, Lao Tse lived about this time.
539	Cyrus founded the Persian Empire.
525	Asclepius raised to rank of God of Medicine in Greece.
522	Democedes founded a medical school at Athens.
521	Darius I ruled from the Hellespont to the Indies.
500	Later Iron Age (La Tène culture).
490	Battle of Marathon.
484	Herodotus.
480	Thermopylae and Salamis.
460-361	Hippocrates.
431-404	Peloponnesian War.
429-347	Plato.
384-322	Aristotle.
370-286	Theophrastus of Eresos.
338-323	Alexander the Great.
146	Carthage, Corinth destroyed.
120-63	Mithridates VI.
44	Julius Caesar assassinated.
4	Birth of Jesus of Nazareth.
31 B.C.-14 A.D.	Augustus Caesar.

A. D.

14-37	Tiberius. Celsus.
30	Jesus of Nazareth crucified.
23-79	Pliny the Elder.
54-68	Nero. Dioscorides.
61	Boadicea of Britain massacred by Romans.
79	Plague following eruption of Vesuvius. Pompeii destroyed.
117-138	Hadrian; Roman Empire at height. Aretaeus. Soranus of Ephesus.
130-201	Galen.
161	Marcus Aurelius rules Rome.
220	End of Han Dynasty in China.
303	Martyrdom of Saints Cosmas and Damian.
306	Constantine the Great becomes Emperor of Roman Empire.
369	Hospital of St. Basil erected at Caesarea by Justinian.
395-1453	Byzantine Empire.
400	Fabiola founds first nosocomium (hospital) in Western Europe.
451	Attila raided Gaul.
476	Fall of Western Roman Empire.
527-565	Justinian I. Aëtius of Amida.
528	Monte Cassino founded.
542	Nosocomia founded at Lyons by Childebert I and at Arles by Caesarius.
568-774	Establishment of Lombards in Italy.
571-632	Mohammed.
622	Mohammed's Hegira.
651	Hôtel-Dieu founded by Saint Landry, Bishop of Paris.
711	Moslems invaded Spain from Africa.
749-1258	Eastern Caliphate.
768-814	Charlemagne.
786-802	Reign of Haroun al-Rashid in Bagdad.
820-1517	Rise of Venetian Republic.
848-856	School of Salerno first heard of.
865-925	Rhazes (smallpox and measles).
871-901	Alfred the Great.
980-1036	Avicenna.
1020-1087	Constantinus Africanus.
1066	Battle of Hastings.
1096-1272	Crusades.
1099	Order of St. John of Jerusalem founded.
1110-1113	University of Paris founded.
1126-1198	Averroës, Arab philosopher, in Cordoba. Avenzoar.

THE CODE OF HAMMURABI

THE rich lands which lie between the Euphrates and Tigris rivers, Mesopotamia, now part of Iraq, often have been called "the cradle of civilization." Contemporary with Egypt, there were organized communities in the twin valleys as long as 6,000 years ago, with evidence of the existence of physicians as early as 3000 B.C. When Mesopotamian peoples began to record the happenings of their day on clay tablets or stone, Medicine was a well-recognized profession.

Unlike Egypt, the peoples, the languages, and the governments of Mesopotamia underwent many changes throughout the years during which ancient civilization flourished there. Although various groups such as the Sumerians, Akkadians, Amorites, Assyrians, Elamites, and Chaldeans, paraded across the historicopolitical stage of this ancient land, the ancient indigenous culture prevailed and absorbed each group of newcomers. In spite of political vagaries, there was basically one Mesopotamian civilization, which is often loosely called Babylonian. Social, religious, and way-of-life patterns varied little, and the practice of the healing arts seems not to have changed considerably throughout the millennia. In ancient Mesopotamia, the basic concepts concerning disease and its treatment were apparently religious.

Seals of Sumerian physicians, at least 5,000 years old, and ancient Sumerian prescriptions are known. Also, there is a rather extensive documentation on Mesopotamian medicine written in cuneiform script on clay tablets. However, one of the oldest documents, and one of significance to medicine, is the Code of Hammurabi. This is one of the oldest known law collections, promulgated by the Babylonian King Hammurabi, toward the end of his reign. There is no agreement among authorities as to the time of Hammurabi's reign. Dates as early as 2123 B.C. and as late as 1686 B.C. are given. Therefore, the origin of the Code can be placed only in the general area of 2000 B.C. Obviously it is a codification of much older laws and customs.

This extremely interesting document, preserved on a pillar of black diorite standing now in the Louvre, in Paris, France, deals with all phases of economic and family life in ancient Mesopotamia. Of its 282

14

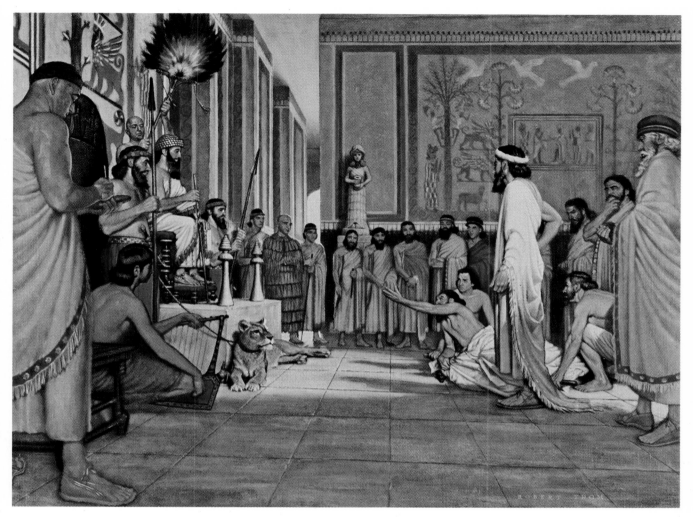

THE CODE OF HAMMURABI

The clay tablets of ancient Mesopotamia document the practice of medicine as early as 3000 B.C. Of significance to medicine, too, is one of the oldest regulatory laws, the Code of Hammurabi, promulgated by that Babylonian ruler about 2000 B.C. In a Babylonian throne room, a physician is defending with dignity his professional practices against the complaints of a dissatisfied patient who seeks invocation of the drastic penalties of the Code. The King, the scribe, court attachés, guards, priests, friends of plaintiff and of defendant, comprise the cast of this critical drama of law and of medicine 4000 years ago.

paragraphs, 11 refer to the practices of physicians and veterinarians. Several substantially similar translations are available. Excerpts of one by Charles Edwards, of London, paragraphs 215-224, follow:

"If a doctor has treated a Freeman with a metal knife for a severe wound, and has cured the Freeman, or has opened a Freeman's tumor with a metal knife, and cured a Freeman's eye, then he shall receive ten shekels of silver.

"If the son of a plebeian, he shall receive five shekels of silver.

"If a man's slave, the owner of the slave shall give two shekels of silver to the doctor.

"If a doctor has treated a man with a metal knife for a severe wound, and has caused the man to die, or has opened a man's tumor with a metal knife and destroyed the man's eye, his hands shall be cut off.

"If a doctor has treated the slave of a plebeian with a metal knife for a severe wound and caused him to die, he shall render slave for slave.

"If he has opened his tumor with a metal knife and destroyed his eye, he shall pay half his price in silver.

"If a doctor has healed a Freeman's broken bone or has restored diseased flesh, the patient shall give the doctor five shekels of silver.

"If he be the son of a plebeian, he shall give three shekels of silver.

"If a man's slave, the owner of the slave shall give two shekels of silver to the doctor.

"If a doctor of oxen or asses has treated either ox or ass for a severe wound, and cured it, the owner of the ox or ass shall give to the doctor one sixth of a shekel of silver as his fee."

Here is rather grim evidence of a regular, recognized medical profession existing 4,000 years ago that attempted at least minor surgery, observed its legal responsibilities, and operated on a government-controlled sliding fee schedule, all based on the social status of the patient. The influence of this Code spread far beyond Babylonia, as is demonstrated in the Old Testament and in ancient Jewish philosophies of "an eye for an eye and a tooth for a tooth." Abraham, originally a citizen of the Mesopotamian city-state of Ur, founded the Hebrew nation at about the same period that Hammurabi ruled Babylon. "Through Judaism, Christianity and Islam, ancient Mesopotamian

16

institutions have survived to the present day in the West and in the East," says Sigerist.

Ancient Mesopotamians believed that the air was filled with disease-producing demons who could attack humans when the gods, offended by some sin of the patient, stopped protecting him. Also, sorcerers could mobilize these demons. Hammurabi's code provides ordeal, and even the death penalty, for such acts by sorcerers.

Divination was developed to an extraordinary degree by Mesopotamians. Many techniques were used. Their systems of dream interpretation still influence the superstitious today. Their stargazing, though done for magical rather than scientific reasons, acquainted them with a number of important astronomical facts. They left amazingly precise clay models of sheep livers, because the livers of sacrificed animals were another source of prophecies and divinations. Priests were trained to be specialists in the observation of this organ.

Divination also was used for the "diagnosis" of disease. That is, practitioners attempted to determine what sin the patient had committed, what god had to be pacified, and what demon had to be driven out. Treatment then consisted primarily of prayers and animal sacrifices to the gods, and of exorcism (the recitation of spells) to drive out the spirits. Often great poetic beauty was achieved in these chants. In addition, drugs and physiotherapeutic measures were employed.

The separation of medicine and priestcraft seems not to have advanced as far in Mesopotamia as it did in Egypt, yet there is evidence of a tendency in this direction. In the famous book on prognosis, "*When the incantation priest goes to the house of a sick man . . .*" the observation of symptoms may be found replacing the observation of omens. Case histories set down on the clay tablets of Babylonia are less elaborate, but similar in style and content to those of Egyptian papyri. They consisted of descriptions of symptoms, prognosis, and indications for treatment. Certain pathologic conditions, such as migraine, otitis media, jaundice, pleurisy, and kidney stones, may be recognized from the texts of the clay tablets.

The armamentarium of the ancient Mesopotamian physician was very rich in drugs—even though the drugs were credited with magical rather than pharmacodynamic values. Hyoscyamus, hellebore, hemp, mandrake, opium, and belladonna, as well as mineral and animal substances have been identified as elements of Babylonian prescriptions. Thompson reports having found 250 vegetable substances and 120 minerals in an "Assyrian Herbal" reconstructed from cuneiform tablets found in King Ashurbanipal's library. Even by modern standards, some of the therapy prescribed seems quite rational. For instance, poppy and mandrake were used to relieve pain and to produce sleep; mustard for counterirritation; elaterium for catharsis; sulfur for scabies; cannabis for neuralgia and mental depression; belladonna as an anodyne, to relieve bladder spasm and dysmenorrhea, and for asthma.

Like that of ancient Egypt, ancient Mesopotamian medicine, especially its drug lore, undoubtedly had a certain influence on early Greek medicine, and thereby, indirectly on modern medical practice. Of incomparably greater medical importance, however, as Ackerknecht points out, was the powerful influence that Babylonia exerted on Judaism, transmitting to it many of its myths, theories, and laws, including the ideas of contagion and isolation, and of the weekly day of rest. It is from Judaism that the world's Western civilization inherited these concepts. Both of these ideas have been of immeasurable importance over the centuries in the prevention of disease.

WORLD EVENTS AND MEDICAL HISTORY

Dates, persons, and events of significance to the evolution of Medicine include:

1131	Council of Rheims forbid clerics to practice medicine.
1135-1204	Moses Maimonides.
1137	St. Bartholomew's Hospital (London) founded by Rahere.
1140	King Roger II of Sicily restricted medical practice to licentiates.
1158	University of Bologna founded.
1180	University of Montpellier founded.
1198	Frederick II (aged 4) became King of Sicily.
1193-1280	Albertus Magnus.
1198	Hospital movement inaugurated by Innocent III.
1201	Oxford first called a university.
1204	Innocent III opened Santo Spirito in Sassia Hospital (Rome).
1210	Collège de St. Côme founded at Paris by Jean Pitard.
1211	Innocent III recognized University of Paris.
1212	Children's Crusade.
1214-1294	Roger Bacon.
1215	Magna Charta signed in Britain.
1215	St. Thomas's Hospital founded.
1222	University of Padua started.
1223	Cambridge became a university.
1227-1274	Thomas Aquinas.
1231	Medical school at Salerno.
1235-1311	Arnold of Villanova.
1240	Law of Frederick II favoring dissection and regulating practice of medicine and pharmacy.
1244-1245	University of Oxford chartered.
1246-1248	University of Siena started.
1252-1517	Mameluke Dynasties (Egypt).
1257	Sorbonne founded at Paris.
1260-1320	Henri de Mondeville.
1266	End of Western Caliphate.
1270-1280	Spectacles introduced by Venetians.
1271	Marco Polo began travels.
1280	Kublai Khan founded Yuan (Mongol) Dynasty in China.
1300-1368	Guy de Chauliac.
1303	Universities of Rome chartered.
1319	First criminal prosecution for body snatching.
1330	Gunpowder used in warfare.
1336-1453	Hundred Years' War.
1345	First apothecary shop in London.
1347	University of Prague chartered.
1348	Gonville and Caius College (University of Cambridge) founded.
1348-1350	Black Death (magna mortalitas).
1368	Ming Dynasty succeeds Yuan Dynasty in China.
1376	Board of medical examiners in London.
1385	University of Heidelberg chartered.
1402	University of Würzburg chartered.
1429-1431	Syphilis first mentioned.
1440-1450	Invention of printing.
1443	Hôtel-Dieu de Beaune, France, founded.
1452-1519	Leonardo da Vinci.
1454	Gutenberg Bible printed.
1457	Gutenberg Purgation-Calendar (first medical publication).
1477	Universities of Tübingen and Upsala founded.
1478	Spanish Inquisition.
1479	First edition of Avicenna printed.
1490-1553	Rabelais.
1492	Discovery of America by Columbus.
1493-1541	Paracelsus.
1497	Scurvy on Vasco da Gama's voyage.
1498	Florentine *Receptario* (first official pharmacopoeia).
1505	Royal College of Surgeons of Edinburgh chartered.
1505	University of Seville chartered.
1509-1547	Reign of Henry VIII in England.
1510-1590	Ambroise Paré.
1514-1564	Andreas Vesalius.
1517	Luther propounded his theses at Wittenberg.
1518	Royal College of Physicians (England) founded (September 23).
1519-1556	Charles V, King of Spain and Emperor of Germany.
1524	Cortes erected hospital in Mexico.
1526	Paracelsus founded chemotherapy.
1530	Collège de France (Paris) founded.
1536	Paracelsus' *Chirurgia Magna* published.
1538	Vesalius published his *Tabulae Anatomicae Sex*.
1538	University of Santo Tomas (San Domingo) founded.
1540	English barbers and surgeons united as "Commonalty of the Barbers and Surgeons."
1540	Valerius Cordus discovered sulfuric ether.
1543	Copernicus described revolution of planets around the sun.
1543	Vesalius published the *Fabrica*.
1543	English apothecaries legalized by Act of Parliament.
1544	Albert III founded University of Königsberg (August 17).

TREPHINING IN ANCIENT PERU

ONE of the more important of medical phenomena, historically speaking, is that of trephining—a "surgical operation in life on the head and skull." Skulls 8,000 to 10,000 years old, bearing the marks of trephination, are about the only evidence available of the medical activities of prehistoric man in the Old World. Such skulls also provide the earliest evidence of medical activities in the New World Stone Age —which in most areas lasted until the coming of white men in the 1500's A.D.

Whether the practice of trephining originated independently in various parts of the world, or stemmed from some original center in the Old World, remains undetermined. Evidences of the practice of making openings in human skulls by artificial surgical means may be traced from prehistoric days until the present. Trephined skulls have been found in France and in other parts of Europe, in northern Africa, Asia, New Guinea, Tahiti, and New Zealand. In the New World the practice had extensive distribution, evidences having been found from Kodiak Island in Alaska, among both inland and west coast Indians, and on through the Americas to the Andes regions of South America. There is a school of anthropologists and ethnologists who believe that the ancient peoples of North and South America crossed a once-existing natural land bridge across the Bering Strait, bringing with them techniques and cultures from Eurasian sources. These people are thought to have penetrated as far south as the Strait of Magellan, where, according to Junius Bird, nomadic hunters existed in the seventh millennium B.C. Hrdlicka states his belief that "with a procedure of such complexity [as trephining], it would seem much more probable that it had spread from some original center in the Old World until finally it was transmitted to America. Its extensive distribution [in the Western Hemisphere] speaks strongly for its Asiatic transmission."

Peru apparently was the center of intensive practice of trephining in the New World. In this area, use of the operation can be traced

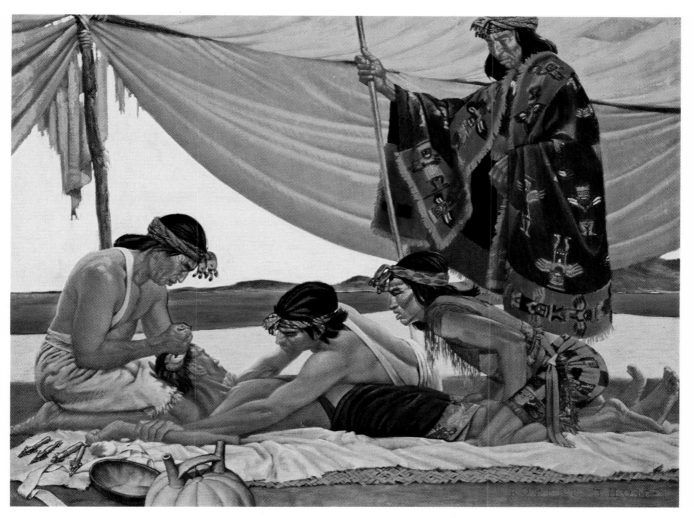

TREPHINING IN ANCIENT PERU

On the dry, sun-swept Pacific coastline of the Paracas peninsula, a first-century Peruvian surgeon is beginning a trephining operation with the aid of knives of glass-hard obsidian, a crude plant narcotic, cotton, and bandages. Assistants immobilize the patient, and a priest seeks supernatural intervention through incantations and prayers as the slow and highly hazardous operation proceeds. Peru was the center of intensive practice of trephining in the New World, where the operation (opening of the skulls of living patients) can be traced from well before dawn of the Christian era to the twentieth century.

from well before the beginning of the Christian era until the twentieth century.

The ancient Peruvians had no written language, in the manner of ancient European and Asian civilizations, and we are unable to read the knotted strings (quipus) that probably served them as records and documents. Therefore, most information about the Peruvians stems from the examination of mummies and the funereal bundles that surrounded them, and from their magnificent pottery, on which were represented many figures of persons having diseased conditions, including mutilations resulting from such infections as uta (leishmaniasis) and Carrion's disease. Medical scenes and procedures also are depicted on these ancient Peruvian ceramic "documents," which were fashioned with great skill, artistry, and no small degree of native humor.

Although nomads existed much earlier, and definite centers of civilization can be identified in South America as early as 2500 B.C., it was among the sedentary peoples along the narrow western coastlines that evidence of trephining is most abundant. The Chimu and Mochica civilizations, dating from about 500 B.C., show such evidence. Their graves contain many trephined skulls, and their pottery, into the shaping of which went reflections of almost every daily activity, shows trephination scenes. The richest source of data on the subject, however, comes from the Paracas, a small group of well-advanced civilized people who occupied an area around the Paracas Peninsula, south of Lima. This civilization preceded the founding of the Inca empire by several centuries, and it had been forgotten by the time the Incas were conquered by the Spaniards.

"The people of Paracas were not only artistic geniuses [as demonstrated by their exquisite, intricate weavings, feather art, and fire-engraved pottery] but men of science, as well," says Rebeca Carrion Cachot. "Great conquests were made in the field of medicine and especially that of surgery . . . There are audacious trephinations which cover extensive areas of the skull. The openings were covered with gold plates."

The percentage of successfully trephined skulls in Peruvian collections is unique. These ancient Peruvians succeeded in an operation

22

that, up to the end of the nineteenth century, was regarded by Western surgeons as highly dangerous. Evidence of repetition of the operation on an individual has been found: one skull bears five trephination holes. That the patient survived is demonstrated in many instances by evidence that postoperative healing processes had taken place.

Frequent employment of trephination in Peru might have been associated with several common disorders. Wounds of the head undoubtedly were a primary reason, as Muñiz and McGee point out: "If we take into account the class of offensive weapons [slings, large wooden clubs, star-maces, stone clubs and hatchets] used by the ancient Peruvians in their terrible conflicts, almost hand to hand, it will easily be comprehended that complex fracture of the skull with depression of its bony plates must have been very common." Many trephined skulls indicate that such comminuted fractures preceded the operation. Yet trephination probably was used also in attempts to relieve headaches or mental disease. The prevalent practice of artificially deforming the skull (occipital flattening, and fronto-occipital flattening) may have given rise to a higher frequency of these affections than would have been found in areas where such practices were not customary. Possibly the operators sought to free demons and devils rather than to relieve cranial pressure.

"Whatever the reasons were," as Wakefield and Dellinger point out, "they must have appeared to be adequate to those concerned, for the operation was tremendously dangerous under the conditions with which primitive man was forced to contend . . . a certain authority in favor of the operator and his assistants must have been a necessary qualification."

Peruvians used sharp knives of obsidian, stone, and bronze for trephination, as well as bone instruments, bandages, native cotton, and other auxiliary items. Procedures included trimming, scraping, sawing, and cutting. Some openings were made by crisscross cutting; others were square, polygonal, circular or oval. Drilling also was employed. No part of the cranial vault was sacred. Hrdlicka wrote: "The primitive surgeon not infrequently dared more than would the modern. Some of the operations, and successful at that, were performed directly over the blood sinuses . . . Andean primitive surgeons used various objects for 'stoppers.' In some cases these consisted of a gourd, or perhaps a bone; in others they used portions of shell; rarely, beaten silver."

Ancient surgeons also evidently realized the dangers of exposure of wounds to open air, and applied dressings. Trephined skulls have been found with dressings in place.

Trephining was only one of the accomplishments of ancient Peruvian surgeons. They also opened inflamed sinuses, excised tumors, amputated limbs and replaced them by prostheses. Amputation was carried out not only as a surgical procedure, but also as a punitive or ritual procedure in ancient Peru.

In spite of these advances, Peruvian medicine remained strongly allied to religious practices. Disease was thought to be largely the consequence of sin. Confession, accepted by a special group of priests, and purification rites were prominent forms of treatment. Disease also was diagnosed and treated by a strange type of transference rite. That, says Ackerknecht, is how the guinea pig, a native of Peru, started its unhappy career in medicine. Guinea pigs were first held over the affected part of the patient to absorb the disease-causing principle, then slaughtered and studied for diagnosis. Sacrifice to the gods, including human sacrifice, was another form of treatment.

Gradual passage from supernaturalistic to naturalistic explanations for disease is to be found in the Peruvian belief that winds and seasons produced certain diseases. The disease-producing winds originally were thought of as wind-spirits and wind-gods; but gradually they became regarded as regularly operating natural forces. This concept had an important influence on Peruvian preventive medicine, probably the next greatest accomplishment of ancient Peru.

Some procedures were magico-religious rites; but clean water supplies, good drainage, and legal regulation of diets, sex life, and working hours were effective far beyond the religious sphere. As in Europe, the clyster was traditionally employed as a therapeutic measure.

An original practice of Peruvian medicine, in looking out for the general welfare of the populace, was careful consideration of geographical origins of troops and populations when sending expeditions either to highland or lowland locations and climates. In a country of such diverse altitudes, rapid changes of habitat could not be made safely.

Healers of Incan Peru were supported by products of the Emperor's fields, or the "fields of the sun." The sick and crippled were fed with produce from the "land of the clan." In an attempt to discourage primitive specialization, Incan law required that surgeons, bleeders, and other healers also should be competent herbalists.

One of Peru's greatest contributions to civilization was its outstanding collection of medicinal plants, many of which were unknown in Europe prior to the Spanish expeditions of the sixteenth century. Among the better known were coca leaves, source of cocaine; and cinchona bark, source of quinine. Evidence indicates that these drugs were known and employed for many centuries before Europeans came to the New World. In addition to medicinal plants, Peruvians used remedies derived from animal and mineral sources.

Without question, ancient Peruvian medicine may be compared very favorably with medical practices of such Old World civilizations as Egypt and Mesopotamia.

PRIMITIVE MEDICINE

PRIMITIVE MEDICINE is timeless. It is as old as the palaeolithic cave dwellers. It is as new as today. Early evidences of its practice can be traced back 10,000 years. Yet it is being practiced in some part of the world at this very hour—in certain remote areas of Africa, Asia, South America, Australia, the islands of the Pacific; or among some of the Indian tribes and Eskimos in North America. The pace of advancement of medicine from its beginnings has not been even. In some societies living in today's world, cultures remain at near Stone Age levels; and it is reasonable to assume that in their medical practices they have retained many characteristics of their prehistoric predecessors.

Tribes or social units having no written language and very simple forms of technology are sometimes designated as "primitive" by archeologists and ethnologists. Though existing primitive cultures vary greatly, practice of medicine among them seems to consist of a comparatively small number of elements. These fundamentals are very much the same in all native cultures, varying only in their combination. They are quite different, however, from those constituting scientific systems that have evolved with advancing degrees of civilization.

Members of a primitive society do not distinguish between medicine, magic, and religion. They, first of all (very much as do we), will deal with disease in a matter-of-fact way, using various household remedies, without special theories or employment of practitioners. But when these measures fail, they will resort to measures very different from those we would take. While we assume that disease and death result from natural causes, primitive men regard them almost entirely as work of supernatural agents: gods, holy people, ghosts, or sorcerers. Spirits and ghosts are provoked into action by neglect, or by the breaking of one of the sacred rules (taboos), either by the patient or by one of his family. Sorcerers are motivated by property conflicts or by jealousy. Disease is produced by projecting magic objects or spirits into the body of the sufferer, by abducting one of his several souls, or by some other nonrational means. It follows logically that diagnosis of disease from

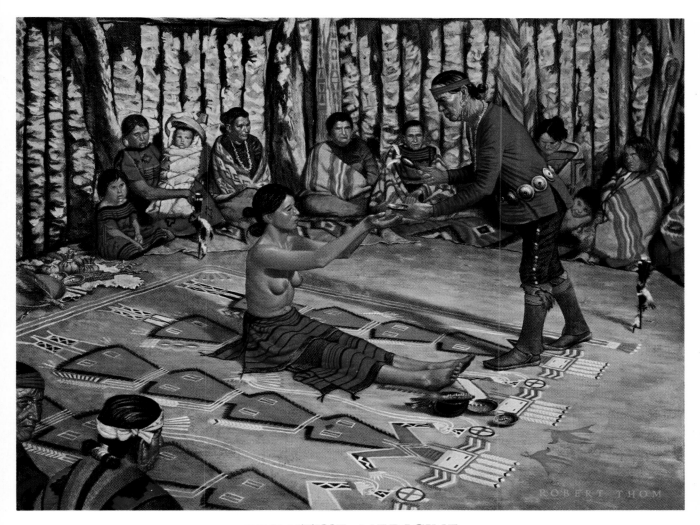

PRIMITIVE MEDICINE

Primitive medicine is timeless. It is as old as the cave dweller, yet in many remote parts of world its practice is as new as today. The sandpainting ceremonies of American Navaho Indians are unusually beautiful examples of primitive medicine, embodying all its elements—physio- and psychotherapy, religion, magic, singing, and drug lore. In a medicine "hogan," family and friends join in the Mountain Chant's nine-day ceremonies, in which this sandpainting has an important part. The "singer" (medicine man) sings, prays, and manipulates magico-religious artifacts. Herb preparations given the patient are shared by the "singer" and by the spectators too in this primitive health-seeking rite.

27

such supernatural causes cannot be made by mere observation and examination of the patient. The medicine man must use supernatural techniques. All the time-honored techniques of divination (still practiced by the superstitious in our own society) are brought to bear, including: magic, trance, stargazing, crystal gazing, bone-throwing, confession of sin, hand-trembling, and interpretation of dreams.

With equal logic, primitive men feel that treatments to combat, to placate, or to overcome such supernaturalistic causes, must themselves be primarily supernatural, magico-religious ceremonies. As a rule, these consist basically of prayers and incantations. However, they contain also elements which we would designate physiotherapeutic and psychotherapeutic, although they are interpreted in magico-religious terms. Primitive man is extraordinarily subject to suggestion, which explains his strong response to spells, to charms, and to other magic; and his fears of violation of taboos. On the physical side, baths, emetics, purging, massage, bleeding, and cupping are to be found. Herbal medicines also are employed during the course of many ceremonies.

Primitive drug lore is a most puzzling mixture of a few very effective drugs, and a wide variety of those which probably are utterly ineffective. Some drugs, about which modern medicine first learned from primitive peoples, still are used extensively in present-day practice. These include: cascara, coca, picrotoxin, strophanthin, emetine, curare, ephedrine, and, quite recently, reserpine. It must be realized, however, that crude forms of these were employed by primitive medicine men, not from the empirical point of view, but entirely because they worked powerful magic as part of a complex ritual. Often they were administered equally to family members and to guests, as well as the patient, and partaken of by the medicine man himself.

Unquestionably, primitive medicine achieves no small part of its results through psychotherapy. Confession and suggestion, which loom large in native practice, lately have enjoyed a considerable comeback in our own medical system. Primitive medicine does not differentiate between bodily and mental disease. Certainly, the patient must derive considerable sense of security from magic and religious ceremonies, both with family and with community participation. Corresponding improvement in morale and in physical response might well be expected; and, with upsurge of the body's own defense mechanisms, perhaps even bacterial invaders might be somewhat thwarted.

Preventive medicine is not absent from primitive practice. Again, it relies mainly on magico-religious forms (ceremonies, amulets). Some ceremonial practices, such as sweat baths, purgatives, circumcision, sex and food taboos, and hiding or burial of excrement, unquestionably contribute to personal and to community health. Ritual scarification sometimes includes real inoculation against smallpox.

The medical practitioner in primitive society, the medicine man, is primarily priest or shaman. He is a learned man, comparatively speaking, because he knows more than other people about the transcendental world, so much so that he sometimes has power over it. He very often is the only professional man in an undifferentiated society. He is neither fraud nor psychopath, as sometimes has been assumed erroneously. His magic or illusionary practices are done symbolically and in keeping with a strict code and well-established ritual. What he does, he does in sincerity; anthropologists believe he is just as sincere as the modern doctor.

All elements of primitive medicine—religion, sacred dances, magic, prayers, hymns, mythology, together with certain rational elements—are to be found today in the beautiful, colorful, sacred song ceremonials which have been practiced, virtually unchanged, for at least a century, possibly more, by the Navaho Indians of the Southwestern United States.

Navahos are a deeply religious people of Athabascan stock (closely related to many tribes of northwestern Canada) who ranged down from the north into what is now the southwestern part of the United States around 1000 A.D. According to one school of anthropologists, Navahos, like all North and South American Indian tribes, are descendants of people who crossed a land bridge from Asia and Siberia, beginning some 10,000 years ago. At present, Navahos live principally in a semiarid region located in parts of New Mexico, Arizona, and Utah.

Most Navaho rituals are performed with certain aims in mind: restoration of health, and insuring immunity to further disease. With these rituals they hope to supplicate, propitiate, or coerce the Holy

People—supernatural Beings who have great powers over people on earth. Navahos fear death and everything connected with it—the dead, they believe, may return as ghosts to plague the living; when death of a patient becomes inevitable, the Navaho medicine man withdraws.

Navaho chants, or "sings," always have mythologic sanction. Each ceremonial has certain songs, prayers, and herbal medicines peculiar to it; and many of these have their own particular sandpaintings. Around 600 different sandpaintings have been recorded, each representing certain divinities or associated events in Navaho mythology. Technically, these pictures, made on a clean sand base, or occasionally on a buckskin or cloth substitute, usually inside a *hogan* (the Navaho dwelling, or on occasion, specially built medicine hut), perhaps should be called drypaintings, for various crushed minerals and vegetable materials also are used for certain types of ceremonials. Patterns, retained in memories of medicine men, or "singers," are handed down from one to another. Many years of apprenticeship and study are required of the Navaho tribesman who aspires to become a practitioner of religious ritual.

Though the chants may vary greatly as to songs, prayers, and sandpaintings, the Navaho's basic procedure is nearly always the same: family and friends gather in the hogan; they participate with the patient in ceremonies; when a sandpainting has been done, the patient sits down upon it, and treatment by the singer begins, to the accompaniment of song and of prayer. When treatment is completed, the patient leaves the hogan, the sandpainting is destroyed, and the sands carried out and disposed of according to ritual.

Of Navaho healing "sings" or ceremonials, one of the more elaborate and colorful is the Mountain Chant, or the Mountain Top Way. Dr. Washington Matthews described this chant in great detail in a report to the Director of the Bureau of Ethnology of the Smithsonian Institution, published in 1887. Several later reports substantially corroborate Dr. Matthews' observations, indicating the changeless nature of these rituals.

The Mountain Chant is based on a myth, which in briefest expression describes the captivity among the Utes of a culture hero called "Reared In The Mountains," his escape by intervention of the supernaturals, his travels, sufferings, adventures, and initiation under divine guidance into religious rites that were to be communicated to his people.

Of the Mountain Chant ceremony, Dr. Matthews says its purposes are various. "Its ostensible reason for existence is to cure disease; but it is made the occasion for invoking the unseen powers in behalf of the people at large for various purposes . . . It would appear that it is also designed to perpetuate their religious symbolism . . . The last night . . . is an occasion when the people gather and have a jolly time. The patient pays the expenses and, probably in addition to the favor and help of the gods and the praise of the priesthood, hopes to obtain social distinction by his liberality."

The first four days' ceremonies (of nine in the Mountain Chant) were perhaps less colorful than the others. Early each morning, before eating, the patient, the singer, and all others who desired, men and women, entered the ceremonial hogan. Seated around a fire, they took a hot emetic infusion of many different kinds of plants mixed together, and sweat profusely. Small sandpaintings sometimes were made around the fire, and other procedures, such as asperging with a fragrant herb lotion, were involved.

On the fifth day, according to Washington Matthews' description, the first of the holy pictures was drawn in sand and pigment on the floor of the hogan. On the sixth day, another sandpainting was made. One of the more interesting paintings was made on the seventh day. The painters' work began soon after 6 A.M. and was not completed until 2 P.M. About a dozen men assisted the medicine man, who did little of the manual labor but watched the work and frequently criticized and corrected it. When the painting, featuring four "tall gods," was finished, the singer applied sacred corn pollen to brow, mouth, and chest of each of the gods. A whistle was blown, the sick woman and a companion entered and cast corn meal on the floor. The patient took off her moccasins and upper garments and sat on the form of the white god, and the singing and rattling resumed. Without interrupting his song the chanter sprinkled the picture with a cold decoction of herbs he had previously prepared. He then applied the moistened sprinkler to each of the gods, then administered the decoction to his patient in two draughts, to her companion, to himself in the same manner, then gave the dregs to the onlookers to pass from one to another. He applied pigments from different parts of the figures to corresponding parts of the patient. This was followed by fumigation rites by sprinkling pungent, aromatic herbs on hot coals, fumes of which the patient inhaled. Then the patient left the lodge, the painting was erased, and the sand was carried out.

A less elaborate sandpainting followed on the eighth day (although in some ceremonies the last painting is the most elaborate), accompanied by rituals much like those of the preceding three days. While this was going on inside the medicine hogan, a great stack of wood was being assembled in the center of the corral outside. At this time, too, a great number of people began to assemble. Much food was prepared, and games developed for pastime. On the ninth day, until sunset, preparation of certain properties for use in the coming ceremonies went on. Just after sunset, the old chanter posted himself in the east of the corral and began a song. The corral itself, a huge circle, was built of branches. Then people assembled inside the corral, the great fire was lighted, and many dances, remarkable for their daring and endurance, followed. At least a dozen dances took place, lasting throughout the night—and the singer chanted on through it all!

Shortly after sunrise, the corral was razed. The chanter packed his sacred utensils and left. The patient greeted and thanked her friends for having attended and aided in her treatment.

The technique of sandpainting is an art. Pictures are drawn to an exact system. According to the medicine men, designs are transmitted from teacher to pupil, and for each ceremony are unaltered from year to year and from generation to generation. Colored powders are taken from bark trays or other containers into the painter's palm and allowed to pass out between his thumb and forefinger. The degree of accuracy achieved by this freehand method is astounding.

Logic of primitive man differs from ours. While his medicine appears strange, if not absurd, to modern observers, in the framework of the outlook upon life of a native society it is meaningful and logical. It is effective enough, too, to be retained by many primitive peoples even when in competition with modern medical concepts brought to them by medical missionaries, government clinics or administrators.

WORLD EVENTS AND MEDICAL HISTORY

Dates, persons, and events of significance to the evolution of Medicine include:

1545	Giambattista da Monte gave bedside instruction at Padua.
1549	Anatomical theater at Padua.
1550	Paré's essay on podalic version published.
1558-1603	Reign of Elizabeth I.
1561	Fallopius published *Observationes Anatomicae* (fallopian tubes).
1561-1626	Francis Bacon.
1564-1616	Shakespeare.
1564-1642	Galileo.
1578-1657	William Harvey.
1582	University of Edinburgh chartered.
1584	Sir Walter Raleigh brought curare from Guiana and introduced the potato.
1590	Compound microscope invented by Hans and Zacharias Janssen.
1599-1660	Velasquez.
1604-1609	Galileo elucidates law of falling bodies (1589).
1606-1669	Rembrandt.
1607	Settlement of Jamestown, Virginia.
1609	United Netherlands.
1609	Henry Hudson anchors "Half Moon" in New York Bay.
1609	Galileo invented telescope.
1609-1618	Kepler stated laws of planetary motion.
1610	Galileo devised microscope.
1611	University of Santo Tomas (Manila) founded.
1613	University of Cordova (Argentina) founded.
1615-1616	Harvey lectured on the circulation of the blood.
1617	Guild of Apothecaries of the City of London founded.
1618	First edition of *London Pharmacopoeia*.
1618-1648	Thirty Years' War.
1620	Landing of the Pilgrims at Plymouth, Massachusetts.
1620	Van Helmont stressed chemical role of gastric juice in digestion.
1622-1673	Molière.
1624-1689	Thomas Sydenham.
1628	Harvey published *De Motu Cordis*.
1630-1638	Treatment of malarial fever with cinchona bark known in Peru.
1632-1723	Antony van Leeuwenhoek.
1636	Harvard College founded.
1639	First hospital in Canada.
1639-1650	Juan del Vigo introduced cinchona into Spain and Italy.
1643	Sir Edward Greaves described typhus fever as a "new disease" in England.
1644	Hôtel Dieu in Montreal.
1645	Royal ("Invisible") Society founded in London.
1648	Van Helmont's *Ortus Medicinae* published.
1648	Francesco Redi disproved theory of spontaneous generation.
1649-1660	Commonwealth in England.
1654-1715	Reign of Louis XIV.
1660	Willis described puerperal fever.
1661	Malpighi published first account of capillary system (*De pulmonibus*).
1661	Robert Boyle defined chemical elements and isolated acetone.
1661	Descartes published first treatise on physiology (*De homine*).
1661	De Graaf showed that ova arise in the ovary.
1665	Newton discovered binomial theorem (published 1669) and law of gravitation.
1665	Great Plague of London.
1666	Great Fire of London.
1669	Lower showed that venous blood takes up air in the lungs.
1670	Malpighi discovered malpighian bodies in spleen and kidneys.
1670	Willis discovered sweet taste of diabetic urine.
1672	Le Gras brought ipecac to Europe from America (Piso, 1648).
1672	De Graaf described the graafian follicles in the ovary.
1673	Leeuwenhoek began making microscopes.
1675	Leeuwenhoek discovered protozoa.
1681	Royal College of Physicians of Edinburgh founded.
1682-1725	Peter the Great ruled Russia.
1682-1771	Giovanni Battista Morgagni.
1683	Sydenham's treatise on gout published.
1683	Leeuwenhoek described and sketched bacteria.
1685-1750	Johann Sebastian Bach.
1690	Locke's "Essay Concerning Human Understanding" published.
1693	College of William and Mary founded, Williamsburg, Va.
1698	Statute of Montpellier required students to visit hospitals.
1702	Stahl stated phlogiston theory.
1708-1777	Haller.
1710	Charité Hospital opened at Berlin.
1713	St. Côme merged into Académie de Chirurgie (Paris).

THE TEMPLES AND CULT
OF ASCLEPIUS

LIKE THAT of all peoples of antiquity, the beginning of Greek medicine dates back beyond recorded history. It emerges upon the world scene as a curious mixture of mythology and rationality. While paying obeisance to the gods favored by their people and times, Greek medical practitioners seem to have been relatively free of the religious handicaps which affected the thinking of their colleagues in some other lands. They approached their practice from a more rational, naturalistic point of view, which, though not always correct, had at least some degree of scientific background.

Side by side with Greek scientific medicine, however, there grew up a religious medical cult which became the most famous of its kind in all history: the cult of Asclepius. At an even earlier date, certain groups of Greek physicians identified themselves as Asclepiads ("son of," or, "of the family of," Asclepius).

First mention of Asclepius in Greek literature is in the Homeric poem, the *Iliad*. Here Asclepius is represented as one of the aristocrats of old, a tribal leader, physician, and father of physicians. At that time he is referred to as a man; a skilled physician; and a student of Chiron (a Thessalonian physician whose equestrian skill gave him the reputation of having been a centaur—compound of man and horse). According to Homer, Asclepius' sons, Machaon and Podalirius, served both as military leaders and physicians in the historic siege of Troy (about 1180 B.C.). Whether they were true sons, or "sons" by virtue of following the calling of Asclepius, is not clear. Though by no means verified, some ancient scholars believed that Asclepius' death took place in the year 1237 B.C.

Ancient writings, particularly Homer's, credit Asclepius with superior knowledge and ability in medicine. While not the originator of Greek medicine, as is sometimes claimed, apparently he was responsible for markedly improving it. Legend slowly developed around the great

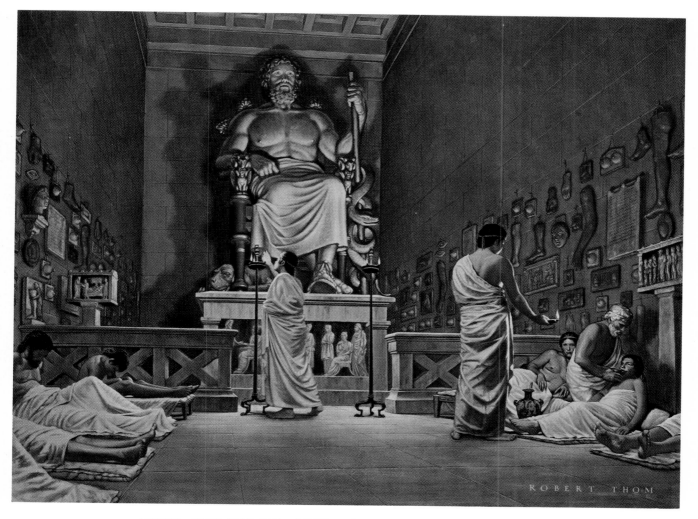

THE TEMPLES AND CULT OF ASCLEPIUS

Every night for nearly a thousand years (500 B.C.-500 A.D.), sick and afflicted pilgrims flocked to the Grecian Temples of Asclepius to take part in a ritual called incubation. The ancient, kindly god of medicine was expected to visit them during a dream-state and either heal them or prescribe drugs, diet, and modes of treatment. Only requisites were that they should be clean and "think pure thoughts." To show their appreciation, recipients of Asclepius' favor caused votives (stone or terra cotta images of the afflicted parts which supposedly had been healed) to be made, suitably inscribed, and presented to be hung as testimony on the temple walls. More than 200 such temples existed.

healer. He became thought of as a half-god, the son of Apollo and a mortal woman. Rescued from the womb of his slain mother by Apollo, an early god of medicine, legend states that he was turned over to Chiron, who raised and educated him. Eventually the god of gods, Zeus, is supposed to have killed Asclepius with a thunderbolt because he had revived the dead—threatening prerogatives of the deities.

The stature of Asclepius continued to grow in Greek thought over the centuries, and around 525 B.C., popular opinion seems to have raised him to the rank of a god. It was then thought that, by grace of a remorseful Zeus, Asclepius had been granted immortality after his violent death, and had taken over his father's position as god of medicine. His legend was adapted to this new role, and by 450 B.C., Asclepius had been supplied with a large mythical family, which included not only the sons Machaon and Podalirius, but a third, Telesphorus; and daughters Hygeia, Panacea, and Iaso, who symbolized other aspects of their father's calling.

The cult of Asclepius gradually spread throughout Greece until more than 200 temples, or Asclepieia, were known. These probably began with, or at least centered about, the Asclepieion at Epidaurus, in central Greece. Other temples of exceptional fame were located at Cos, Tricca, Pergamum, Lebena, Aegae, Corinth, and Athens. The cult was carried to Rome in 293 B.C., when at the request of the Romans, an Epidaurian mission sailed up the Tiber. A sacred snake is said to have sprung from the vessel and to have swum ashore on Tiber Island, and a temple to Asclepius was built on the spot. More and more Asclepius became accepted as the most important Greco-Roman god of healing—a position he was to hold until about 500 A.D.

Earlier temples of Asclepius seem to have been patterned after those devoted to the worship of other Greek gods. Later, they became much more elaborate institutions, usually situated, like the modern spa or health resort, in a favorable spot with good air, springs of pure or mineral water, and woods, though some were located in large cities.

The Asclepieia were large, sprawling groups of buildings, courtyards, groves, and watering places. Their scope was somewhat broader than that of the modern sanitarium. Centrally, of course, was the temple of Asclepius, ornate with magnificent works of art, and other treasures, many of gold. Close by was a second important building, the *abaton*, where pilgrims retired to sleep and to be visited by the god in their dreams. Smaller temples, devoted to other gods, might be found on the premises. Usually a holy well and a hallowed grove were a part of the grounds. In addition, there might be hostels, baths, and gymnasiums. At Epidaurus, a magnificent outdoor theater and a stadium in which games were periodically featured, were parts of the Asclepieion. A large corps of priests, helpers, choirboys, musicians, and others, was required. Sacred animals, especially dogs and snakes, roamed about the grounds. Numerous stone tablets and steles, bearing stories of miraculous cures, were located on the grounds; and on the walls were many votive offerings of stone, terra cotta, or other materials, some of which paid tribute to Asclepius and to his mythical family. More frequently, these votives reproduced in relief some part of the patient's body which had been healed, along with suitable laudatory statements and prayers of thanks. Inscribed tablets told of pious monetary donations. About the grounds also were statues, altars, benches, and other conveniences contributed by grateful, wealthy patients for the convenience and comfort of visiting pilgrims, who frequently numbered in the hundreds.

Visitors to the Asclepieia included, of course, the sick, in various stages of seriousness of illness. In addition, perhaps even greater numbers of healthy persons came to worship, to insure their good health, and, likely, to enjoy holidays, much as at today's spas. Certainly games, plays, periodic festivals, recreation and amusements of other sorts were afforded. Then too, worship services, sermons, and singing were used to help put pilgrims in proper mental mood for the steps to follow. Troubled persons might enter temples to pray at any time.

The cult was not restricted to the poor. The great Sophocles wrote a hymn for Asclepius. The last words of Socrates dealt with Asclepius; and numerous emperors, including Alexander the Great, Marcus Aurelius, and Julian, were devotees of the healing god. In keeping with the spirit of their god, however, keepers of the Asclepieia seem not to have been motivated primarily for profit, and the poor, the indigent, the rich, and the mighty were received with equal kindness. In fact, the poor and indigent might even have received financial help in the temples. Unlike most other Greek deities, Asclepius was considered a kind, sympathetic god, a physician first of all, to whom anyone, in suffering or in trouble, might turn. Those who could afford it were expected to pay, and cheats were punished; but no worthy persons were denied, the only requisite being that "Pure must be he who enters the fragrant temple; purity means to think nothing but holy thoughts." Only those near death, and parturient women, were denied entrance; neither birth nor death was permitted within the temple areas.

Those who came in quest of the god's help were required to bathe and to offer sacrifices (cakes or animals). Apart from this nothing further is mentioned as required of pilgrims, not even an admission fee.

At night, patients went to places where they were supposed to wait for the god. Usually, these would be the *abaton*, although in some Asclepieia patients were allowed to sleep in the temple. Dressed in their usual apparel, they lay down on the bare floor, or on a pallet; lights that were burning when the patients assembled were then extinguished.

This practice, called incubation, was a standard custom. The god was seen by the pilgrim in his sleep, or in a strange state between sleeping and waking. Asclepius is reported to have come in the form in which he is portrayed in statues—as a bearded man, his face gentle and calm; or as a youth of beautiful and fine appearance. In his hand he held a rustic staff, about which a serpent twined. There was nothing to terrify the patient. If the god did not visit the patient the first night, incubation was continued on following nights. Once personal contact was made, the god proceeded either immediately to heal the disease brought to his attention, or to advise treatment to be followed. While many miracles are attributed to Asclepius, they seem to have been associated with reports of earlier times, with the latter form of care taking precedence in later chronicles. Serpents, too, are reported to have appeared to patients in their dreams, and to have healed them by licking their wounds.

According to inscriptions, the god cured paralysis, epilepsy, blindness, baldness, dropsy, wounds, headaches, sterility, worms, tuberculosis, dyspepsia, gout, and many other afflictions. Not only did Asclepius effect cures, he also was thought to protect health, and to protect families. His temples were places of asylum for fugitive slaves and for warriors eluding capture. He was thought of as a kind of supernatural family doctor; and his close personal relationship with his worshipers, his kindness, which was not shared by other ancient gods, might explain survival of his worship and of his cult during early centuries of the Christian era. Asclepius was considered the principal and the most serious competitor of Jesus Christ by the early Christian church fathers. Though they attacked Asclepius with vigor and bitterness, early church leaders had to recognize many parallels between the old god and Jesus Christ, who in early gospels appeared to be a physician, a healer of diseases, and a performer of miracles. Such a god indeed must have been very attractive to a society which was as concerned with health (hypochondriac) and as afraid of death as was the ancient Greek society. Strange as it might appear today, the Asclepieia seem not to have been places of pretense, fraud, or trickery; but temples of a cult based on sincere belief, in which many people found relief through their faith. No enmity appears to have existed between regular Greek physicians, of whom there were many, and priests of Asclepius, who dealt largely with the incurable and with the poor. Because of this practice and because of limitations of science, undoubtedly large numbers of ill persons turned to Asclepius as a last resort. From among these, might it not be reasonable to expect to find a percentage who would respond to spiritual and to psychosomatic influences found in the Asclepieion?

No longer regarded as a deity, Asclepius still is revered in medical circles, and many societies bear his name. His staff, entwined by a serpent, still is the symbol of medicine, used and worn in many ways. (This symbol, of course, is not to be confused with the so-called caduceus, which originally was associated with the god Hermes.) The serpent, however, may be found in the lore of many ancient peoples, including that of Babylon and that of the Hebrew tribes.

SUŚRUTA—SURGEON OF
OLD INDIA

THAT ancient land, India, nurtured man to its breast early in the dawn of civilization. The dry sands of Sind, now in West Pakistan, have revealed to archeologists remains of civilizations going back 5000 to 6000 years, and perhaps further—peoples whose well-constructed cities included houses with adjoining bathrooms and wells, and elaborate public drainage systems. Some scholars believe that it was these early people, whose civilization dates from a period contemporary with the early Egyptians and Babylonians, that were conquered by Aryans during their invasion from the north, about 1600 B.C. From them, the Aryans learned many civilized ways, and from this amalgamation developed the Aryan-Hindu people. The conquering Aryans brought with them a group of dialects belonging to the Indo-European linguistic family; one of these dialects, to which the name Sanskrit was later applied, came to be the polished instrument of literary composition and the vehicle of Hindu civilization through the ages. Centuries later the Aryan Indians migrated and planted colonies in different parts of the world, chief among which were in the countries to the east of India —Burma, Thailand, Cambodia, Laos, Viet Nam, and the great archipelago now called Indonesia.

The literature of the Hindus is rich in lore of many fields. As a means of "painless" training of princes and highborn in social and diplomatic manners, they composed fairy tales in which beasts took the part of human beings. These in turn were translated into Pahlavi, Arabic, Syriac, Hebrew, Latin, Spanish, Italian, German, French, and English, and adapted as children's stories into almost every society of the world.

The oldest and most sacred books of the Hindus are collectively called the Veda, a word literally signifying knowledge, but in view of the fact that religious knowledge was considered knowledge *par excellence*, the word Veda should be taken in this specialized sense. The oldest and foremost portion of the Veda is the Rig Veda, consisting of hymns of praise to the various deities of the large Hindu pantheon. There are also

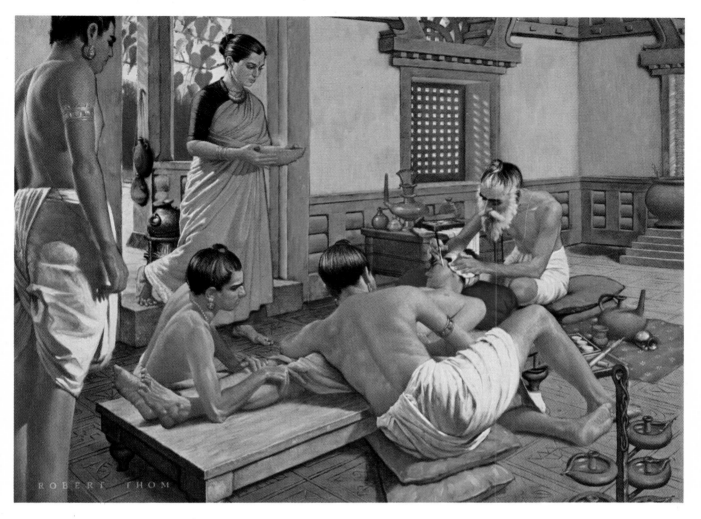

SUŚRUTA—SURGEON OF OLD INDIA

Suśruta, famed Hindu surgeon, is depicted in the home of a noble of ancient India, about to begin an otoplastic operation. The patient, drugged with wine, is steadied by friends and relatives as the great surgeon sets about fashioning an artificial ear lobe. He will use a section of flesh to be cut from the patient's cheek; it will be attached to the stump of the mutilated organ, treated with hemostatic powders, and bandaged. Details of this procedure, and of Suśruta's surgical instruments, are to be found in the Suśruta-saṁhitā, *ancient Indian text. Plastic surgery was practiced in India more than 2000 years ago.*

41

some very remarkable hymns of a philosophical and speculative character. The most recent of these collections, and the last to attain canonicity, the Atharva Veda, for the most part consists of various charms and spells designed to ward off the effects of diseases and the incursions of enemies. The Atharva Veda is the earliest document in India in which there may be found allusions to medical subjects, although they are of a somewhat primitive character, and largely permeated by magic and sorcery.

In the course of the centuries, the Hindus greatly improved upon and supplemented the primitive beliefs about medicine in the Atharva Veda, and came to apply to the art of healing the same subtlety of intellect and penetrating study that characterize the many other technical branches of Indian learning. The body of literature that gradually grew up on the subject of medicine is called the Āyur Veda—literally, the "knowledge of life," or, the knowledge by which life may be improved and prolonged. Āyur Veda was regarded as an Upaveda or subsidiary Veda and ancillary to the Atharva Veda which was, after all, its basis and out of which it had largely grown. In India, to this day, the practices of the Āyur Veda which have prevailed through recorded time still hold sway to a considerable extent, particularly in the villages and in the bazaars of the modern cities. There are schools for the study of Āyur Veda in various parts of India today, where the ancient lore is studied, usually in conjunction with modern Western medicine. Also, considerable research is being carried on currently to determine the value to modern scientific medicine of many of the ancient, traditional Indian medicines and remedies. The treatment for leprosy which persisted until very recent modern times in the West, involving the use of chaulmoogra oil, was known to the Hindus centuries ago. Likewise, Indian snakeroot, or rauwolfia, was employed for centuries by the Hindus for relieving various disorders, before reserpine was extracted from the root and found spectacularly useful in the treatment of hypertension and of mental disorders. But the connection of medicine with magic has never been forgotten in India, and the scientific treatises have references to demons as one of the sources of disease and incantations as remedies. Even to this day one may still hear talk in India of curing snake bites by the use of incantations. It is interesting to note that organic life was divided into four great classes: Svedaja or "sweat-born," which embraced the insect world; Aṇḍaja or "egg-born," comprising birds, snakes, etc.; Jarāyusa, or "membrane-born," including mammals of various kinds and human beings; and Udbhissa or "sprout-born," embracing the whole of the vegetable kingdom.

The most important medical manuals grouped under the generic name Āyur Veda are: the *Charaka-saṁhitā* or "Compendium of Charaka," supposedly compiled by the physician of that name attached to the court of the Kushān Emperor Kanishka whose queen he allegedly cured; the *Suśruta-saṁhitā* or "Collection of Suśruta," whose name is traditionally one of the most illustrious in the whole galaxy of Indian physicians; the *Ashṭāṅga-saṁgraha* or the "Compendium of the Eight Branches," which has reference to the eight topics under which Indian medical science was generally treated; the *Ashṭāṅga-hṛdaya-saṁhitā* or "Collection of the essence of the Branches"; and the *Nidāna* of Mādhavakara, the chief Indian work on pathology.

Among the many distinguished names in Hindu medicine, that of Suśruta stands out in particular. Unfortunately, the dates of Suśruta's lifetime, like those of so many other figures in India's long history, are not definitely assignable. From mention of his name by the famous Arab physician, Rhazes, as well as from accounts of the Chinese Buddhist pilgrim, I-tsing, and his inclusion among medical authorities mentioned in the famous Bower manuscript (about 350 A.D.) found in Chinese Turkestan in 1890, there can be no doubt that Suśruta flourished prior to the fourth century A.D. Certainly this is the very latest period that can be assigned to him. However, several writers have placed him at a much earlier date—sometimes as early as 400 B.C. There is no agreement on this point.

Suśruta's fame rests for the most part on the famous compilation known in Sanskrit as the *Suśruta-saṁhitā*, or "The Collection of Suśruta." Though this work is mainly devoted to surgery, it also includes medicine, pathology, anatomy, midwifery, biology, ophthalmology, hygiene, and not a little psychology and understanding of what would today be called the "bedside manner." Suśruta attempted to arrange systematically experiences of older surgeons, and to collect scattered facts about medicine into a workable series of lectures or manuscripts.

The accuracy of Suśruta's descriptions and classification of diseases is really remarkable. Much of his great compendium has a modern feeling about it. Of course, the original autographic manuscript of the *Suśruta-saṁhitā* has not survived. Extant only are copies of copies and revisions of revisions, so that the original work of Suśruta has been much obscured by centuries of emendation, supplementation, and various kinds of alteration. However, from beneath the layers of all the incrustations of later men's ideas the original lustre of Suśruta still shines forth.

Suśruta begins his *Saṁhitā* with an allegorical description of the beginning of medical teaching, but he quickly gets into some very practical suggestions about how a medical student should be selected, how he should be initiated, and the oath he should take (which is strikingly like the Oath of Hippocrates). He also sets forth quite plainly the qualifications of a physician about to enter practice— rules of personal and of professional conduct singularly parallel to those of today. Suśruta also urged upon his students continual practice, and outlined many ways for them to perfect their skills before using instruments on patients. His philosophy is well expressed in his *Saṁhitā:* "A physician, well versed in the principles of the science of medicine [Āyur Veda] but unskillful in his art through want of practice, loses his wit at the bedside of his patient, just as a coward . . . On the other hand, a physician, experienced in his art but deficient in knowledge . . . is condemned by all good men as a quack, and deserves capital punishment at the hands of the king. Both these classes of physicians are not to be trusted, because they are inexpert and half educated. Such men are incapable of discharging the duties of their vocation, just as a one-winged bird is incapable of taking flight in the air . . . A physician well versed in the principles of surgery, and experienced in the practice of medicine, is alone capable of curing distempers, just as only a two-wheeled cart can be of service in a field of battle."

Among other observations made by Suśruta in this volume, having to do generally with medicine, is the following:

"An intelligent physician should preserve the state of health in the healthy individual, while he should increase or decrease the quantity of bodily humours, vital fluids, or excrements in a sick patient according to the exigencies of the case until his health is perfectly restored."

On physical types, he observed that: "A lean frame should have preference to a stout one . . . "

There is no lack of understanding of the value of psychology in treatment of patients to be found in the *Suśruta-saṁhitā*. For example, after describing the type of room and bed in which a patient suffering with an ulcer (infected wound) should be placed, Suśruta directs that: "Thus the patient shall lie in comfortable posture, attended upon by his sweet-talking friends and relations . . . [who] shall alleviate the pain of his ulcer with pleasant and interesting topics, and by solacing him with the prospect of a speedy recovery."

Piercing the lobes of ears of infants (to protect them from evil influences, and for purposes of ornamentation) apparently was a common minor surgical procedure. Here, Suśruta directs that: "The child should be placed on the lap of its nurse, and benedictions pronounced over it. Then having soothed it and lured it with toys and playthings, the physician should draw down with his left hand the lobules of its ears with a view to detect, with the help of reflected sunlight, [the closed up] apertures that are naturally found to exist in those localities. Then he should pierce them straight through with a needle held in his right hand . . . Plugs of cotton-lint should be then inserted into the holes of the pricked ear lobules, which should be lubricated or rubbed with any unboiled oil . . . "

Bhishagratna states that "To Suśruta may be attributed the glory of elevating the art of handling a lancet or forceps to the status of a practical science." Suśruta devotes considerable space to description of proper surgical instruments, emphasizing that they should be made of "pure, strong and sharp iron." He describes some 125 surgical instruments, frequently likening them to some well-known object, as in the case of forceps, two of which are called "lion's jaw," and "heron's bill." Included are tongs, hooks for the removal of nasal polyps, the rectal speculum, and magnets for removal of metallic foreign bodies.

Surgical procedures are classified in eight groups; among them: incision, excision, scraping, puncturing, extraction, secreting fluids, and suturing. Hindus also practiced chemical surgery with alkalies and cautery. Suśruta also describes 14 types of bandages and dressings and discusses when and when not to use them. He describes at great length treatment of suppurating swellings and ulcers; and surgical procedures for lithotomy, amputations, and ophthalmic operations. He and his associates were superior in performance of cataract operations; and in suturing of intestines, in which they employed heads and mandibles of large ants as clamps. Suśruta also describes in detail various obstetric procedures, indicating skill in this field that was not achieved in the West until many centuries later. Operations for hemorrhoids, for fistula in ano, and for abdominal obstructions are described.

In Hindu society, as in many contemporary ancient societies, punishment of wrongdoers frequently took the form of physical mutilation. Cutting off the nose was the usual punishment for adultery. Such judicial demolitions may perhaps be looked upon as the chief cause for the introduction of plastic surgical measures for repairing disfigured ears or noses. Suśruta describes otoplasty in detail: "A surgeon well versed in the knowledge of surgery should slice off a patch of living flesh from the cheek of a person so as to have one of its ends attached to its former seat [cheek]. Then the part, where the artificial ear lobe is to be made, should be slightly scarified [with a knife] and the living flesh, full of blood and sliced off as previously directed, should be adhesioned to it [so as to resemble a natural ear lobe in shape] . . . " He then directs that the part shall be anointed with honey and clarified butter, and covered with a cotton and linen bandage, tied neither too loose nor too tight, and dusted with powders of baked clay. He gives full directions for postoperative care, and for shaping the new lobe.

A rhinoplasty is also described by Suśruta:

"Now I shall deal with the process of affixing an artificial nose. First the leaf of a creeper, long and broad enough to fully cover the whole of the severed or clipped part, should be gathered; and a patch of living flesh, equal in dimension to the preceding leaf, should be sliced off [from down upward] from the region of the cheek and, after scarifying it with a knife, swiftly adhered to the severed nose. Then the cool-headed physician should steadily tie it up with a bandage decent to look at and perfectly suited to the end for which it has been employed. The physician should make sure that the adhesion of the severed parts has

46

been fully effected and then insert two small pipes into the nostrils to facilitate respiration, and to prevent the adhesioned flesh from hanging down. After that, the adhesioned part should be dusted with [hemostatic] powders; and the nose should be enveloped in Karpasa cotton and several times sprinkled over with the refined oil of pure sesamum . . . "

Disease was defined by Suśruta as follows: "Man is the receptacle of any particular disease, and that which proves a source of torment or pain to him, is denominated as a disease. There are four types of disease such as, traumatic or of extraneous origin, bodily, mental and natural." Disease was explained as a disturbance in the equilibrium of the three humors (called Dhātus or Doshas); wind (vāta); gall (pitta); and mucus (kapha); when these were in perfect balance and harmony, a person was said to be healthy. Wind was further subdivided into five varieties: udāna, the seat of which is in the throat, moves upwards and produces speech; prāṇa, lodged in the heart, issues from the mouth and is responsible for breathing and helps in introducing food; samāna in the stomach is supposed to fan the fire of digestion and thus assist in "cooking" or digesting the food and also to separate the food into chyle, urine and feces; apāna, located in the lower bowels, is said to expel the feces, urine, semen and the fetus; vyāna is generally diffused throughout the body, and among other things, keeps the blood and sweat active.

Disease could be explained equally well as a consequence of sin committed in a former existence (Hindus believe in transmigration of the soul), or of possession by demons. Symptoms indicated loss, absence, or derangement of humors. The body was alleged to consist of seven elements—chyle, blood, flesh, fat, bone, marrow, and semen, and each of these is transferred into the following after five days. The heart was thought to be the seat of intellectual processes and was described as shaped like an inverted lotus flower, closed during sleep and open during waking.

As has been observed by Keith, "The striking similarity in many points between the Greek and Indian medical systems has long been well known. We find in both such things as the doctrine of humors, whose derangement explains disease, the three stages of fevers, and other disorders which correspond to the Greek . . . It must, however, be confessed that it is very difficult to determine how much is due to Greek influence and how much is merely parallel development."

While omens, good and bad, were considered important by Hindu physicians, Suśruta gives extensive directions concerning diagnosis. Questioning of the patient, and examining him with all five senses, were directed. Pulse was studied. Tasting of urine to determine presence of diabetes by the sweetness of the liquid was practiced by Hindu physicians a thousand years before Europeans became aware of this method.

Hindu physicians were good observers, too. They determined constitution by comparing body proportions; and arrived at prognoses not only from omens but from the patient's features. The description of a dying patient clutching at his bedclothes in the *Suśruta-saṃhitā* is very similar to the classic description in Hippocrates' *Prognostic*. His writings include also excellent descriptions of pulmonary tuberculosis; skin diseases, including leprosy; diabetes and urinary diseases; ascites, with reference to liver cirrhosis; and fevers. Hindu doctors were familiar with epilepsy and with other convulsive disorders; with tetanus; hemiplegia; elephantiasis; abscesses; osteomyelitis; and with puerperal fever. They knew scrofula and goiter; and they described venereal diseases. In fact, Suśruta mentions no less than 1120 diseases.

Therapy among the Hindus always included prayers and incantations. They used "cleaning" procedures, such as cathartics, emetics, and venesection; but were well aware of dangers involved therein. Diet too, was considered important. In fact, Suśruta seems to have been close to modern nutritional concepts, for he stated that: "Plants should be regarded as partaking of the virtues of the ground they grow upon."

Drugs derived from plant, animal, and mineral kingdoms were employed extensively. Suśruta mentions no less than 760 vegetable drugs; Charaka, some 500. Hindus also had extensive knowledge of poisons, and were specialists in treatment for snake bites.

In the medical texts of the Hindus, there is no mention of a general anesthetic, from which it may be inferred that none was known in ancient days. Suśruta, however, distinctly directs that "wine should be used before operation to produce insensibility to the pain of the operation." The Hindus also inhaled the fumes of burning Indian hemp (cannabis) as an anesthetic at a period of great antiquity.

Hindu medical literature devotes a great deal of attention to hygiene and to prevention of disease. Tooth-brushing twice a day, washing, massage, physical exercise, proper food, well-regulated sex life, and rest were recommended. Sleep during the day was to be avoided, as were fly-infested foods. In times of epidemics, people were advised to migrate to healthier locations, to pray, and not to use water or vegetables from questionable sources. Physicians employed variolation against smallpox; it was from Hindus that the Western World first learned of this method of prevention, which paved the way to discovery of vaccines in the nineteenth century A.D. Suśruta gives a good description of hay fever in this sentence: "Sometimes the pollens of poisonous flowers or grasses, wafted by the winds, invade a town or village, and produce a sort of epidemic cough, asthma, catarrh, or fever, irrespective of all constitutional peculiarities or deranged bodily humors agitated thereby."

Hindu physicians were carefully trained in apprenticeships; and like Greek physicians, they were advised to be honest, clean, and of good and dignified appearance.

In his foreword to Kashikar's English translation of Dr. Julius Jolly's *Indische Medizin*, J. Filliozat says: "Indian Medicine has played in Asia the same role as the Greek Medicine in the West, for it has spread in Indo-China, Indonesia, Tibet, Central Asia, and as far as Japan, exactly as the Greek medicine has done in Europe and the Arab countries . . . The importance of Indian medicine had already been realized by the Greeks of Alexander [331 B.C.]." Yet, through its continuous connection with theology, Hindu medicine tended to remain static. As a whole, Greek medicine had greater influence on the world, because Greeks developed medicine through a completely secular approach to growing science.

In conclusion, it may be noted that the *Saṁhitās* of Charaka and Suśruta were translated into Persian and Arabic about 800 A.D., and since Arabic medicine became the chief authority for European medicine down to the seventeenth century, Indian ideas undoubtedly have indirectly entered modern Western medicine. Certain it is, in any case, that British physicians learned the art of rhinoplasty from Indian surgeons in the days of East India Company.

HIPPOCRATES: MEDICINE
BECOMES A SCIENCE

THE ART of medicine in the ancient world developed to its highest point in Greece, during the millennium between 500 B.C. and 500 A.D. However right or wrong their theories might have been, Greek physicians of this period showed great clinical acumen. Early in this period, practitioners of Greek medicine generally made the decisive turn (despite the cult of Asclepius) from supernaturalism to acceptance of exclusively naturalistic and scientific explanations of, and methods of, treatment of disease. Medical principles established during this period dominated medicine during the following one thousand years; and their influence on present-day medicine is evidenced by the predominance of Greek terminology.

Centuries before this bright millennium, Greek medicine followed the usual pattern of magico-religious practices. Then came a period during which philosopher-physicians transformed medicine to a somewhat scientific, naturalistic, but highly speculative and theoretical (and frequently inaccurate) profession. However, most Greek physicians, unlike their contemporaries in some other nations, were not priests, but craftsmen. Thus were combined empirical knowledge of craftsmen and speculative theories of philosophers.

Best known of these pseudoscientific principles was the humoral theory. The human body was thought to consist basically of four humors: blood, yellow bile, black bile, and phlegm. In a state of health these four humors were balanced. Unbalance in their proportion resulted in disease, and nature made efforts to restore this balance by throwing off matter. It was the physician's job to assist nature in these efforts. Remnants of this old humoral theory of more than 2,600 years ago still survive in such everyday words as sanguine, melancholic, phlegmatic, and bilious.

Greatly as philosophers influenced Greek medicine, early in the fifth

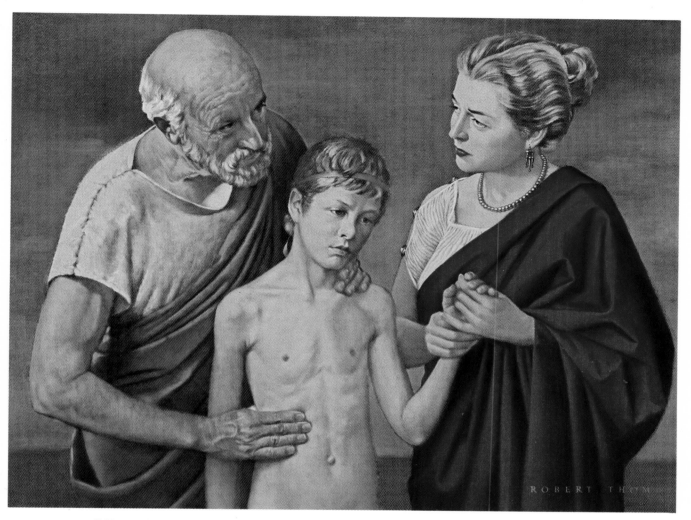

HIPPOCRATES: MEDICINE BECOMES A SCIENCE

The art of medicine in the ancient world developed to its highest point in Greece, during the millennium between 500 B.C. and 500 A.D. This creative period is symbolized by Hippocrates, the "Father of Medicine," whose name has come to represent the beauty, value, and dignity of medicine for all times. Hippocrates' kindliness and concern are embodied in his aphorism, "Where there is love for mankind, there is love for the art of healing." These qualities are reflected in the face of this great practitioner, scientist, and teacher, as he palpates a young patient and attempts to soothe a worried mother sometime late in the fifth century B.C. His name is still revered in medical circles.

century B.C., another change in course began in a swing from speculation to rationalism, with increasing emphasis on clinical observation.

The greatness of this creative period of Greek medicine is symbolized by Hippocrates, a contemporary of immortals such as Pericles, Sophocles, and Socrates. In his hands, medicine became an art, a science, and a profession. Hippocrates' name has been synonymous with "Father of Medicine" for more than two thousand years. His name has come to represent the beauty, value, and dignity of medicine for all time.

Very little is known about Hippocrates' life history. He was born on the little island of Cos, in the Aegean Sea, about 460 B. C. Hippocrates seems to have been a relatively common Greek name; the great physician's grandfather also bore the name. Hippocrates was the second of seven sons of a physician named Heracleides, who professed to be one of the Asclepiads, a group of physicians claiming Asclepius as their patron. According to tradition, Hippocrates began the study of medicine at the Asclepieion of Cos, later studying at the Asclepieia at Cnidus, at Thasos, at Thessaly, and, according to some biographers, in Egypt, in Lydia, and in Scythia. He is said to have returned to practice in his home community on the island of Cos, but it is evident that he traveled widely. He visited many cities in Greece and in foreign countries, practicing his profession and collecting ideas. His medical reputation spread, and he soon came to be regarded as the outstanding representative of the Coan School, which concerned itself primarily with prognosis and with treatment of the patient as a whole. Hippocrates disapproved of the school at Cnidus, which emphasized diagnosis, localistic explanation of disease, and active treatment of individual organs. (The age-old question of the general practitioner versus the specialist!) The writings of Aristotle and of Plato indicate that Hippocrates achieved great renown during his lifetime. He must have been a physician of wide experience and of common sense. Hippocrates is reported to have died at Larissa, a town near Thessaly, in the year 361 B.C., at the age of 99 years.

Hippocrates, it is recorded, had two sons, Thessalus, and Draco, both of whom became physicians of note, and a physician son-in-law, Polybus. They were founders of the school of Dogmatism, based on

52

Hippocrates' aphorisms. They carefully preserved Hippocratic principles, and their writings bore the name of their illustrious father.

While authenticity of Hippocrates as a person cannot be seriously challenged, authenticity of collected writings known as the Hippocratic Corpus or Collection is subject to considerable question. Which among threescore pieces of literature were written by Hippocrates, and which by admirers who, following the customs of the day, attributed their work to their more famous predecessor, is debatable. These writings seem not to have been those of one man, perhaps not even of one group. This circumstance, however, does not invalidate the fact that they summarize the first great peak in Greek medicine. Despite their variances, all Hippocratic manuscripts stress the naturalistic approach and put great emphasis on the value of observation of disease processes rather than on study of the cause of disease, relegating speculative theories to a minor position. Therein also is to be found medicine's first "Declaration of Independence," in the first lines of *On the Sacred Disease* (epilepsy): "It is thus with regard to the disease called Sacred: It appears to me to be nowise more divine nor more sacred than other diseases, but has a natural cause from which it originates like other affections. Men regard its nature and cause as divine from ignorance and wonder, because it is not at all like other diseases." According to Celsus, Hippocrates was first to emancipate medicine from trammels of superstition and delusions of philosophy.

In Hippocratic aphorisms are to be found such important statements as "Fat persons are more exposed to sudden death than the slender"; "Spasm supervening upon a wound is fatal" (tetanus); "Spinal deformity often coexists with cough and tubercle of the lungs" (Pott's disease); and "Diarrhea in pulmonary tuberculosis is a mortal symptom." Among his sayings, which later became favorites with physicians, were these: "Life is short, the art long, the occasion fleeting, experience fallacious, and judgment difficult," and "You must not only do the proper thing, but do it at the right time." For those who aspired to become physicians, Hippocrates had this advice: "Whoever is to acquire a competent knowledge of medicine ought to have the following advantages: a natural disposition; instruction; a favorable position for study; early tuition; love of labor; leisure. First of all, a natural talent is required, for when Nature opposes, everything else is in vain; but when Nature leads the way to what is most excellent, instruction in the art takes place, which the student must appropriate to himself by reflection, early becoming a pupil in a place well adapted for instruction. He must also bring to the task a love of labor and perseverance, so that the instruction, taking root, may bring forth proper and abundant fruits. . . Physicians are many in title, but very few in reality. . ."

Greek physicians were apprentice trained, and the oath by which they were bound to their masters reflects the high ethical standards of the profession. Though it has borne his name for more than two thousand years, scholars seriously question whether the Oath of Hippocrates was actually written by the great physician himself. Revered though it is and has been by physicians down through the years, evidence seems to indicate that this document was the product of medical groups that developed in the century following Hippocrates' lifetime. Nevertheless, it is certain that this document embodies principles and precepts of the great physician, and that it deserves wide acceptance as the oath to be taken by all who are about to enter upon practice in the profession of medicine.

Hippocrates and Greek physicians who followed him believed that treatment was intended primarily to assist nature. Therefore, it was mild and, in the light of present-day thinking, considerably more reasonable than were methods used by medical men in later periods. Of primary importance both in health and in disease was diet. Only when diet failed were drugs used, and only when drugs failed was surgery applied. Greek books on surgery reveal that great skill was used in treatment for wounds, fractures, and dislocations. Operations for fistula of the anus and for hemorrhoids were prescribed, and daring operations, such as trephining of the skull and opening of empyemata, were reported.

Materia medica of Hippocrates was limited; he employed few drugs, but he did use cathartics and sedatives.

Development of prognostics in all likelihood rose through the social status of Greek physicians as traveling craftsmen who could not afford to assume responsibility for treatment of incurables. For prognosis,

Greek physicians often referred to climatic data; disease and health were thought to be dependent to a large extent on local climate.

Observation became the physician's most useful tool—observation based on inspection and examination of the patient. Palpation was employed—innumerable patients with large spleens caused by malaria provided ample reason for use of this technique. Auscultation in crude form also was employed. Greek medical writings abound with valuable observations on such well-known diseases as malaria, pulmonary tuberculosis, mumps, pneumonia, anthrax, and apoplexy. Diabetes, diphtheria, leprosy, plague, tetanus, as well as mental and dermatologic diseases, were described later. Some facts and observations cited in these early writings were not rediscovered by medical men of the Western World until many centuries later.

From Hippocrates through Rufus and Aretaeus to Galen, Greek physicians remained great observers.

The second great peak of Greek medicine was reached in the third century B.C. in Alexandria, the city founded by Alexander the Great. Humoral theories of disease were less predominant at that time than in earlier and in later periods, and disease was explained as due to changes in solids of the body. The study of anatomy also was actively pursued.

The third great peak in Greek medicine developed in Rome in early centuries of the Christian Era. This period is symbolized by Galen, physician and pharmacist, who served two emperors. Under Galen's influence, science prevailed over art in the concept of medicine. While politics of the world became Roman, medicine remained Greek. Great as Romans were as conquerors and administrators, they never reached comparable levels in medicine. Greek physicians led in practice and development of medicine in Rome, as they did elsewhere, during the great millennium that began with Hippocrates.

GALEN, INFLUENCE FOR FORTY-FIVE GENERATIONS

TWO great names—Hippocrates and Galen—stand out in the history of Greek medicine, towering over all other pinnacles of achievement surrounding them. Hippocrates dominated the beginning of a period of remarkable scientific creativity, which lasted more than seven hundred years. Galen, near the end of the period, both furthered scientific knowledge and crystallized it in an amazing volume of written works.

While next to nothing is known of Hippocrates as a person, many facts concerning Galen's life are well documented; and the facets of his personality are interjected repeatedly into his voluminous writings.

Galen's writings and teachings—marked by brilliant observation and wise therapeutic application as well as colossal error and insufferable dogmatism—dominated medical thinking and practice for fifteen hundred years—an occurrence unique in world experience. More than a few of Galen's astute observations are in accord with modern medical beliefs. His errors were not seriously challenged in medical thought and teaching until the anatomist Vesalius, in 1543, and the physiologist Harvey, in 1628, courageously questioned the infallibility of Galenic authority and effectively substantiated their findings through demonstration.

Galen was born in 130 A.D., in the Greek city of Pergamon in Asia Minor (now Turkey), seat of one of the largest temples of Asclepius and also of one of the "seven churches which are in Asia," addressed by the Christian Saint John (*Revelation 2*) in the first century. Galen was the only child of the architect, Nikon, a mild, just, and comparatively wealthy man who took a deep interest in the boy's education. His mother, on the contrary, was a difficult woman, subject to fits of anger toward servants and ready to quarrel with her husband. Galen's writings reveal scant regard for her; but her influence apparently was manifested in his temperament.

Named *Galenos* (meaning calm or serene), the boy's education was supervised by his father on the family farm until he was 14; then he

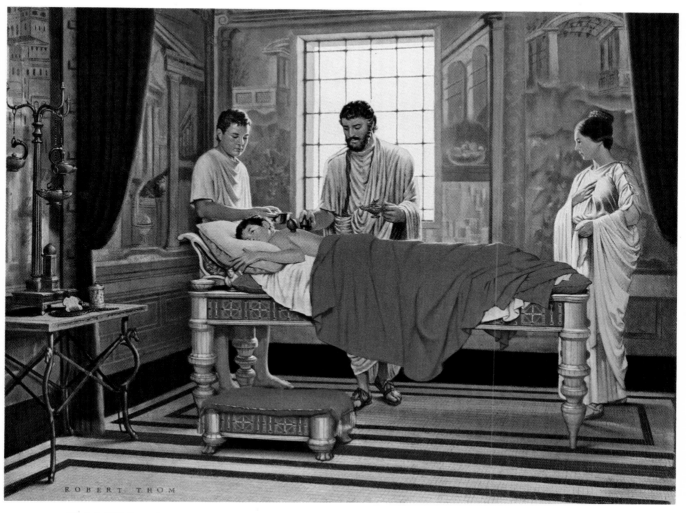

GALEN, INFLUENCE FOR FORTY-FIVE GENERATIONS

Galen was a pillar of medicine; the last important pillar in the millennium of Greek domination of the medical world. Physician to emperors as well as commoners in the Roman Empire, Galen (130-200 A.D.) traveled extensively, lectured widely, wrote prolifically. The great Greek was a shrewd observer who gained much experience through experimentation. Cupping was among the forms of treatment which he advocated. Pharmacy as well as medicine benefited from his formulas, called "galenicals;" he was a leader in the health sciences of his day. Galen's teachings were accepted as dogma by both teachers and practitioners of medicine for fifteen hundred years.

57

was taken to Pergamon to attend lectures in philosophy and in mathe-matics. To preserve a spirit of impartiality, his father directed him to attend courses given by representatives of the four leading philosophic systems of the day. Then, according to Galen's own writings, Nikon had a dream, influenced by Asclepius, directing that his son study medicine.

Galen began the study of anatomy in Pergamon at about age 17, continuing there until his father's death; this was followed by study at great centers of learning of the Greek world at Smyrna, Corinth, and Alexandria, during which he added medical subjects to his growing store of knowledge. Nor was philosophy neglected. About the year 158, Galen, at age 28, returned to his home town of Pergamon. The head priest at the Asclepieion appointed him physician to the gladiators. This provided him a great opportunity to study not only practical applications of hygiene and medicine, but living anatomy, as revealed by terrible wounds suffered by contestants whom it was his duty to treat.

Four years later, the restless young physician departed for Rome, then capital of the world. There, despite numerous charlatans, com-petitors, and enemies, he soon acquired great fame through spectacular diagnoses and modes of treatment, public lectures, discussions, physi-ologic demonstrations, and writings. His reputation grew to the point where he was called to examine the Roman emperor-philosopher Marcus Aurelius. Galen's shrewd diagnosis that the Emperor was suffering from indigestion, as opposed to the complicated theories of other physicians on the scene, won him an appointment as court physician.

Galen frequently absented himself from Rome on lengthy research and study trips which took him throughout many lands. One of these came, very conveniently, during a "plague"—an attitude not regarded as unethical among physicians before the eighteenth century. However, he soon was recalled from Pergamon by Marcus Aurelius to a military camp at Aquileia; then shortly thereafter he was ordered to return to Rome to take over medical supervision of the Emperor's son, Com-modus, whom he continued to serve as physician even when the latter succeeded his father as Emperor. About 192 A.D., however, the Roman political climate became unhealthy for scholars and philosophers, and

Galen returned to his home town of Pergamon. Presumably he continued to travel and to write until his death at 70, at the dawn of the third century.

The medicine and pathology Galen practiced, and about which he wrote, were based mainly on the speculative Hippocratic theories of the four humors, on critical days, and on fallacious theories regarding pulse and urine. These did not give way to more realistic approaches until the sixteenth, seventeenth and eighteenth centuries. Despite his mixture of rational science with philosophic speculation, Galen was a good observer and shrewd clinician. With pride he tells how he explained a patient's puzzling sensory disturbances in the fourth and fifth fingers as due to infraction of a vertebra in the neck resulting from a fall from a horse, treatment of which cured the condition. He tried to differentiate between bloodspitting and bloodvomiting, between colic from kidney stone and colic from the intestines. He also understood well the psychosomatic element of illness. Called to treat a noblewoman who was declining rapidly in a nonfebrile melancholic condition, he observed sudden reddening of the cheeks and increase in pulse rate when the name of Pylades, an actor, was mentioned accidentally. After experimenting for a few days by having names of other actors mentioned in her presence, but never obtaining the change in pulse except on mention of Pylades, he correctly diagnosed her case as an unsatisfied passion for the actor.

In the fields of therapy and of pharmacy, Galen is remembered mainly for his schematism and extremely complex prescriptions, sometimes containing dozens of ingredients. Formulas of this type make up a class of pharmaceuticals still called "galenicals." Yet he followed Hippocratic tradition by treating patients for numerous conditions by using diet and physiotherapy alone. He was extremely interested in hygiene and prevention of disease, the importance of which he put above treatment, and about which he wrote several books.

Galen was an able surgeon in his youth, but gave up surgery at Rome, since fashion regarded such manual activity as no longer proper for a learned physician. Though his followers learned from him the theory of laudable pus, he himself tried to heal wounds without suppuration.

Galen was a scientist as well as a practitioner. As a matter of fact, there is good evidence that medicine, which primarily was an art with Hippocrates, primarily was a science with Galen. Though he did not dissect humans, even in dissecting animals Galen cleared up a great number of basic anatomic problems; among them was the origin of blood vessels in the heart and of nerves in the central nervous system. His description of anatomy of bones and muscles is excellent, considering that it was gained from monkeys and pigs; and, even though its errors had to be cleared away by Vesalius, it helped to attain a basic understanding of human anatomy.

Harvey, some fourteen hundred years later, overthrew Galen's physiologic ideas on the tidal ebb and flow of the blood. However, this cannot obscure the fact that Galen was the greatest experimental physiologist before Harvey. He demonstrated the nature of arteries, of ureters, of recurrent nerves, and of the spinal cord; he had ideas concerning function of motor and sensory nerves; and he appreciated states of tonus and of contraction.

Galen's physiology was vitiated by his philosophic bent, and by his Aristotelian teleology; that is, by his conviction that the Creator had given to every organ a purpose, and that if he could figure out this purpose he would know how the organ functioned. But while Galen's speculative, dogmatic, and dialectic inclinations, which endeared him to the Middle Ages, often irritate modern readers, one cannot avoid being impressed by the acuteness of his mind. In taking up a problem, he thoroughly considered every possible implication and ramification. "Reason," he wrote, "finds the answers most quickly, but experience confirms our confidence in them."

Galen's accomplishments were so manifold and his written works so numerous that they defy cataloguing. His subjects covered dietetics, pathology, therapeutics, pharmacy, anatomy and physiology, hygiene, medical philosophy, and Hippocratic commentaries—indeed a universe of thought. Written in Greek, this Galenic treasure did not reach the Latin Western World except through an Arabic detour. Byzantine physicians built up Galen's glory, and admiration of his teaching was

60

transmitted to Oriental Christians and to Moslems. His works were translated from Greek into Syriac, and from Syriac into Arabic. Then, in the eleventh and twelfth centuries, Arabic versions and commentaries were translated into Latin. Some of Galen's original treatises are completely lost; and some have been recovered only from these Arabic translations.

The profession of medicine gained a wealth of facts and ideas from Galen. Despite confusion in influence of medical schools and of philosophic sects, he gave to the world a synthesis of medical thought and knowledge solid enough to last nearly fifteen hundred years. His mind was quick and well organized; he was well informed on many subjects. In the earlier period of his life, he continually insisted on experiments and on demonstrable proofs; but the open-minded young Galen later became one of the great dogmatists of all times. However, the magnitude of his dogmatism was increased by his followers and commentators. During the Middle Ages, when thinking for one's self was not fashionable, Galen was accepted and perpetuated as the infallible master. This, as George Sarton says, "was a creation of the disciples, rather than of the master himself." Blame for the slavish submission of later generations to his authority cannot be placed upon him.

Galen was a pillar of medicine; the last important pillar in the millennium of Greek domination of the medical world. He was a topflight scientist in his day.

RHAZES AND ARABIC MEDICINE

PREDOMINANCE of Greek influence on world medical thought covered the millennium from 500 B.C. to 500 A.D. The next millennium, between 500 A.D. and 1500 A.D., may be characterized as the medieval period of medicine—a time of great strife, of sociopolitical change, of regression and progression. It was a time-crucible in which classic traditions of the defunct Roman Empire, practices of barbaric paganism, philosophies of rapidly growing Christianity, and the vigorous thirst for knowledge that followed the dramatic rise of Islam were amalgamated. Medieval medicine borrowed elements from all these sources in varying degrees, and passed on to succeeding eras a *corpus medicus* the better for this wedding of widely divergent systems.

During the early Middle Ages, Western Europe was engulfed in wave after wave of conquering barbarians, who ruthlessly destroyed libraries and centers of learning. No less destructive to life and morale were waves of epidemic plague that swept the Western World. During these centuries, Greco-Roman medicine, grown sterile following the time of Galen, was virtually lost to the Western World. Only those works laboriously copied and preserved by the monks in Christian monasteries remained—and these were hidden behind the walls of scattered cloisters. Although carried on as an accessory to their sacred mission, writings of monks reflected the more practical aspects of monastic medicine, and were helpful in maintaining cloister infirmaries and herb gardens. The period of monastic medicine was officially closed when the Council of Clermont in 1130 forbade the practice of medicine to monks.

The force which was to change the course of medicine in the Western World, and to restore to it the lost legacy of the Greco-Roman period, was the impact of Arabic science.

In little more than one hundred years after Mohammed's flight from Mecca (622 A.D.), Moslem Arabs had conquered the Near East, North Africa, and Spain; and by 737 A.D. they had reached the banks

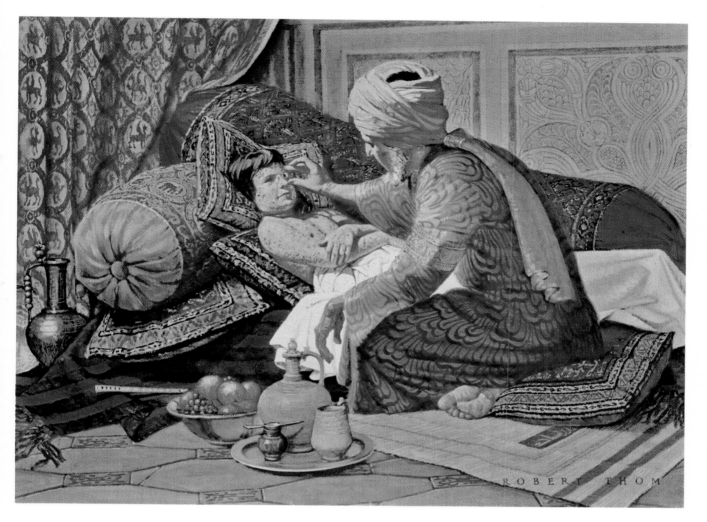

RHAZES AND ARABIC MEDICINE

The West is deeply indebted to medieval Arabs for preservation of ancient Greco-Roman knowledge during the Middle Ages, and for improving on it. Our numeral system and many words, such as alcohol, came from the East, as did many medical advances. Leaders in Arabic medicine were the Persians, Rhazes and Avicenna. Rhazes (865-925 A.D.), noted for keen observation and inventiveness, was first to describe measles and smallpox; to observe pupillary reaction to light; to use mercurial purgatives; and to publish a text on children's diseases. His teachings were very highly regarded for many centuries.

of the Loire in France. Their ideologic conquest of Greek legacies of science and classics was no less rapid.

Knowledge of the Greeks, in medicine as in other fields, came to the Arabs through Christian sectarians (such as the Nestorians) who were driven out by the Byzantine Empire, center of learning when Rome declined and Christianity became the dominant religion. Scholars among these early displaced people translated Greek authors' writings into Semitic languages, first Syriac and Hebrew, then Arabic. Thus Arabs became familiar with, and enthusiastically embraced, the teachings of Hippocrates and of Galen. By the tenth century all essential Greek medical writings had been translated in Damascus, Cairo, and Bagdad, as had more Greek classics than the West knew of before the Renaissance. The Arabs then began adding their own discoveries and observations to the written body of Greek tradition.

There is little doubt that Arabic medieval civilization was more highly developed than was that of the contemporary West. One of the reasons therefore might have been the great tolerance wisely exhibited by Arabs during their earlier medieval period. Many famous "Arabic" physicians actually were Syrians, Persians, Spaniards, Jews, or Christians, writing in Arabic. This was true not only in great centers of the eastern Arabic world, but also in Arabic kingdoms in Spain. Constant traffic between the Eastern and Western Caliphates kept both areas well informed on translations of old ideas and on new developments. It was by this long detour through the Near East, North Africa, and Spain, that Greek medical lore returned to Western culture, carrying with it the cumulative contributions of Arabic scientists.

How greatly the West profited from its contacts with Arabic civilizations in all fields is evidenced by the fact that we still use the numeral system which Arabs adapted from India; and many of our everyday words, such as algebra, alcohol, and the like, are of Arabic origin. In the twelfth century, especially through schools in Sicily and Spain, Latin translations of great Arabic medical books based on Galen and on Hippocrates became available to the West; and up until the sixteenth century, Arabic authors were the highest medical authorities in new Western universities, such as Montpellier and Bologna. Arabs, Jews, and Christians, alike, regarded Avicenna and Rhazes as the greatest Arab medical authors. Today, the works of Rhazes generally are considered of somewhat greater significance than those of Avicenna, because of Rhazes' greater inventiveness and attention to observation. This evaluation, however, is opposed to that given these writers during the Middle Ages.

Abu Bakr Muhammad ibn Zakuriyya, or al-Razi, known to the West as Rhazes, was born in the Persian city of Rai, about 865 A.D. Up until his thirtieth year, he seems to have been primarily concerned with music, physics, and alchemy. During a visit to a Bagdad hospital, he is said to have become so interested in medicine that he decided to devote the remainder of his life to this profession. He studied with the Jewish physician, Ali ibn Sah al-Tabari, who was well versed in Greek, Persian, and Hindu medicine. After having been director of the hospital in his home town, in about 907 A.D. Rhazes became director of a large hospital at Bagdad and a court physician as well. He seems to have traveled widely, visiting Cordova, Jerusalem, and various cities in Africa. He became famous as practitioner, teacher, scholar, and benefactor of the poor.

Rhazes is supposed to have written 237 books, of which only 36 have survived. Therein he dealt with all the sciences, but his greatest interest was medicine. In his theories, Rhazes was a Galenist; in practice, he seems to have been guided more by the principles of Hippocrates. He showed great independence and originality, and his texts were spiced with descriptions of personal observations.

Most famous of Rhazes' works was the *Continens*, a kind of medical encyclopedia, put together from his notes after his death. A shorter encyclopedic work is the book dedicated to Persian Prince Almansor. However, the work most highly regarded today is Rhazes' little book on smallpox and measles—one of the few to have been translated into English. The great merit of this book is that it offers the first medical description of these two important infectious diseases. Although humoral theories cited impress today's reader as queer, and although Rhazes did not fully differentiate the two diseases, the clinical descriptions are clear and concise. The volume is concerned mainly with therapeutics.

Writings of Rhazes contain ingenious and penetrating observations on topics as widely variant as hiccough, purgatives, spinal injury, and embryotomy. He made other practical contributions to medicine, such as introduction of mercury compounds as purgatives (after having tried them on monkeys); introduction of lead ointment; and ligature with sutures made from animal gut. He was perhaps the first to observe and to record reaction of the pupil to light. Rhazes urged use of cold water in inflammatory fever, and insisted that treatment for fever be based upon its causation. His book on the "habit which becomes natural" might be regarded as an early though imperfect sketch of conditional reflex.

Evils of quackery were subjects of bitter attack, and Rhazes wrote much about them. He also discussed careless practices of physicians which sometimes caused patients to turn to quacks.

Rhazes contributed the first known book on children's diseases, and a book on "cure within the hour" which must have been immensely popular. He described an instrument for removal of foreign bodies from the esophagus, and invented a lead catheter which he preferred because of its flexibility. His treatise, "A Dissertation on the Cause of the Coryza which occurs in the Spring when the Roses give forth their Scent," is one of the earliest known descriptions of hay fever.

A man of deep sympathy, Rhazes could not endure poverty and suffering; and, though he earned large fees, he gave away so much that he himself died in want and in poverty. During the later years of his life he was blind, supposedly as a consequence of a blow on the head delivered in anger by Prince Almansor. Apparently he suffered from cataract, but refused operation, saying that he had seen so much of the world that he was weary of it. Though records are vague, Rhazes is believed to have died around 925 A.D.

Even after more than a thousand years of medical progress, Rhazes' works and accomplishments command admiration of medical scholars of today.

The torch of Arabic medicine was carried to further heights by Avicenna (ibn Sina, 980-1037), another Persian writing in Arabic—physician, pharmacist, poet, philosopher, and stormy career politician. His great *Canon,* called the most famous medical textbook ever written, was but one of more than one hundred medical treatises which he wrote.

In the Western Caliphate, the names of Averroes (ibn Rushd, 1126-1198) and of the Jewish physician and philosopher, Maimonides (Musa ibn Maimun, 1135-1208) were among the brilliant lights of medieval medicine.

Capture of Cordova in 1148, by primitive, bigoted, and rigidly orthodox Moslem Almohades, sounded the death knell of Arabic science and medicine in the West; and, in turn, the Eastern Empire fell before merciless Mongols under Hulagu Khan, in 1258. Not only were accumulated intellectual treasures destroyed, but nearly all scholars and learned men were pitilessly murdered. In the West, however, the Almohades in turn fell before Christians. Fortunately, Christians did not destroy the culture of Islam, but absorbed most of it, to the benefit of succeeding generations of medical men.

"Islamic medicine and science," says Meyerhof, "reflected the light of the Hellenic sun, when its day had fled, and they shone like a moon, illuminating the darkest night of the European Middle Ages. Some bright stars lent their own light, and that moon and stars faded at the dawn of a new day—the Renaissance."

MEDIEVAL HOSPITALS

MEDIEVAL times (500 A.D. to approximately 1500 A.D.) are noted, insofar as science and medicine are concerned, as a period of sterility, of inertia. Yet out of this troubled millennium came a significant contribution to the welfare of mankind: the hospital.

In the Western World, cultural breakdown brought about by political upheavals, ravages of epidemics, growing pains of new religious concepts, and slavish adherence to ancient teachings, set back man's progress for a thousand years. Universities, established during the second half of the Middle Ages, for several centuries served only to repeat Greek and Galenic observations, theories, and prescriptions, weighted down by ponderous additions of highly speculative discussions and philosophic interpretations. Medieval medicine received its inspiration, not from physicians in sickrooms, but from clergymen in libraries.

Hospitals in the Western World were largely the creations of Christianity. However, institutions of a similar nature had existed in other parts of the world long before the birth of Christ. Records tell of hospitals in Ceylon as early as the fifth century B.C., and in India as early as 260 B.C. Arabian hospitals, with large and liberal endowments, came long after the beginning of the Christian era. Whether the Mohammedans got the idea from Buddhists or from Christians is subject to conjecture.

Romans created hospital-like institutions when they established large buildings for treatment of troops stationed on distant frontiers, and when they opened *valetudinaria* for care of civilians who were sick.

Early European hospitals were more like homes for the aged, or hospices. The sick found their place in these hospitals only insofar as they were a part of the group of helpless individuals, including paupers, pilgrims, travelers, aged persons, orphans, and others destitute. For such as these, Christian charity provided "hospitality," especially food and shelter. Early medieval hospitals rarely specialized in treatment of the sick. Usually the sick were received for the purpose of supplying

68

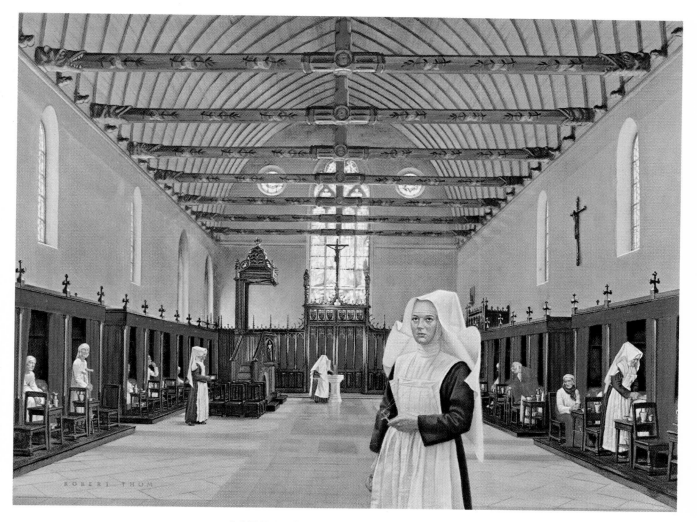

MEDIEVAL HOSPITALS

The Great Room of the Poor (La Grand' Chambre des Povres) is believed to be the world's oldest edifice to have been in continuous use as a hospital. Representative of medieval hospitals, it is a part of the Hôtel-Dieu of Beaune, France, founded in 1443. Combined with modern professional hospital service it carefully preserves the atmosphere of the fifteenth century. A small chapel is located at the end of the room. Sisters of the Congregation of Sainte Marthe, garbed in habits traditional to their ancient order, have cared for the sick, the aged, and the indigent in this hospital for more than five hundred years, uninterrupted by wars, by economic upheavals, or by political changes.

their bodily wants and of ministering to their spiritual needs until they were well enough to return to work.

Famous early Christian hospitals were the "Basilias" in Caesarea in Asia Minor, and the hospital of Edessa in Mesopotamia, both founded around 370. Fabiola founded a hospital in Rome around 400. The great hospital in Constantinople (now Istanbul) dates from the sixth century.

The oldest actual hospital in France seems to have been the Hôtel-Dieu, founded in Lyons about 542 by Childebert I, king of the Franks. The famous Hôtel-Dieu of Paris was founded about 652 by St. Landry, the twenty-eighth Bishop of Paris. The oldest hospital in Italy is believed to be Santa Maria della Scala in Siena, established in 898.

Impetus was given to development of hospitals in the twelfth century by the Crusades; and further stimulation during the fourteenth century by the spread of the plagues. Large groups of people were moving by various routes to the Holy Land, and stragglers, sick, and wounded were returning. In fact, the first written provisions for regular medical care are to be found in statutes issued by the Order of St. John to its Jerusalem hospital in 1181. This movement of thousands of individuals under almost primitive circumstances provided most favorable conditions for spread of disease and for epidemics.

Leprosaria, frequently known as lazarettos (a name derived from St. Lazarus), had been established outside the walls of thousands of European cities. The average leprosarium, however, harbored only about a dozen persons. Though many of these institutions disappeared after leprosy began to decline in Europe in the fourteenth century, others continued, having been adapted to the care of sick and of indigent persons.

Foundation of the Order of Hospitallers of the Holy Ghost in 1180 stimulated a new wave of founding of hospitals. In a short time, Holy Ghost hospitals were opened within cities all over Europe. Pope Innocent III (1198-1216) sponsored the founding of such a hospital in Rome, in 1198, at the old Tiber bridge. Innocent summoned Guy of Montpellier and put him at the head of the Order and of the Roman hospital. This institution, the Ospedale di Santo Spirito, continues in operation today. In Florence, the Ospedale di Santa Maria degli Innocenti, established as a foundlings' hospital, has operated continuously since 1421.

Many hospitals founded by the Order of the Holy Ghost were established in Germany. In that country, however, it was common practice for hospitals to be established or operated by municipalities.

The first hospital of record in England was built in York, in Saxon times, 937 A.D. After the Conquest, many more were founded. Others of early days include: St. Gregory's, dating from 1084; St. Cross', at Winchester, from 1123; and St. Thomas', from 1215. One of the most important of English medieval hospitals, and still a distinguished institution, is St. Bartholomew's, of London, founded in 1123.

In Spain, Madrid's General Hospital traces its foundation to three Moorish hospitals, combined by Philip II in 1566. The Saracen cities of Spain also had large, well-managed hospitals.

Moslems were no less zealous than Christians in promoting works of charity. In fact, Arabians were far ahead of their European contemporaries in adopting kindly treatment toward mentally ill persons. Numerous hospitals were erected in Mohammedan cities in Asia Minor. As early as 707 A.D., the Caliph El Welid is reported to have founded a hospital in Damascus; another was established at Cairo in 874; two at Bagdad in 918; and three more in Egypt, between 925 and 977. By 1160, Bagdad is reported to have had 60 operating hospitals.

One of the greatest of Moslem hospitals was Al-Mansur, founded in 1283, in Cairo. This hospital is reported by a medieval chronicler to have had incomes of as high as $100,000 a year from the landed property assigned to it. Separate wards were provided for patients with important diseases, as were wards for women and for convalescents; lecture rooms, an extensive library, outpatient clinics, diet kitchens, a separate room for compounding medicines, and an orphan asylum were included; and the staff included both male nurses and female nurses. Admission of patients was unlimited, every sick or poor person who came to its doors was accepted; duration of stay was not restricted; and each convalescent, on discharge, was given a suitable sum of money so that he might not have to return to work before fully recovered.

Spaniards, according to Prescott, reported having found flourishing hospitals in Mexico at the time of the conquest. The Western Hemisphere has a number of hospitals which date back to early colonial times. Oldest among these is believed to be the Hospital of the Immaculate Conception in Mexico City, established in the early 1500's. In Canada, the oldest are the Hôtel-Dieu du Précieux Sang, in Quebec, founded in 1639, and the Hôtel-Dieu de St. Joseph, founded in Montreal in 1644. In what is now the United States, the first hospital founded as such was the Pennsylvania Hospital in Philadelphia, which was brought into existence with the help of Dr. Thomas Bond and Benjamin Franklin, in 1751. There are a number of institutions which were established at an early date as almshouses or workhouses, later becoming hospitals in the present sense. Among them were the Philadelphia General Hospital (1751), Bellevue Hospital in New York (1735), and Charity Hospital in New Orleans (1736). In the Philippines, the Hospital de San Juan de Dios was founded in Manila in 1596.

In addition to the Hôtels-Dieu of Lyons and Paris, several other old French hospitals still operate. In 1260, Louis IX founded the Hôpital des Quinze Vingts as a home for the blind. It is now a general hospital, but specializes in ophthalmology. Louis XIII founded La Salpêtrière as an asylum for indigent women; it later became a hospital for patients with mental and nervous diseases, and today is an immense rambling institution providing general hospital services.

One of the most charming old hospitals in France, and one quite typical of hospitals established in medieval times, is the Hôtel-Dieu of Beaune. It is reputed to be the oldest existing hospital which has continuously occupied its original building. Set in the midst of the ancient walled city of Beaune, in the heart of Burgundy's *Côte d'Or*, some 250 miles southeast of Paris, this hospital has a history as colorful as its steep, gabled roofs.

Severe times preceded its establishment; the Hundred Years' War was just drawing to a close; and the French kingdom of Charles VII, and the Duchy of Burgundy, under Philip the Good, had just become reconciled by the treaty of Arras (1435). When soldiers were not plundering the countryside, professional robbers were. Terrified country people fled for refuge to castles and to walled cities. Famine and pestilence further compounded their miseries. The pitiful needs of the poor, the destitute, and the sick were too much for small cities to cope with.

This situation stirred charitable emotions in the chancellor to the Duke of Burgundy, Nicolas Rolin. Wealthy in his own right, high in diplomatic circles, Rolin and his wife, Guigone de Salins, agreed to devote their fortune to building a "hostel of God" for the poor and the sick. The chancellor had approval for his project from Pope Eugene IV and from Duke Philip. Beaune, because of its fortifications and its situation at the crossroads of fifteenth-century travel routes, was the site chosen. Land was acquired adjoining the market place. On August 4, 1443, under the portal of Beaune's Church of the Notre Dame, in the presence of eminent churchmen, civic leaders, and citizens, the charter was drawn for the Hôtel-Dieu de Beaune.

The hospital followed the Flemish style of architecture. The first structure was completed and dedicated in December, 1451, and the first patient was admitted January 1, 1452. Six sisters were assigned to care for the poor and the sick who sought shelter in "la Grand' Chambre des Povres"—the Great Hall of the Poor.

The great, or main, ward indeed is an edifice of magnificence and beauty: it is 236 feet (72 meters) from the entrance to the stained glass windows at the far end; 46 feet (14 meters) from wall to wall; and 52 feet (16 meters) from the beautifully flagstoned floor to the tip of the soaring roof. This roof is shaped like the hull of a ship, turned upside down (symbolizing charity going about the world as a ship sails on the sea). Eleven six-sided wood beams span the structure from eave to eave, with king posts ascending from their centers to the peak of the roof. The beams are exquisitely carved with gargoyles and symbolic figures, brightly painted; and escutcheons of the founders decorate the central joints. Along the sides, each bed is enclosed in a separate cubicle, with draw curtains for privacy. The motif of dark red and gold is carried throughout—curtains, drapes, and bed covers, each adorned with initials and symbols of the founder and his wife who made possible this project. Outside each bed-cubicle there is a small table and chair, each with its individual pewter goblet, bowl, and copper basin—to this day preserving style and grace of the fifteenth century.

Across one end, and a part of la Grand' Chambre des Povres, is a small but beautifully appointed chapel. It is so arranged that, when the dividing curtains are drawn, patients may attend Mass and follow the service without moving from their beds. This arrangement is similar to that to be found in many fifteenth-century French hospitals.

Since its building, begun in 1443, many additions have been made to this hospital. Among these are: several wards, a great kitchen, a pharmacy, a museum; also added were gardens, courts, and precious pieces of art. Innovations of yesteryear are museum pieces today, supplanted for practical purposes by new and modern equipment; but these are preserved for their nostalgic and historic significance.

Like its contemporary institutions, the Hôtel-Dieu de Beaune gradually changed from a hostel for the poor and the aged to proffer services of a modern hospital. Despite vicissitudes of time, economic changes, and numerous wars, this hospital has continued to serve the poor, the sick, and the needy, day in and day out, for over 500 years. The ancient buildings with gay, varicolored tiled roofs that belie the grief and the pain they shelter, have been maintained in good repair; and, while modern methods have supplanted those of old, the air of fifteenth-century France has been preserved. Even the costume of the good sisters of the Congregation of Sainte Marthe (known in the old days as the "Dames Hospitalières de l'Hôtel-Dieu de Beaune"), who have given devoted and loving attention to those entrusted to their care, has remained virtually unchanged since the day the first great ward opened, January 1, 1452.

Here, in this little provincial city in the heart of the *Côte d'Or*—sun-bathed slopes whose vineyards produce France's famed Burgundy wines—one may see and experience the beauty and atmosphere of long-gone centuries, yet feel pulsing the life, the compassion, and the devotion that has permitted hospitals, of all of man's establishments, to have enjoyed an honorable place in history longer than most contemporary institutions.

As previously pointed out, little or no provision was made for medical care in early European medieval hospitals. First provision for medical service seems to have developed in institutions on the Moslem-Christian frontier of the Holy Land during the Crusades.

74

In Paris at the Hôtel-Dieu, about 1221, Maître Hubert, surgeon, was engaged to treat the poor and the sick. At Marseilles in 1331, a definite medical service was organized in the Hospital of the Holy Ghost; and evidence has been uncovered of similar services in Bruges, Belgium, and in some cities in Germany. In Spain and in the Byzantine Orient, however, this practice was centuries old at the time it began in Germany and France.

Not even in the Hôtel-Dieu of Paris, however, was any teaching use made of this wealth of clinical material during the first thousand years of its existence. Any practical experience the medical student got was obtained by attaching himself to some obliging physician who acted as an extramural teacher and took the student along on his rounds. To Italian physicians della Monte and Oddi belongs credit for establishing bedside teaching in hospitals. Della Monte (1489-1552) is said to have given very popular practical courses in the Hospital of St. Francis in Padua. A medical school was created in connection with St. Bartholomew's in London about 1662. Names of great physicians and surgeons are to be found associated with this school, including those of Percivall Pott, John Abernethy, William Harvey, Sir James Paget, and David Pitcairn.

Even at best, medieval hospitals left much to be desired. The Hôtel-Dieu in Paris in the fourteenth century had grown to a capacity of 800 to 900 patients; and it probably doubled in size within another century. However, the number of beds actually was much less, for it was the practice of those days to use enormous beds holding four to six patients. Included in this hospital's equipment in the fifteenth century were two portable bathtubs mounted on wheels.

Crude and medically deficient though they must have been, and without sanitary facilities, medieval hospitals shaped a solid foundation of compassion upon which today's modern hospitals are built. From wards, operating rooms, and laboratories of hospitals of the nineteenth and twentieth centuries has come a stream of decisive clinical discoveries. Viewed in perspective, the conclusion is inescapable that modern medical practice owes much indeed to charitable and humanitarian principles laid down in the hospitals of medieval times.

PARACELSUS—STORMY PETREL OF MEDICINE

No FIGURE in the long history of medicine bequeathed it a greater heritage of controversy than Paracelsus. To this day, more than 400 years after his death, he is praised, and condemned; revered, and vilified; raised to the pedestal of sainthood, and damned as quack of quacks. By some persons, his mystical writings are regarded as evidence of an advanced mind, far ahead of its time, capable of thoughts and of insights lofty beyond interpretation by minds of ordinary contemporaries; according to others, his crabbed phrases, written as with a pen dipped in vitriol, are but a fabric of crudity and of vanity cloaking ignorance and superstition. In fact, our very word, bombast, is said to stem from Paracelsus' name, Philippus Aureolus Theophrastus Bombastus von Hohenheim. His pen name, Paracelsus, defiantly flung in the faces of the academicians—meaning "better than Celsus"—is typical of his boastful attitude. Pachter wrote that he was either king or beggar, never a gentleman.

Paracelsus without doubt reflected the violent and confused aspirations of the common man of the early sixteenth century. Strange as his ideas seem today, when viewed against the background of his century, they are no more revolutionary than were those of his contemporaries. Ackerknecht says of him: "He was more modern than most of his contemporaries in his relentless and uncompromising drive for the new and in his opposition to blind obedience to authoritarianism and books. On the other hand, he was more medieval than most of his contemporaries in his all-pervading mystic religiosity." He is remembered, not so much for his achievements, but for his fight against orthodoxy.

Paracelsus was born at an interesting time: "when Europe stretched her limbs after a sleep of a thousand years in a bed of darkness." He came into the world just after Columbus had discovered America; during his lifetime Luther was to cleave catholicism in twain; and Copernicus was to recast astronomy. Two years after Paracelsus' death, Vesalius was to publish his *Fabrica*, the revolutionary atlas of anatomy that added to

76

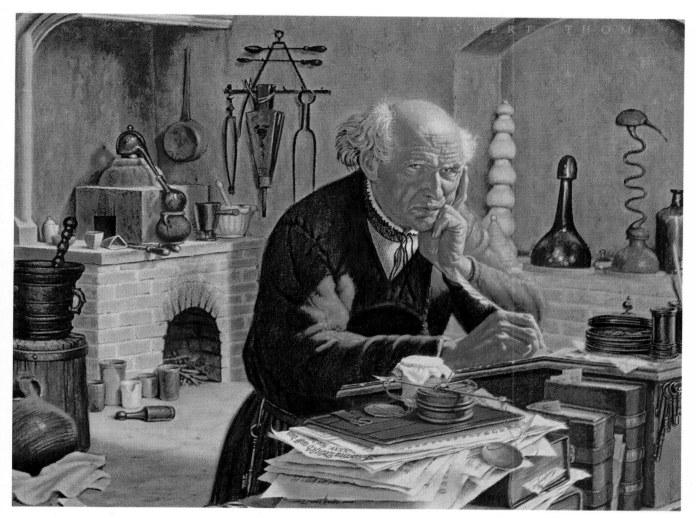

PARACELSUS—STORMY PETREL OF MEDICINE

In the Renaissance "chemical kitchens" of Theophrastus Bombastus von Hohenheim (1493-1541), who boastfully called himself Paracelsus, many things were brewed: chemicals, polypharmacal mixtures, serious medical writings—and vitriolic, abusive attacks upon medical colleagues, religionists, and political officials. Swiss-born Paracelsus' controversies forced him to travel widely, move frequently. Labeled genius by some, quack by others, his medical efforts got results, and patients liked him. He attacked medieval "sacred cows," Galen and Avicenna, helped turn medicine from them to rational research. He attempted to manufacture new remedies, and he advocated use of chemicals in medicine.

77

Galen's decline from authority, which was initiated by Paracelsus.

Paracelsus was born in Einsiedeln, Switzerland, in 1493, the son of an illegitimate offspring of the noble German Hohenheim family. His father, Wilhelm, practiced medicine. His mother was a local serf who apparently was inclined toward mental depression and committed suicide when the boy was but nine years old. The father then moved with his rachitic child to Villach in Carinthia, where the elder von Hohenheim cared for the personnel at mines owned by the famous banking family of Fugger. A great deal of alchemical work was being done at the mines (alchemy was the chemistry of the time). Impressions gained there by youthful Paracelsus were to dominate his entire life.

His interest shaped by his father's instruction, Paracelsus in 1507 became a traveling scholar. Along with his taste for medicine he seems also to have acquired an appetite for alcoholic beverages—an appetite often to bring him reproach in later life. On the other hand, sexual activities seem to have been conspicuously absent in his life. According to some authors, he was an eunuch. Paracelsus' studies took him to the universities of Heidelberg, Freiburg, Cologne, Tuebingen, Vienna, Erfurt, and across the Alps in 1513, to Ferrara, Italy.

Greatly disappointed with the Galenic, old-bookish knowledge then offered by the universities he attended, Paracelsus soon scorned venerated volumes and proceeded to invent his own particular brand of medical practice. He further shocked his contemporaries and the faculties of the universities by lecturing and writing, not in the Latin of the learned world, but in the vernacular of his Swiss homeland.

From this point on, Paracelsus became a traveling doctor (though his enemies declared he had no formal degree), going from town to town, sometimes in dirty rags, and others in flamboyant finery. Constant companion was his large sword, in the handle of which he hid his most precious medicines. Up and down southern Europe he went, applying his new science. Despite his unorthodoxy, his results appear to have been excellent. In wayside hostels and in palaces his art won fame and acclaim. He was asked to see patients whom other doctors had given up. His cures were called miraculous. His successes made him suspect of black magic—a reputation that was to cling to his name for centuries. Paracelsus no longer sought learning from old books; he sought knowledge from all peoples: peasants, alchemists, fortunetellers, thieves, musicians, midwives, barbers, bathkeepers, gypsies, loafers, old women, and, on occasion, from other physicians. He sought to know, not what does this drug do, but what "virtue" within it accomplishes the desired results. These "virtues" or secret forces, he called *arcana*. "God has not permitted any disease without providing a remedy," he proclaimed. He studied the human body as a whole, its physiology rather than its anatomy; its working, growth, and decay, rather than its individual parts by themselves.

Yet through it all, despite his successes, Paracelsus managed to antagonize persons of authority, in medicine, in education, and in politics. There seems to have been in him a martyr urge which set up chain reactions of controversies and misfortunes. Community after community found his presence intolerable. He was forced to move on, again and again. He had a streak of clownishness in him; at times his behavior was that of a buffoon. One author wrote sarcastically that Paracelsus often was as gross as were aristocrats of his time. His self-advertising and self-acclaim were distasteful; he ruthlessly and obscenely attacked other medical men. Though sometimes the guest of kings, he kept faith with the commoners and serfs. Though a religious man, he was more at home in the local taproom than in cloistered halls. Not infrequently, his unkempt dress more closely resembled that of a teamster than of a renowned physician.

Numerous wars of the early 1500's provided Paracelsus with opportunities to practice surgery. Though modern readers find his works a collection of superstitious and repellent folk remedies; nevertheless out of his surgical experience came certain principles (strongly opposed by his contemporaries) far in advance of his time. Among these was insistence that wounds be kept clean. "If you prevent infection, Nature will heal the wound by herself," he wrote. Illogical though his "weapon ointment" might have been (a balm thought to be most effective when applied, not to the wound, but to the instrument that made it), this method of sparing the wound from aggravation may have saved the lives of many soldiers in these European conflicts. Paracelsus also was among the first to have tried to determine dosage scientifically. "The right dose makes the difference between a poison and an arcanum," he asserted.

Following active service in Italian wars, Paracelsus visited Spain, France, and England, only to return to wars in Holland and in Sweden. After their conclusion, he traveled through Russia to Constantinople, to Egypt, and back through the Greek islands and the Balkans, visiting mines and alchemists associated with them. To alchemists, whom he considered to be kindred souls, he often urged: "Stop looking for gold; instead, find medicines." His role in development of medical chemistry, as an originator and as a publicist, was significant.

In 1524, Paracelsus, rich in experience but poor in cash, returned for a time to his father's house and to the valley of mines, again to work in mines and in smelters. Lung affections common there gave Paracelsus abundant opportunities to help patients and to study disease. The fruit of these experiences was the first book ever written on an occupational disease: *On Miners' Consumption*.

Paracelsus tried to settle in nearby Salzburg. Unfortunately, he became involved on the side of the peasants in a local uprising, and had to leave town abruptly. From a period of voluntary travel, Paracelsus now entered upon a phase in his life wherein travel frequently became both necessary and hasty. The people of no city seemed willing to accept him for long as a resident. Then come his hour of triumph.

The famed Renaissance publisher, Froben, was ill with a persistent infection of his leg. Local doctors had proposed amputation—at that time a dangerous, likely fatal, procedure. Mutual friends suggested that the famous doctor see the famous patient. Froben sent for Paracelsus and gave him living quarters in his house in Basel, Switzerland (now preserved as a museum of pharmaceutical history). With his lucky star shining its brightest, Paracelsus rapidly succeeded in curing his patient's infection. The doctor's success, it seemed, was at last established. It was in Froben's house, too, that Paracelsus met another leader in Renaissance thought, Erasmus of Rotterdam, "prince of the humanists." The publisher and the philosopher influenced Basel's city council to offer Paracelsus the office of municipal doctor and professor at the University. He promptly accepted.

The faculty of the University, however, was in no mood to accept this rebel who failed to produce evidence of an earned medical degree and who lectured in Swiss vernacular rather than in learned Latin. His lectures were well attended, but the faculty was outraged. Paracelsus immediately set about adding fuel to the flame of his own destruction: he upset local physicians, pharmacists, and civic leaders with his rough, dictatorial authority; and he publicly insulted fellow professors.

At the peak of his opportunity for a respectable career in Basel (a comparable opportunity was not to occur again), Paracelsus staged a symbolical act that has gone down in history associated with his name. It was St. John's Day, June 24, 1527. Students, celebrating Midsummer, had built a great bonfire. Paracelsus, accompanied by students carrying the heavy, venerated *Canon* of Avicenna, joined the throng. At his command, they hurled the great book into the fire. "Thus the realm of medicine has been purged," Paracelsus wrote.

Though loved by those whom he had healed, by act after act and with pamphlet after pamphlet Paracelsus tore from himself the shreds of respectability. The city council's patience was exhausted. Police were sent to fetch the culprit. Alerted by a friendly warning, Paracelsus fled.

He went to Colmar, to Esslingen, and on to Nuremberg. His apparently miraculous cure of nine of fifteen inmates in the Nuremberg leper asylum (likely they were syphilitics rather than lepers) laid the foundation once again for a promising career. Characteristically, Paracelsus almost immediately attacked the powerful Fuggers for selling guaiac wood, their quack remedy for syphilis. He soon was forced to leave Nuremberg and resume his travels. Again he roamed through Switzerland, southern Germany, Bohemia, and Austria. For a time, in 1532, Paracelsus experienced a profound religious crisis and turned to writing mystical theological treatises. Then once more he returned to medicine —on occasion well off, with friends, patients, money and prestige; then, again, in disgrace, fleeing, nearly destitute. No authority—professional, ecclesiastical, or civil—was too powerful to be immune to attack from Paracelsus' tongue or pen; however, his prestige never had a chance to rise to a level that would protect him from retaliation. His only alternative was to move on, time after time.

At last, in 1540, the Prince Bishop of Salzburg offered asylum to Paracelsus, and, exhausted, he spent his remaining days in relative quiet in the town that had once expelled him. His years, though not great in number, had not treated him well physically. He wrote his will, probably on his forty-eighth birthday; and three days later, on September 24, 1541, he died, likely victim of fatigues and stresses of his restless and wretched life.

It is difficult to arrive at fair judgment of a personality so contradictory. Paracelsus undoubtedly was one of the most arrogant and irregular individuals in medical history. Though often called a quack, he does not fit that category: the average quack is irregular because he has not the capacity to meet formal requirements; Paracelsus in many ways was far ahead of the medical men of his day. The quack, too, has but one aim—to get rich quickly; Paracelsus was always poor. Had he been willing to conform, he might have been wealthy. His extraordinary success as a physician cannot be attributed to his personality, but must have been due to real ability as a healer.

Wherever he went, Paracelsus left a trail of "chemical kitchens." When his patrons were generous, he built them to suit his alchemical taste; when in poor circumstances, he brewed his drugs on the charcoal beside his hostess' soup. Experimenting was his exacting pastime, and in exercising it Paracelsus spared neither himself nor his neighbors. In his experiments and in their medical applications, Paracelsus inaugurated an era of iatrochemistry—forerunner of twentieth century chemotherapy. In so doing, Paracelsus challenged not only Galen's venerated system of body humors, but also the search for a medical cure-all—so popular in the sixteenth century.

It was Paracelsus who introduced powdered tin as an anthelmintic; brought antimony into vogue; introduced zinc and zinc salts to medicine; used mercury compounds instead of metallic mercury for syphilis, and sought to establish definite dosages therefor. He employed lead, arsenic, copper, and iron compounds; he was familiar with sulfuric acid. His advocacy of the use of pure chemicals for specific diseases was perhaps one of his greater contributions to medicine. Characteristically, his contemporaries bitterly fought these revolutionary suggestions; but succeeding generations of medical men profited by them and carried forward experiments with chemicals in medicine.

Many forward-looking ideas are to be found buried in the mystical chaff of Paracelsus' writings. His great book on surgery concentrated not so much on operations as on how to avoid them; and, a generation before Paré, he condemned the barbarous practice of cautery of wounds. His theory that diseases sprang from seeds was an early version of the germ theory; and his "tartaric" diseases, the first inkling of metabolic disorders. His sympathetic attitude toward patients with mental disease reveals an insight into psychiatry and psychosomatics. Though idolized by faith healers, Paracelsus wrote: "Nobody can be cured by faith unless the disease was imaginary in the first place," and again, "The curing power of medicines consists not so much in the spirit that is hidden in them but in the spirit in which they are taken." Doctors of his day held it beneath their dignity to do the work of midwives; yet Paracelsus braved their prejudices and helped many women in childbed. In the presence of the sick, he was a changed man. "His arrogance and bombast turned to humanity and charity. His heart was naturally noble," a biographer avers.

Another difficulty in evaluating Paracelsus' contributions is the distortion to which they have been subjected both by detractors and by disciples. As medical men, his disciples contributed little credit to Paracelsus. Their surgery was crude. Their use of strong chemicals was not tempered by dosage precautions, an essential of Paracelsus' methods. To his name, however, went the blame for their errors.

To bring Paracelsus into proper perspective, it must be kept in mind that a personality as strange as his was by no means unique in the early Renaissance period. There were many irregulars, all exponents of profound revolutionary ideas, in religion, in economics, in politics, in science, and in medicine. But revolutions do not tend to proceed in orderly or reasonable ways. Foundations for the future, which such revolutions often create, frequently are obscured by rubbish and ruins of older structures destroyed in the process.

Paracelsus himself perhaps put his finger on the key to the success he enjoyed, despite his handicaps, when he wrote: "They drove me out of Lithuania, and Prussia, and Poland . . . The Dutch did not like me either, nor the schools . . . but thank God, the patients liked me!"

VESALIUS—AND THE ANATOMY OF MAN

IT TOOK Andreas Vesalius only five years to undercut the foundation stone of infallibility from beneath Galen, medieval medicine's idol, and to raise the study of human anatomy to a science based upon the solid rock of direct observation. The work Vesalius did during this period has been called "one of the greatest treasures of Western civilization and culture." His masterpiece, *De Humani Corporis Fabrica*, declared by Sir William Osler to be the greatest medical book ever written, is not only one of the more remarkable known to science, but one of the truly noble and magnificent volumes in the history of printing. When it came off the presses in Basel in 1543, it revealed courage and independence of thought in keeping with the resurgent spirit of the Renaissance.

There had been anatomists before Vesalius. Galen had written extensively on anatomy, but his writings teemed with errors. Unable to dissect human bodies, Galen drew his opinions from anatomic structures of monkeys and of pigs. Although dissection of human bodies was begun in the thirteenth century, belief in Galen's authority was so strong that for centuries his errors were neither discovered nor denounced. Among the pre-Vesalian anatomists who made significant contributions to man's knowledge of man were: Mondino of Bologna, who in 1315 made the first public anatomic demonstration upon a human body, and whose students carried on his traditions; Guy de Chauliac of France, who followed Mondino's methods; Marc Antonio della Torre, first professor of medicine at Padua, who began a comprehensive work on anatomy prior to his death in 1506; Leonardo da Vinci, whose drawings, made in the early 1500's, lay hidden for many years, but excited admiration and praise of later generations; Berengario da Carpi, first to make a comprehensive attempt at anatomic illustrations from nature (1521); Giovanni Batista Canano of Ferrara, an active dissector and discoverer of the valves in the veins (which perhaps inspired Harvey's research a hundred years later); and Charles

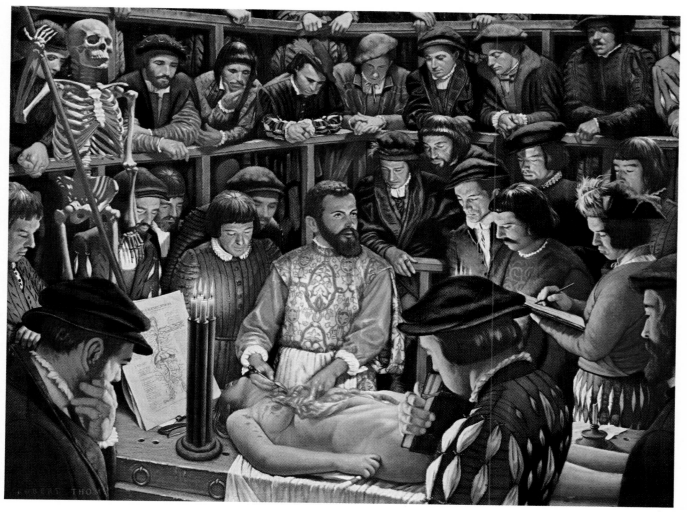

VESALIUS—AND THE ANATOMY OF MAN

Andreas Vesalius of Brussels, the first great teacher of anatomy from natural observations, conducted many anatomical demonstrations on human bodies while Professor of Surgery and of Anatomy at the University of Padua, 1537-1543. Highly successful, these were attended by medical students, physicians, interested civic officials, sculptors, and artists. First to break with Galen's 1400-year-old anatomical texts, Vesalius published Tabulae Anatomicae Sex *in 1538, and in 1543, the monumental* De Humani Corporis Fabrica. *Though reviled and ridiculed by Galenists, the validity of Vesalius' works soon overcame detractors and they became classic in medical literature.*

Estienne, whose text, begun in Paris in 1530, follows Galen, but was first to portray the whole arterial, venous, and nervous systems.

Professional artists played important roles in the early development of anatomy. In addition to Leonardo da Vinci, there were Dürer, Donatello, Verrocchio, Michelangelo, Raphael, Tintoretto, and Titian. Sculpturing and figure painting of truly great artists were based quite solidly on dissection and on natural observation; and attendance of artists and sculptors at dissection demonstrations became commonplace in the sixteenth century.

The most commanding figure in European medicine after Galen and before Harvey, Andreas Vesalius, was born in Brussels, December 31, 1514, of a long line of medical men. The family originally came from Wesel in the Duchy of Cleves, and took the name Wesele or Wessale after the name of the town. Latinized, this became Vesalius. The three weasels (Flemish, wesel) which appear on Vesalius' coat of arms refer to this origin. Peter, his great-great-grandfather, was a physician of reputation who wrote a commentary on Avicenna. John, Peter's son, taught medicine and served as physician to the city of Brussels and as advisor to the Duke of Burgundy. Evarard, John's son and Vesalius' grandfather, was physician to Mary of Burgundy, who became the wife of Emperor Maximilian I. Everard was author of a commentary on the *Ad Almansorem* of Rhazes, which inspired young Andreas Vesalius' graduation thesis. Andreas, father of the anatomist, was apothecary to Margaret of Austria and later to her nephew, Emperor Charles V. To the wife of this Andreas, Isabella Crabbe, was born Andreas Vesalius of Brussels.

Vesalius spent early years of his life in his native city. Encouraged by his mother and by the extensive family library, he early acquired the habit of reading and of studying ancient authors. He is said also to have exhibited intense interest in anatomy at an early age, and to have dissected many small animals. In 1528, he entered the University of Louvain, where he received a thorough grounding in Latin, an acquaintance with Greek, and continued to pursue writings of medieval authors on scientific subjects.

From Louvain, Vesalius went on to study at the University of Paris, probably in 1533. Possessed of a great name, this institution was highly conservative, an attitude which was embraced by the medical school, placing students at a disadvantage in relation to scientific progress that was being made, especially at Italian universities. Vesalius' teachers included Johann Guinther of Andernach (Guinterius), and Jacques du Bois of Amiens (Sylvius), both old-fashioned anatomists whose knowledge was acquired by reading Galen. Of the former, Vesalius once wrote, rather maliciously, that he had seen him using a knife only at the dinner table. Sylvius was said to have remarked that any structure found in contemporary man which differed from Galen's description could be due only to a later decadence and degeneration in mankind. "If you trust Galen, why dissect?" was a favorite professional cliché.

Like other young students of the times, Vesalius at first accepted Galenic anatomy, since there was no other. He had reason to complain that students learned less in the anatomic theater than a butcher might learn in his shop. Nevertheless, Vesalius acquired considerable knowledge of anatomy on his own initiative. By surreptitiously visiting old Parisian cemeteries and the gallows, he gathered an abundance of material—to the point where he dared wager with fellow students that he could identify any bone blindfolded. His teachers began to request his assistance in demonstrating anatomy, and in 1536 he conducted a demonstration singlehanded.

After some three years in Paris, Vesalius returned to the University of Louvain. Here, at great personal risk, he secured from a gallows a nearly complete skeleton which he proceeded to articulate. His reputation was growing, and in 1537 he was granted permission to conduct the first demonstration of human dissection to have been seen in Louvain in eighteen years. In February, 1537, he published his baccalaureate thesis, *Paraphrase on the Ninth Book of Rhazes*.

Dispute over the old controversy about venesection (whether it should be conducted near the wound, or far from it) ended Vesalius' stay in Louvain. He journeyed to Basel, where he had his thesis reprinted by Robert Winter. He then went on to Italy, where there were greater opportunities for study of anatomy and of medicine. He went to Venice, and from there on to the then Venetian city of Padua. One of the centers of scientific renaissance was the University of Padua, founded in 1222. By the sixteenth century its medical school was noted for its progressive and critical spirit. Under tutelage of the Professor of Medicine at Padua, J. B. della Monte, who introduced a type of clinical instruction that had hardly been seen since the days of Hippocrates, Vesalius made frequent visits to the sick both in Padua and in the capital city of Venice. Probably it was on one of these trips that Vesalius became acquainted with a fellow countryman, the artist Jan Stefan van Kalkar, a student of Titian, who later was to illustrate some of Vesalius' work.

Vesalius had not long to wait for recognition in Padua. At a solemn convocation, December 5, 1537, he was examined by the faculty and granted the degree of Doctor of Medicine "with highest distinction." On the following day, after performing a dissection, he was nominated by the Senate of Venice to be Professor of Surgery at the University of Padua, an appointment which carried with it also responsibility for teaching of anatomy and of botany. Vesalius at this time was in his twenty-third year.

Now, with a free hand, and with characteristic energy, the ambitious young professor began serious anatomic studies and demonstrations, breaking sharply with tradition. Instead of remaining seated, as had been the custom, in a lofty chair while assistants demonstrated and barbers cut, Vesalius descended into the operating theater to dissect and to demonstrate personally as he lectured. Students, physicians, and other men of learning crowded his classes. Many came to dispute, only to be convinced by the undeniableness of the young professor's demonstrations. To clarify his discussions, in 1538 Vesalius introduced large charts delineating various anatomic systems. Students received these so enthusiastically that, to prevent use and distribution of inferior copies, Vesalius was led to publish his drawings. To his own three sketches of the vascular system were added plates of his skeleton, drawn from three standard aspects by van Kalkar. The six plates were issued in 1538; today they are known as *Tabulae Anatomicae Sex*. They proved to be an instantaneous success, and were at once plagiarized in many countries. Not only were Vesalius' anatomic annotations unusual in accuracy and clarity; the woodcuts set a new standard in anatomic illustration as well as in the printing art.

Other publications followed rapidly. They were not free of Galenic errors, however, for it was not until 1539 and later that Vesalius became thoroughly convinced of errors in Galen's anatomic writings. Engaged on one hand in bitter controversy with one of his former teachers, Drivère, over venesection, and on the other in serving as one of the editors of an *Opera Galeni*, a complete edition of the works of Galen, Vesalius encountered many puzzling questions. He intensively sought answers in human bodies under his knife. As he learned, he lectured, wrote down his findings, and made, or caused to be made, hundreds of new drawings. This work grew and grew, finally culminating in publication of his masterpiece, *De Humani Corporis Fabrica*, in 1543. Printing of this work was undertaken by Johannes Oporinus, of Basel, erstwhile pupil and much-abused secretary of Paracelsus. Vesalius himself journeyed to Basel to supervise printing of this work. An excellent blend of format, typography, and illustration, Vesalius' *Fabrica* has been called: the greatest contribution ever made to human anatomy; the greatest single contribution to medical sciences; and the milestone marking the beginning of modern medical science.

Along with the *Fabrica*, Vesalius also published a smaller companion volume, known as the *Epitome*. This book was written in simpler style— intended to help orient students and other readers before attempting the more formal and advanced *Fabrica*—as "a pathway beside the highway" of the major work.

As might be expected, the revolutionary *Fabrica*, which made the anatomy of the revered Galen look like a colossal collection of gruesome errors, aroused a storm of vilification and abuse, hurled at Vesalius by most of his contemporaries. Sylvius, his former teacher, turned against his brilliant pupil with a storm of coarse abuse, calling Vesalius a madman. Colombo, his former assistant, sought to discredit and to deride his teacher. Not insensitive to these criticisms, Vesalius in rage and disappointment was reported to have burned notes that he was preparing for another publication.

Vesalius was not without friends, however, despite the vehemence of his attackers. According to Fallopius, the great majority of Italian physicians supported Vesalius and adopted his new teachings. His dissections and lectures were in considerable demand. The anatomist spent a year or two in travel, conducting courses in anatomy at the universities of Pisa and of Bologna. In Basel, he articulated a skeleton that may be seen to this day.

Insofar as his contributions to science, to medicine, and to anatomy are concerned, Vesalius' career ended with publication of the *Fabrica* and the *Epitome*, though he was to live another twenty years. Whether his change in choice of careers resulted from disappointment over slow acceptance of his work, or from desire for more conventional living, Vesalius forsook university halls for more lucrative practice. Says Robinson: "His numerous enemies did not silence him, the Inquisition did not smite him in his prime, but the siren of aristocracy seduced him from science."

War broke out in 1544, and Vesalius became court physician to Charles V of Spain. In this capacity, he served at Saint-Dizier, where he applied his surgical art and performed autopsies to determine causes of deaths. It was at Saint-Dizier, too, that Ambroise Paré, attached to the opposing French forces, was to make observations supporting his great contribution to surgery—disproving that gunshot wounds were poisonous, and discarding the barbaric use of boiling oil. Paré also was to popularize the *Fabrica* and teachings of Vesalius by writing an epitome of them in the vernacular of Parisian France.

During the winter of 1543, Vesalius' father, the imperial apothecary, died, leaving his son a substantial inheritance. After the halt of hostilities in September, 1544, Andreas Vesalius returned to the family residence in Brussels, married Anne van Hamme, and fathered an only child, a daughter named Anne. His professional stature was growing, and when Emperor Charles V arrived in Brussels in 1545, Vesalius was called upon to treat his imperial employer. He continued to enjoy royal favor, though his beliefs, that medicine should be regarded as a whole and not as separate specialties, and his personal methods in practice both of medicine and of surgery, aroused the ire of his contemporaries.

The second folio edition of *De Humani Corporis Fabrica* made its appearance in August, 1555. The volume was far more elegant than the earlier edition, the paper was heavier, the type larger. A new title page was prepared, and there were many improvements in the text. New material was added and corrections made. Strangely, original woodcuts, from which these editions of the *Fabrica* were printed, remained in existence in one place or another, in Europe, for 400 years, finally to be destroyed in the bombing of Munich during World War II.

On January 16, 1556, Charles V completed arrangements for his abdication and turned his Spanish and Sicilian kingdoms over to his son, Philip II of Spain. To Vesalius he gave a life pension and permission to enter the service of the new ruler.

From this point on, Vesalius' career was neither particularly significant nor happy. He complained that, in Inquisition-ridden Spain, not even a dry skull was available. There are many stories about his last years in Spain, none of which can be verified. However, in 1564, he undertook a pilgrimage to the Holy Land, stopping off at Venice, to learn that his friend Fallopius had died, leaving the chair of anatomy at Padua vacant once again. Whether Vesalius considered returning to the Paduan post is not known. He departed from Venice in April of 1564 for Palestine. On his return trip, it is believed he was shipwrecked on the small Greek island of Zante, and died there October 15, 1564.

Andreas Vesalius of Brussels has been called "the first man of modern science." Certainly he was the first physician to break openly with tradition, to study anatomy and to write of it directly from observation. However, he was not the only one: his contemporary, Eustachius, and his pupil, Fallopius, were his peers in discovery and in description of anatomic structures. Vesalius' great work, the *Fabrica*, after having been slandered, rapidly became a classic text in medical education; the work was pirated extensively; and, having freed anatomists of the fetters of Galenism, it stimulated other men to greater strides in anatomic research during the following centuries.

AMBROISE PARÉ
SURGERY ACQUIRES STATURE

WHAT tempestuous, revolutionary Paracelsus did for medicine, and brilliant, bold Vesalius did for anatomy—quiet, kindly, observant Ambroise Paré did for Renaissance surgery: he raised it from a scorned, antiquity-shackled trade to professional stature. His example and his writings influenced many of his contemporaries and pupils toward scientific and humane methods, and won for surgeons and for surgery new respect in the turbulent world of the sixteenth century.

Starting in late antiquity, learned physicians more and more frequently abandoned surgery, leaving performance of operations to manual workers, especially barbers. Separation of medicine and surgery was virtually complete in the Middle Ages—a situation that was to prevail in some places until well into the nineteenth century.

Surgery was held in low repute until its rebirth in the fifteenth and the sixteenth centuries. Only in Italy and in some centers in France did surgery even then gain grudging respect among practitioners of medicine, and among learned persons of the period. This rebirth was hastened by several factors: the general rise of the importance of the common man in the cultural and political growth of the period; technical developments, such as gunpowder; and spread of syphilis. These new conditions confronted medical men with problems that had to be faced without reliance on reference to classical authorities of antiquity.

The man to whom surgeons owe a debt of gratitude came from lowly origin, and, by standards of his day, was not well educated. He learned by observation in the great school of experience, under tough, grueling conditions of military conflict. Yet he came to know intimately most great figures of his century in social, military, and political circles in France. As Packard points out, Ambroise Paré was more than a great surgeon: his reputation for honesty and for sagacity was such that he became confidant and counselor to many of those with whom he

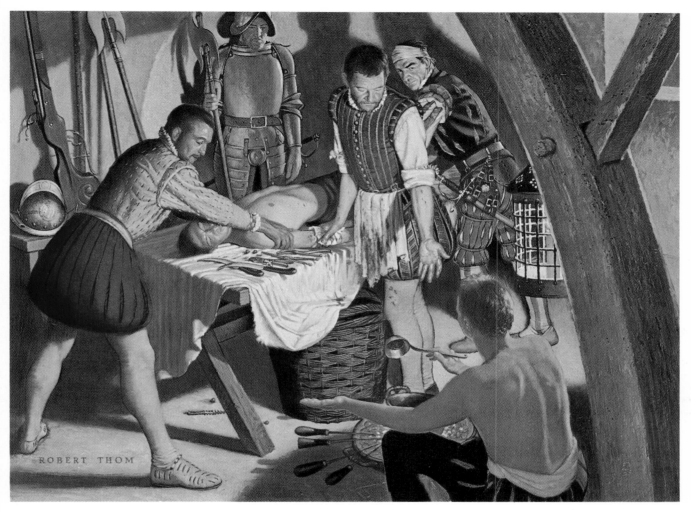

ROBERT THOM

AMBROISE PARÉ: SURGERY ACQUIRES STATURE

Ambroise Paré, young French army surgeon with troops of King François at Turin, in 1536, had his first experience treating men for arquebus wounds. Running out of boiling oil (traditional treatment for gunshot injuries), he improvised, discovered that unburned patients healed much better, and resolved never to use hot oil again. Countless soldiers and citizens benefited from this rule. It was some years later, in 1552, that Paré put aside cautery irons used to stop bleeding in amputations and reintroduced ligatures for tying blood vessels. During his life (1510-1590), practical, inventive, observant, compassionate Paré served as surgeon to four French kings; earned the title: "Father of Surgery."

came in contact, including kings, courtiers, and common soldiers. In an age when religious hatred was most intense, nonconformist Paré was sheltered by the King in his private chamber during the bloodiest massacre of Huguenots in Paris' history.

Not only did Paré attend heavy duties of an enormous civilian practice as well as demands made upon him as a military surgeon, but he also wrote voluminously, and found time for scientific research and for study. He loved his fellow men and liked their company. His gentle humanity was demonstrated repeatedly: in his compassion for his patients; in his willingness to comfort them though he knew their condition to be hopeless; in his determination and persistence in treatment, which restored many men to health when other physicians had given them up as bound for the grave. His writings, all in French, are narrated in simple language, and they convey the impression of exact observation and of truthful reporting. The only attacks made upon him were due to professional jealousy.

Ambroise Paré was born at Bourg Hersent, a little village near Laval, about 1510. His father is said to have been *valet de chambre* and barber to Sieur de Laval. Several of his near relatives were in medical occupations. A brother, Jean, was a master barber-surgeon at Vitré, and a brother-in-law, Gaspard Martin, a master barber-surgeon in Paris. Ambroise Paré apparently began his studies under his brother, Jean, and later became apprenticed to a barber-surgeon in Paris, in 1532 or 1533.

At that time the medical profession in Paris was sharply divided into three classes: physicians, members of the Faculté de Médecine, who tried to control all persons who practiced the healing arts; surgeons, belonging to the Confrérie de Saint Côme, who would not condescend to operate, but who treated patients for surgical conditions with plasters, ointments, and cautery; and barber-surgeons, who practiced venesection, cupping, and leeching, who shaved their customers, and who constantly tried to extend their activities by attempting operations, dressing wounds, and the like. These barber-surgeons were usually unlettered and unfamiliar with Latin, and therefore unfamiliar with the classic literature of medicine. However, they were almost the only practitioners of surgery in Paris. Paré's textbooks were the

94

works of Guy de Chauliac and of Jean de Vigo, which had been translated into French.

Paré did not remain for long in the barber's shop. Soon he became *compagnon chirurgien* at the Hôtel-Dieu, a position similar to that of today's intern or resident. At the time, the Hôtel-Dieu was the only public hospital in Paris. Therefore, opportunities for observation and for experience were excellent. After nearly four years, in 1536, Paré left the Hôtel-Dieu, and went off to one of the many French wars as surgeon to Mareschal de Montéjan, colonel-general of the French Infantry. Though Paré did not take examinations for admission to practice in Paris as a barber-surgeon until 1541 (probably because of economic pressures), he plunged into varied and strenuous opportunities for practice afforded by battlefields. It was during this campaign, in 1536, that the young army surgeon made his first great discovery—that boiling oil not only was of no use, but actually was hurtful in treatment for gunshot wounds.

At that time, all authorities on gunshot wounds taught that the victims were poisoned by the gunpowder, and that in order to counteract the poison, they should be treated with boiling oil applied locally. In his account of the incident (in *The Apology and Treatise*, written in later years), Paré describes his observations as follows:

"Now all the soldiers at the Château, seeing our men coming with a great fury, did all they could to defend themselves, and killed and wounded a great number of our soldiers with pikes, arquebuses, and stones, where the surgeons had much work cut out for them. Now I was at that time a freshwater soldier, I had not yet seen wounds made by gunshot at the first dressing. It is true that I had read in Jean de Vigo, first book, 'Of Wounds in General,' chapter eight, that wounds made by firearms participate of venenosity, because of the powder, and for their cure he commands to cauterize them with oil of elder, scalding hot, in which should be mixed a little theriac; and in order not to err before using the said oil, knowing that such a thing would bring great pain to the patient, I wished to know first, how the other surgeons did for the first dressing, which was to apply the said oil as hot as possible, into the wound with tents and setons, of whom I took courage to do as they did. At last my oil lacked and I was constrained to

apply in its place a digestive made of the yolks of eggs, oil of roses, and turpentine. That night I could not sleep at my ease, fearing my lack of cauterization that I should find the wounded on whom I had failed to put the said oil dead or empoisoned, which made me rise very early to visit them, where beyond my hope, I found those upon whom I had put the digestive medicament feeling little pain, and their wounds without inflammation or swelling, having rested fairly well throughout the night; the others to whom I had applied the said boiling oil, I found feverish, with great pain and swelling about their wounds. Then I resolved with myself never more to burn thus cruelly poor men wounded with gunshot."

Upon his return to Paris after this campaign, Paré studied hard, devoting special attention to anatomy. In 1541, after passing his examinations, Paré was admitted to the Community of Barber-Surgeons. That same year he also was married to his first wife, Jeanne Mazelin. Several children were born to this wife, but only a daughter, Catherine, survived to adulthood. The young surgeon's fame was growing. Encouraged by the anatomist Sylvius (Jacques du Bois), professor of medicine in Paris, Paré wrote a classic volume on the treatment of men with wounds made by arquebuses (gunshot wounds). Publication of this volume was not achieved, however, until 1545. In addition to setting forth his ideas about treatment of such wounds, Paré also described his method of locating balls that had caused the wounds: when confronted with a difficult wound, he had the victim reassume the position in which he was at the time he received the wound, then with careful search in the direction of entry the ball might be located.

Paré's second book, written between wars, appeared in 1549. It was a handbook on anatomy, written in simple French text designed for surgeons who were ignorant of Latin and of Greek. While based in part on his own dissections, Paré acknowledged that "a good part has been extracted from the book of André Vésal" (Vesalius). It also dealt with obstetrics and discussed Paré's reintroduction of a method of changing the position of the child in utero (podalic version) when faulty presentation presaged difficult delivery.

For the first thirty years of his professional life, Paré alternated between military service, in one war after another, and brief periods of private practice in Paris. During that time, he served as surgeon to four

96

kings of France. He entered the service of King Henri II as surgeon-in-ordinary in 1552, and served successively Kings François II, Charles IX, and Henri III. The Queen mother, Catherine de Medici, was both his patient and his friend. Under Charles IX, Paré was advanced to the office of first surgeon to the King, January 1, 1562; and he held this high position of trust also in the service of Henri III. In royal service he accompanied the kings or their generals on many campaigns; he was smuggled into the besieged city of Metz to treat wounded beleaguered defenders. In 1553 he was captured by the Spanish, but he practiced medicine while in captivity. When invited to enter the service of the Spanish Emperor, Paré declined. Promised that he would be set free if he could cure the Seigneur de Vaudeville of a leg ulcer from which he had suffered for six years, Paré succeeded, and returned to the service of King Henri II.

In 1554, probably due to his prominence at Court, Paré, though still unversed in Latin, was invited to become a member of the Collège de Saint Côme, thereby becoming a master surgeon—a surgeon of the long robe—instead of a barber-surgeon. However, two years before, in 1552, he had made his most important contribution to surgery, which, during his lifetime, was also the most controversial. Ever thoughtful of the comfort and welfare of his patients, Paré, reluctantly, had used the traditional hot cautery irons to stanch bleeding in patients submitting to amputations. At the siege of Danvilliers, Paré amputated the leg of an officer, using his "new method." In this, he reintroduced the ligature, tying off blood vessels instead of cauterizing the stump with hot irons. Though known to Hippocrates, the ligature had been almost completely abandoned since antiquity, replaced, through Arab influence, by cautery as a means of hemostasis. What Paré's reintroduction of ligatures meant to his patients in being spared pain and suffering may well be imagined; but this was seized upon by Paré's jealous medical contemporaries, especially by an academic professor of medicine, Dr. Étienne Gourmelen. This criticism fortunately stimulated Paré to write his *The Apology and Treatise*, in which he not only answered his opponent's objections by citing specific examples of successful ligations, but went on to give an account of his surgical experiences in various campaigns.

Many other contributions to surgery and to medicine were made by the kindly Frenchman. He invented new surgical instruments, trusses for hernia, artificial limbs, and artificial eyes. He fought superstitions and opposed use of medicines which, though fashionable and expensive, were worthless, such as unicorn and mummy. In Paris, he contended with epidemics of smallpox and plague. He wrote extensively on surgery and obstetrics.

Because of the regard of King Charles IX for Paré, he was one of the few Protestants to have survived the bloody massacre of Huguenots on St. Bartholomew's day in 1572, having been ordered to remain in the King's chamber during the hours of violence.

Over the years, Paré accumulated a comfortable share of worldly goods. A whole block, now bordering the Place St. Michel in Paris, is erected on land once owned by the surgeon. His acts of generosity were many.

Ambroise Paré's last appearance on the stage of history was as dramatic as its predecessors. Characteristically, he thought and acted in behalf of others. Paris in 1590 had been under siege for many months by Henri IV, and the defenders, led by the Archbishop of Lyons, refused to surrender, though conditions within the city were pitiful. Meeting the Archbishop in a public place, the old surgeon courageously called upon the leader to "take in hand the cause of the poor afflicted people." Apparently his words had weight, for within a few days the siege was lifted.

Paré died December 20, 1590, at the age of 80 years. He had lived through world-shattering political and historical events. During his lifetime he had published four editions of his collected works. Editions continued to come out after his death, as his influence continued to spread throughout the world of medicine. On the pages of these volumes, wherein Paré precisely described his experiences, there appears his oft-repeated philosophical summary: *"I dressed him, and God healed him."*

WORLD EVENTS AND MEDICAL HISTORY

Dates, persons, and events of significance to the evolution of Medicine include:

1714-1715	Timoni and Pylarini communicated Asiatic practice of smallpox inoculation to Royal Society.
1716-1794	James Lind.
1718	Lady Mary Wortley Montagu had son inoculated for smallpox.
1718	Geoffroy published table of chemical relationships.
1719	Neumann reported thymol.
1721	Zabdiel Boylston inoculated for smallpox in Boston (June 26).
1722-1809	Leopold Auenbrugger.
1728-1793	John Hunter.
1730	Frobenius described preparation of sulfuric ether.
1740	University of Pennsylvania founded as "College of Philadelphia."
1740	Maria Theresa began reign in Austria.
1740	Thomas Dover invented "Dover's Powder."
1740-1786	Reign of Frederick the Great.
1743	Red Cross arrangement at Battle of Dettingen (June 27).
1743-1794	Antoine Laurent Lavoisier.
1745-1813	Benjamin Rush.
1745-1826	Philippe Pinel.
1746	College of New Jersey (Princeton University) founded.
1747	Marggraf discovered sugar in the sugar beet.
1749-1823	Edward Jenner.
1750	Griffith Hughes gave classic account of yellow fever of 1715 (Barbados).
1751	Pennsylvania Hospital founded at Philadelphia.
1752	Smellie's *Midwifery* published.
1752	Medical Society founded in London.
1752	St. George's Hospital (London) founded.
1753	Lind's *A Treatise on Scurvy* published.
1754	King's College (Columbia University) founded at New York.
1754-1757	Black discovered carbon dioxide.
1761	Morgagni's *De sedibus* published.
1761	Auenbrugger's *Inventum novum* published.
1765	Medical Department of University of Pennsylvania founded.
1767	Kay and Hargreaves invented spinning jenny (beginning of Industrial Revolution in England).
1768	Baumé created the hydrometer.
1768	Marggraf discovered hydrogen fluoride.
1769	Guy's Hospital (London) founded.
1769	Napoleon Bonaparte born.
1769	Scheele discovered tartaric acid.
1770	William Hunter founded school of anatomy in London.
1770	First medical degree in United States conferred upon Robert Tucker by King's College.
1770-1827	Beethoven.
1771-1774	Priestley and Scheele isolated oxygen ("dephlogisticated air").
1771-1830	Ephraim McDowell.
1772	Beginnings of modern Japanese medicine.
1772	Priestley discovered nitrogen and nitrous oxide.
1773	Medical Society of London founded.
1773	Rouelle discovered urea.
1774	Scheele discovered chlorine.
1774	Wiegleb discovered myristic acid.
1774	Rouelle defined chemical nature of a salt.
1775	Lavoisier isolated and defined oxygen; also defined an acid.
1775	Andrew Craigie became first Apothecary General in America.
1775	John Morgan appointed Medical Director General of American Army.
1775-1783	American Revolution.
1776	Declaration of Independence of the United States of America.
1777	Lavoisier described exchange of gases in respiration.
1777	Scheele's experiments with silver chloride laid groundwork for photography.
1778	William Brown published first American pharmacopoeia.
1779	Pott described deformity and paralysis from spinal caries.
1779	Mesmer's memoir of animal magnetism published.
1779	Hôpital Necker (Paris) founded.
1780	Benjamin Franklin invented bifocal lenses.
1781-1826	René Théophile Hyacinthe Laennec.
1782	Medical Department of Harvard University founded.
1783	Scheele discovered glycerin.
1783	DeRozier made first balloon ascension.
1783-1785	Lavoisier decomposed water and overthrew phlogiston theory.
1784	Allgemeines Krankenhaus opened at Vienna.
1784	King's College (New York) rechartered as Columbia College.
1784	Scheele discovered citric acid.

HARVEY AND THE CIRCULATION OF THE BLOOD

WHAT has been called the greatest discovery ever made in physiology—the circulation of the blood—was quietly announced early in the seventeenth century as a part of a series of lectures in anatomy. No fanfare, no impassioned oratory accompanied the matter-of-fact pronouncement which was to shake beliefs in the medical world, to cast off, finally, the revered fetters of Galenism, and to establish an entirely new concept of function of the human body. The man who brought about this revolution was William Harvey, a short, slight, dark-complexioned Englishman, with flashing, spirited eyes and a wealth of nervous energy.

Though Harvey was first correctly to describe and to prove circulation of the blood, he was by no means first to study this marvelous physiologic phenomenon, wherein the heart, a remarkable muscular organ weighing about ten ounces in the adult human, is able to pump approximately twelve pints of blood through a double circular network of thousands of miles of arteries, capillaries, and veins, during a period of a few minutes. Lore concerning the pulse and conjecture about the importance of the heart are to be found in Egyptian papyri written 3500 years ago. Hippocrates, about 400 B.C., considered the pulse to be due to movements of blood vessels. Aristotle, in the next century, attached great significance to the heart, attributing to it many qualities it does not possess. But the erroneous views of Galen, written in the second century A.D., prevailed throughout the medical world for 1500 years. Galen taught that the three principal organs of the body were the liver, the heart, and the brain. Food was absorbed from the intestines and carried to the liver where it was elaborated into blood and charged with (imaginary) natural spirits. The heart, Galen believed, contributed vital spirits; the brain, animal spirits. He believed also that the pulmonary vein carried air from the lungs to the heart; that the septum of the heart was perforate; and that arterial and venous systems were separate. The arteries, he taught, carried vital spirits to the body; the veins carried natural or nutritive spirits, the

100

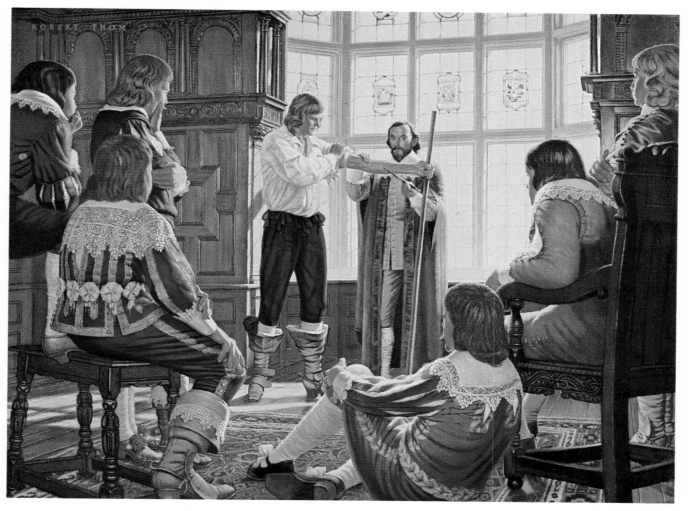

HARVEY AND THE CIRCULATION OF THE BLOOD

William Harvey, slight, energetic, scientific English physician of the seventeenth century, with his famed pointer in hand, used demonstrations to prove his revolutionary theory of the circulation of blood, during his anatomical lectures before the College of Physicians of London. His book De Motu Cordis, *published in 1628, upset traditional followers of Galen, brought entirely new concepts of circulation and of anatomy to medicine. Harvey, a graduate in medicine from Padua and Cambridge, physician to Kings James I and Charles I, was unperturbed by criticism, dedicated to research and to hard work. He died in 1657, after having seen his theory generally accepted by physicians.*

distribution of which was accomplished by tidal ebb and flow of the blood. For medieval and renaissance physicians, the fact that the great Galen had propounded this system was enough!

Early in the sixteenth century, Leonardo da Vinci and Andreas Vesalius questioned Galen's views concerning perforation of the septum of the heart, and primacy of the liver in the venous system. Michael Servetus, in 1553, described the pulmonary circulation; Realdo Colombo, about the same time, demonstrated that the pulmonary vein contained blood and denied that the septum of the heart was porous; and Fabricius of Aquapendente described and demonstrated the valves in veins. But it remained for Harvey, pupil and good friend of Fabricius, to investigate scientifically the circulation of blood and to postulate a sound theory that could be proved by demonstration.

William Harvey was born at Folkestone, in England, April 1, 1578. He was the eldest of a large family fathered by Thomas Harvey, well-to-do merchant and civic official. Several of William's brothers also became wealthy merchants; but William seems to have prepared for the study of medicine early in life. He was given every educational advantage, including King's School at Canterbury and Gonville and Caius College at Cambridge University, from which he received the Bachelor of Arts degree in 1597. Shortly thereafter, Harvey enrolled in the University of Padua. In its famed medical school, where Vesalius had done his most brilliant work, Fabricius of Aquapendente now was at the height of his career, lecturing in the oval, six-tiered amphitheatre which he designed for use in teaching anatomy (and which is still standing). Here, Harvey, one of several hundred students, stood day after day, watching and listening as the master lectured and demonstrated rapidly (lest the reek of unpreserved cadavers become overpowering in the close room). In later years, Harvey was to acknowledge his debt to the great teacher, crediting Fabricius' work on the valves in veins for having stimulated him to investigate the mystery of blood circulation. Galileo, the father of astronomy, also was lecturing at the University of Padua during Harvey's student days, and well may have helped raise the little Englishman's eyes beyond the limits of traditional horizons.

Harvey received the degree of Doctor of Medicine from the

University of Padua in 1602, returned to England, and that year received a second doctoral degree in medicine from Cambridge University. He then settled in London to practice medicine, losing no time in attaching himself to the College of Physicians, to which he was admitted a candidate in 1604. In November of that year he married Elizabeth Browne, daughter of Lancelot Browne, former first physician to Queen Elizabeth. In 1607, the College of Physicians elected Harvey a Fellow. He immediately applied for the post of physician to St. Bartholomew's Hospital. Securing the appointment in 1609, he held this important position until 1643, when he fell from political favor. The articles of his charge demanded of him that: "One day in the week . . . or oftener as need shall require you shall come to this hospital and cause the Hospitaller, Matron, or Porter to call before you in the hall . . . such and so many of the poor harboured in this hospital as shall need the counsell and advice of the physician . . . writing in a book appointed for that purpose such medicines with their compounds and necessaries as appertaineth to the apothecary or this house . . ." Unlike the surgeons, the physician did not visit patients in the wards; and the surgeons were accountable to him regarding the medical treatments which they applied.

Continuing his close association with the College of Physicians, on August 4, 1615, Harvey was appointed to serve as Lumleian lecturer —a position equivalent to that of professor of anatomy. This appointment carried life tenure; and Harvey held the post until 1656, one year before he died. The appointment called for his teaching a course on anatomy requiring six years to complete, consisting of two lectures each week and semiannual anatomical demonstrations on cadavers. At the end of the six-year cycle, the course was repeated.

Harvey began his lectures on anatomy in April, 1616—the same month that Shakespeare died. Lectures were held in the College of Physicians' new headquarters at Amen Corner, at the end of Paternoster Row. In his first lecture of this season, he discussed the abdomen, chest, and head. Lecture notes reveal that, by 1616, Harvey had dissected more than eighty different kinds of animals—a feat the more remarkable in view of his busy private practice.

Of greater significance among these first lecture notes, however, is the first clue to Harvey's convictions concerning the heart and the circulation of blood. The notes, a curious mixture of Latin and English, according to D'Arcy Power, are translated thus: *"It is plain from the structure of the heart that the blood passes continuously through the lungs to the aorta as by two clacks of a water bellows to raise water.*

"It is shown by the application of a ligature that the passage of the blood is from the arteries into the veins.

"Whence it follows that the movement of the blood is constantly in a circle, and is brought about by the beat of the heart. It is a question, therefore, whether this is for the sake of nourishment or rather for the preservation of the blood and the limbs by the communication of heat, the blood cooled by warming the limbs in turn warmed by the heart." The lecturer then went on to other matters.

It was not until twelve years later, in 1628, that Harvey saw fit to publish his great work. This he did in a poorly printed book of only 72 pages, containing a number of errors—but this book became the medium by which the thinking of medical men in anatomy and in therapeutics was revolutionized. His book was titled: *Exercitatio Anatomica de Motu Cordis et Sanguinis in Animalibus*—"An Anatomical Treatise on the Movement of the Heart and Blood in Animals."

The conclusions set forth in *De Motu Cordis* are virtually those written in Harvey's first Lumleian notes, enlarged upon and supported by observations and by demonstrations. Particularly significant, however, is the revelation of Harvey's scientific approach to the problem and his progress to solution. This method involved four steps: observations of facts; thought leading to hypothesis; performance of experiments to prove or to disprove the hypothesis; and finally, conclusions.

In essence, Harvey's observations were: The heart is a muscular organ that contracts and relaxes; contraction (systole) is its active position, expansion (diastole) its position of rest. At each contraction of the auricles, blood is forced into the corresponding ventricles, and thence into the great arteries as the ventricles contract. Once in the arteries, blood cannot return directly to the heart because of the heart valves. Harvey showed that the amount of blood passing through the heart in one hour would have weight three times that of the whole individual man; therefore the blood must pass through the heart again and again.

How does this occur? Harvey then set forth his hypothesis: The blood, he wrote, has "a movement, as it were, in a circle. The blood, forced by the action of the left ventricle into the arteries, is distributed to the body at large..." and, in his opinion, there are paths of communication between the arteries and the veins, whereby the blood is returned to the heart by way of the veins. By the arrangement of valves in blood vessels, he demonstrated that blood in arteries can flow only away from the heart; blood in veins can flow only toward the heart.

Harvey's experiments were at once simple and illuminating. By use of tourniquets he demonstrated that constriction applied to the extremities causes arteries on the side toward the heart to become enlarged and congested; and such constriction causes veins beyond the tourniquet to swell. An even simpler experiment was made by having an assistant grasp a staff firmly in his hand. Harvey, by depressing visible veins with one or two fingers, could demonstrate the single direction of flow of venous blood.

Harvey's conclusions are summed up in his brief Chapter 14. According to Powers' translation they were:

"*Since all things, both argument and ocular demonstration show that the blood passes through the lungs and heart by the force of the ventricles, and is sent for distribution to all parts of the body, where it makes its way into the veins and pores of the flesh, and then flows by the veins from the circumference on every side to the centre from the lesser to the greater veins, and is by them finally discharged into the vena cava and right auricle of the heart, and this in such quantity or in such afflux and reflux, thither by the arteries, hither by the veins, as cannot possibly be supplied by the ingesta, and is much greater than can be required for mere purposes of nutrition; it is absolutely necessary to conclude that the blood in the animal body is impelled in a circle, and is in a state of ceaseless movement; that this is the act or function which the heart performs by means of its pulse, and that it is the sole and only end of the movement and contraction of the heart.*"

In 72 pages, in this simple, direct phraseology, Harvey was to change the course of medical thinking. This was not without opposition, bitter and unreasoning, from defenders of tradition; but Harvey was to live to see his pronouncements become generally accepted throughout the world. Four years after Harvey's death, Malpighi's microscope, in 1661, was to confirm Harvey's postulation of passage of blood from capillary arteries to veins, in the lung; and in 1688, Antony van Leeuwenhoek was to report observation, through his little homemade lenses, of capillary circulation in the extremities.

From 1616 on, Harvey's Lumleian lectures continued; he attended patients at St. Bartholomew's Hospital; and he continued to gain eminence in his profession. In 1618, he was appointed physician extraordinary to King James I (he of King James' translation of the Bible fame). Harvey rose to physician in ordinary to James' successor, King Charles I, who remained Harvey's friend as long as he lived. Harvey became a Censor of the College of Physicians, and later, its Treasurer. On several occasions, the King commanded him to accompany diplomatic delegations abroad. He frequently accompanied his King on hunting trips, having the privilege of dissecting the kill for scientific study. In 1639, he became senior physician to the King, with lodgings at Whitehall. In that year, too, he accompanied Charles I to war in Scotland. That was the beginning of a series of controversies that led to a decade of civil war, travail, downfall of Charles I, and decline of Harvey's political fortunes. He remained loyal to and served his King until Charles was beheaded in 1649. Meantime, however, he found time to conduct and to record many experiments in natural science and in embryology; to become, for a time, a warden of Merton College; and to receive, from Oxford, another doctorate.

Following the King's death and the rise of Cromwell, Harvey retired to a quiet life in the homes of his brothers. Through most of his life, these same brothers had looked after his financial affairs. Afflicted by gout and by arthritis, and heavy of heart, William Harvey now turned his attention almost exclusively to the welfare of the College of Physicians. In 1651, his *De Generatione Animalium*, a work on embryology, was published. In 1654, he refused election to the presidency of the College on grounds of ill health. Two years later, he resigned his Lumleian lectureship and set up a gift fund for an annual dinner and for a commemorative oration.

Death came to William Harvey on June 3, 1657, in his eightieth year. Thus was closed one of the most active, fruitful careers in medicine of the seventeenth century, the contributions of which were to be of benefit to all mankind thereafter.

WORLD EVENTS AND MEDICAL HISTORY

Dates, persons, and events of significance to the evolution of Medicine include:

1785-1853	William Beaumont.
1785	Cod liver oil first used by English physicians.
1785	Lowitz announced decolorizing, deodorizing properties of charcoal.
1785	Minkelers first used illuminating gas in balloons.
1785	Withering's treatise on the foxglove (digitalis) published.
1785	Scheele discovered malic acid.
1789	Klaproth discovered uranium.
1789	Klaproth discovered zirconium.
1789-1799	French Revolution.
1792	Cotton gin (Eli Whitney).
1793	Benjamin Bell differentiated between gonorrhea and syphilis.
1793	Lowitz discovered mono- and trichloroacetic acids.
1793-1794	Reign of Terror in France.
1794	Lavoisier beheaded (May 8).
1794	Thomas Percival's code of medical ethics privately printed.
1795	Joseph B. Caventou, French pharmacist, scientist, born.
1795-1796	Société de Médecine de Paris founded.
1796	Jenner vaccinated James Phipps.
1796	Lowitz prepared absolute alcohol and pure ether.
1796-1815	Napoleonic Wars.
1797	Vauquelin discovered chromium.
1798	Jenner's *Inquiry* published.
1799	Davy discovered anesthetic properties of laughing gas (N_2O).
1800	"Royal College of Surgeons in London" chartered.
1801	Ritter experimented with ultraviolet rays.
1803	Fort Dearborn (present Chicago), Illinois, built.
1803	Klaproth discovered cerium.
1803-1808	Lewis and Clark explored the sources of the Mississippi.
1804-1815	Napoleon Emperor of the French.
1805	Battle of Trafalgar.
1805	Sertürner isolated morphine.
1806	End of Holy Roman Empire.
1806	Proust isolated mannitol.
1806	Vauquelin discovered cinchonic acid.
1809	McDowell performed ovariotomy.
1810	Figuier published qualities of animal charcoal.
1811	Massachusetts General Hospital (Boston) established.
1811	Courtois discovered iodine.
1811	Vauquelin discovered lecithin.

1813-1883	James Marion Sims.
1813-1879	Claude Bernard.
1815	Battle of Waterloo.
1815-1848	Horace Wells.
1815-1878	Crawford Long.
1816	Laennec invented stethoscope.
1817	Vauquelin discovered daphnin.
1817	Robiquet isolated narcotine.
1818	Caventou and Pelletier discovered strychnine.
1818	Meissner coined name "alkaloid."
1818-1865	Ignaz Philipp Semmelweis.
1819	Caventou and Pelletier discovered brucine and colchicine.
1819	Braconnet obtained grape sugar, treating sawdust with sulfuric acid.
1819-1868	William Thomas Green Morton.
1820	First *U. S. Pharmacopoeia* published.
1820	Caventou and Pelletier isolated quinine and cinchonine.
1821-1902	Rudolf Ludwig Carl Virchow.
1821	McGill College and University founded at Montreal.
1821	Runge isolated caffeine.
1821	Döbereiner discovered the process of catalysis.
1821-1894	Hermann L. F. von Helmholtz.
1821	Philadelphia College of Pharmacy founded.
1822	Serullas prepared iodoform.
1822	Louis Pasteur born.
1824	Braconnet discovered pectin, pectic acid.
1825	Jean-Martin Charcot born in Paris.
1825	*American Journal of Pharmacy*, first professional pharmacy periodical in English, published.
1826	Balard discovered bromine.
1827	Serullas discovered ethyl bromide.
1827	Wöhler isolated aluminum.
1827-1912	Lord Joseph Lister.
1829	Daguerre introduced photography.
1829	Tuéry demonstrated antidotal properties of charcoal.
1830	Kahler discovered santonin.
1830-1848	Reign of Louis Philippe.
1831	Guthrie, Liebig, and Soubeiran discovered chloroform.
1831	Soubeiran announced chloroform.
1831	Geiger prepared coniine.
1832	British Medical Association founded.
1832	Robiquet isolated codeine.
1832	Pelletier and Dumas isolated narceine.

LEEUWENHOEK AND THE "LITTLE ANIMALS"

MEDICINE, on its march through millennia, many times has been the beneficiary of men who, uninhibited by the mores of formal education, have allowed their curiosities free rein and have followed leads to basic discoveries that had eluded professional practitioners for centuries. By unorthodox methods, frequently scorned as unscientific, it has been their God-given privilege to come upon revelations that have been boons to all mankind through advancement of the healing arts. Such a man was Antony van Leeuwenhoek.

Leeuwenhoek was not the inventor of the microscope, although it often has been credited to him erroneously. But there is no question that he deserves to be called the father of microscopy, and credited as the man who laid foundations for the sciences of bacteriology and protozoology. With tiny lenses laboriously ground by his own secret methods, Leeuwenhoek became the first man to observe and to report on fascinating, multifarious microscopic forms of life with which, though unbeknown to him, man had coexisted for untold centuries.

Antony van Leeuwenhoek was born at Delft, Holland, October 24, 1632. His father was a basketmaker, his mother the daughter of a brewer. The father died when Antony was five years old, leaving the mother to care for him and his four sisters. Antony's education was scant, and in 1648, at the age of 16 years, he was sent to a linen draper's shop in Amsterdam to learn the business.

After six years in Amsterdam, Leeuwenhoek returned to his native town. Shortly thereafter, Leeuwenhoek married, bought a house and shop, and set himself up in business as a draper and haberdasher. For nearly 70 years, he lived and worked in Delft. Mid-seventeenth century Delft is described as "a fair and populous city, very clean, well built, and very pleasant;" and Holland had risen to front rank among nations in culture, science, and art.

In addition to his drapery business, Leeuwenhoek enjoyed considerable civic success. He held a municipal office comparable to that of

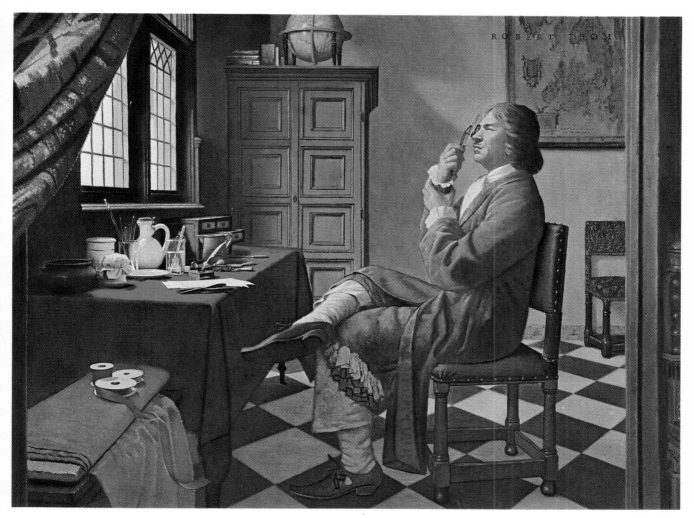

LEEUWENHOEK AND THE "LITTLE ANIMALS"

Antony van Leeuwenhoek, draper of seventeenth-century Delft, Holland, in his spare time retired to his "closet" to observe the wonders of the microscopic world through tiny lenses he laboriously ground and mounted. He was first to report having seen "animalcules"—protozoa and bacteria—and to confirm by direct observation circulation of the blood. Though 200 years elapsed before practical application of his discoveries contributed to medicine, his work laid the foundation for modern medicine's tremendous century-long onslaught against diseases caused by bacteria and other microbiologic entities—a world-wide campaign which has resulted in saving of millions of lives.

alderman; he was official wine gauger; and he was licensed as a surveyor. When Leeuwenhoek's good friend, the now famous artist Jan Vermeer, died, leaving his family an insolvent estate and some of the world's finest pictures, the draper was named administrator to straighten out the worrisome muddle.

There seems to be no record of how or when Leeuwenhoek became interested in grinding lenses and using them to investigate objects too small to be seen by the naked eye. Nor is it clear how he learned the art of lens-grinding. Throughout his life he kept his technical methods secret. Within the confines of his "closet," as he called his workroom, he turned out hundreds of tiny lenses, and mounted them laboriously but crudely between two thin sheets of silver or brass with small openings masking all but the central area of the lens. Most of his instruments were but two to three inches in height, an inch or less in width, and, except for thumbscrews, less than a half inch in depth. Solid specimens were mounted before the lenses on needle points, adjustable with thumbscrews both for height and for distance. Other microscopes were designed to hold small glass vials, or capillary tubes, to bring liquids within extremely short focal ranges. All of Leeuwenhoek's microscopes were made with single lenses; he used no compound lenses. By variations of grinding, he secured lenses of various magnifications. Most of them had magnification factors of not more than 160 diameters, although one in the collection at Utrecht University Museum is reported to magnify 275 diameters.

Of Leeuwenhoek's beginnings, Dobell says: "During the silent period preceding the year 1673, Leeuwenhoek evidently was engaged—in his spare time, when he was not selling buttons and ribbon—in making lenses, mounting them to form 'microscopes' of simple pattern; and after he had acquired much skill in the manufacture of these curious instruments, and had taught himself how to grind and polish and mount lenses of considerable magnifying power, he began to examine all manner of things with their aid."

The first report of Leeuwenhoek's activity in this new and fascinating field came in 1673, when his good friend and fellow-townsman, the famed physician Reinier de Graaf, wrote to the secretary of the Royal Society of London, describing Leeuwenhoek's work and enclosing a letter from the microscopist. This letter was the first of no less than 375 communications written by Leeuwenhoek to the Society over a 50-year period. Evidently Fellows of the Royal Society liked the reports on Leeuwenhoek's observations, for the secretary, Henry Oldenburg, encouraged him to continue his correspondence.

Leeuwenhoek's letters form a unique contribution to the literature of science and particularly of medicine. They were nearly all written in Dutch, the only language he knew; and in a simple, naive, conversational style—sometimes frank and earthy. A native honesty ran through them, however; while Leeuwenhoek's untutored and unscientific interpretations of what he saw led him to erroneous and sometimes ludicrous conclusions, he was most careful to distinguish between description of things he actually saw, and those he conjectured or "imagined." Considering that he was the pioneer in a field without literature or previous observers for his guidance, Leeuwenhoek's reports are most remarkable. He was so intent on telling what he had seen or thought that he had no time to worry about grammar or niceties of literary composition. He worked entirely by himself, receiving no help from contemporary microscopists. He disliked and resented interference, and he distrusted the knowledge—and sometimes the purpose—of persons who went to see him or offered him advice.

In 1680, Leeuwenhoek was elected a Fellow of the Royal Society—a distinct honor and recognition for one living outside England. In 1699, the *Académie des Sciences* of Paris elected him a correspondent. His observations excited great interest, and were widely read—but that was all. Nobody seriously attempted to repeat or to extend them. As the seventeenth century closed, Leeuwenhoek was the only earnest microscopist then living in the world.

Leeuwenhoek's specimens came from his everyday surroundings. No material or substance escaped the insatiable curiosity of the draper of Delft: rain water, scum from the surface of ponds, infusions of peppercorns, unborn mussels, animal and human tissues, scrapings, excreta of all sorts, and all kinds of mineral and vegetable matter, all came before his lenses.

Notable among Leeuwenhoek's peculiar habits was this practice: when he found a specimen particularly to his liking, he left it attached to the microscope and made another instrument. Over the years he accumulated many of these. He placed these in pairs in small lacquered boxes, 12 to 24 boxes in a case. One such case he willed to the Royal Society.

Leeuwenhoek was the first man to discover and to describe protozoa and bacteria (which he called "animalcules"). He used "a grain of sand" (roughly a cube of about 1/30 of an inch) as his standard of comparison, and described sizes of his "animalcules" by estimating that it would take 1,000, 100,000 or 1,000,000 of them to equal the bulk of "a grain of sand." Some of his estimates of identifiable species show a remarkable relation to modern micron measurements. He described with no little wonder the tremendously rapid multiplication of his "animalcules" when samples were allowed to remain standing for a few days; and he was aware of the relative purity of fresh rain water or snow water. Leeuwenhoek made drawings representative of various protozoa, bacilli, cocci, and spirochetes. He studied animal parts, such as blood, bones, eyes, hair, and muscles; he was the first to note striations in muscle fibers; and he is known, particularly, for his study and descriptions of spermatozoa. In his world of microscopic biologic forms, he saw: cellular division, birth, life, and death of his "animalcules"; parthenogenesis of aphids; and budding of hydra. He described how he had witnessed the wonderful branching "tree" which grew when he dropped a bit of copper into a dilute solution of nitric acid and silver. He even tried to observe the explosion of gunpowder under the microscope—an experiment that almost cost him his eyesight.

In one of his letters, after reporting on his observations on microscopic forms both in wine vinegar and in scrapings from between his teeth, Leeuwenhoek revealed a wry bit of sophisticated humor:

"I have had several gentlewomen in my house, who were keen on seeing the little eels in vinegar; but some of 'em were so disgusted at the spectacle, that they vowed they'd ne'er use vinegar again. But what if one should tell such people in future that there are more animals living in the scum on the teeth in a man's mouth, than there are men in a whole kingdom? Especially in those who don't ever clean their teeth? . . . For my part, I judge . . . that all the people living in

our United Netherlands are not as many as the living animals I carry in my mouth this very day . . ."

Leeuwenhoek also reported, in 1686, and frequently demonstrated for visitors, the capillary circulation of blood by placing a very small eel or fish in a glass tube and focusing on the transparent tail. Malpighi had preceded him, in 1661, in this observation, but it is doubtful that Leeuwenhoek knew of Malpighi's work. Leeuwenhoek also concluded that vessels leading away from the heart were arteries, and those toward the heart were veins, bearing out, by ocular observation, facts about which Harvey could only conjecture.

As soon as his discoveries became famous, Leeuwenhoek was visited by all manner of people who wanted to look through his lenses. The list of names of celebrities who called on him is long and impressive: included were travelers, writers, physicians, noted scientists, statesmen, kings, queens, an emperor of Germany, and Czar Peter the Great of Russia. Leeuwenhoek naturally felt flattered, but frankly confessed in one of his letters that he was bored by such interruptions and preferred to be left in peace to carry on his work. Also, he showed such callers only certain of his specimens, refusing to reveal others; and at no time would he disclose his methods of lens-grinding, or sell one of his microscopes.

Naturally, publication of observations of such a multitude of previously unknown things gave rise to attacks from unbelievers, from jealous contemporaries, and from those irked by Leeuwenhoek's lack of formal training. Of such criticisms, Leeuwenhoek wrote: "I am well aware that these my writings will not be accepted by some . . . they're still saying . . . I'm a conjurer, and that I show people what don't exist . . . I well know there are whole Universities that don't believe there are living creatures in the male seed: but such things don't worry me; I know I'm in the right."

In 1716, when Leeuwenhoek was in his eighty-fourth year, the University of Louvain officially sent him a medal in recognition for his work—an act corresponding to conferring an honorary degree.

Though handicapped by failing eyesight and by other rigors of old age, Leeuwenhoek continued his observations and his letters until the end of his life. He dictated the last record within 36 hours of his death. Leeuwenhoek died peacefully on August 26, 1723, in his ninety-first year, and his body was buried in the Old Church in Delft. Maria, his only daughter, true to her father's inclinations, maintained his microscope collection intact until her death.

Neither physician nor surgeon; actually, in formal terms not even a scientist, Leeuwenhoek was recognized by his contemporaries as well as by modern students as one of the most painstaking observers of all time, and the first to report on the great and wonderful world of microbes. Though Leeuwenhoek drew no conclusions regarding the relationship of his "animalcules" to causation of disease or to contagion, other persons soon connected the "little animals" with earlier philosophical speculations regarding the existence of living germs of diseases. Though theoretical implications of Leeuwenhoek's observations were recognized, no one made real or practical use of the knowledge during the next 150 years. Yet Leeuwenhoek's work laid the foundation for Pasteur's pioneering, and for the almost explosive growth of bacteriology and of protozoology in the latter half of the nineteenth century. The revolution in medical thinking and in medical practice which these developments brought about has resulted in prolonging lives of countless millions of people throughout the world during the past 100 years.

WORLD EVENTS AND MEDICAL HISTORY

Dates, persons, and events of significance to the evolution of Medicine include:

1833	Pelletier and Dumas discovered thebaine.
1833	Braconnet discovered dextrin.
1833	Johannes Müller's treatise on physiology published.
1833	William Beaumont published experiments on gastric digestion.
1834	Runge isolated carbolic acid.
1834	Runge discovered aniline.
1834	Dumas obtained and named pure chloroform.
1835	Berzelius coined the term "catalysis."
1837	Gerhard differentiated between typhus and typhoid fevers.
1837	Victoria became Queen of England.
1839	Schwann published treatise on the cell theory.
1840	Henle published statement of germ theory of communicable diseases.
1841	Pharmaceutical Society of Great Britain founded.
1843	O. W. Holmes pointed out contagiousness of puerperal fever.
1844	Rose discovered niobium (Columbium).
1845	Wilhelm Conrad Röntgen born.
1846	Morton introduced ether anesthesia (October 16).
1846	J. Marion Sims devised a vaginal speculum.
1847	American Medical Association organized.
1847	Helmholtz published treatise on *Conservation of Energy.*
1847	Virchow founded *Archiv für Pathologische Anatomie und Physiologie und für Klinische Medizin* (Berlin).
1847	Sir J. Y. Simpson introduced chloroform anesthesia.
1847	Semmelweis discovered pathogenesis of puerperal fever.
1848	Fehling introduced test for sugar in urine.
1848	Claude Bernard demonstrated that glycogen is synthesized in the liver.
1849	J. Marion Sims successfully operated for vesico-vaginal fistula.
1850	Claude Bernard published studies on arrow poisons.
1850	Fehling developed solution for detection of sugar.
1851	Helmholtz invented ophthalmoscope.
1851	Walter Reed born.
1851-53	Pravaz introduced hypodermic syringe.
1852	American Pharmaceutical Association founded.
1852	Santiago Ramón y Cajal born.
1852-70	Second Empire in France; Napoleon III became Emperor.
1854-56	Crimean War: Florence Nightingale.
1854	Paul Ehrlich born.
1855	J. Marion Sims founded hospital for women's diseases (New York City).
1855	Gaedcke announced cocaine from coca leaves.
1856	Sir W. H. Perkin (1838-1907) obtained aniline dyes (coal-tar products).
1858	Virchow's *Cellularpathologie* published.
1859	Darwin's *Origin of Species* published.
1860	Pasteur demonstrated presence of bacteria in air.
1860	Niemann isolated pure cocaine.
1861	Victor Emmanuel became first King of Italy.
1861-65	Civil War in the United States.
1862	Florence Nightingale established training school for nurses at St. Thomas's Hospital.
1862	Dr. Samuel P. Duffield began a small pharmaceutical manufacturing business in Detroit, Michigan.
1863	Old Cook County Hospital (Chicago) started.
1863	American Veterinary Medical Association (Detroit) founded.
1863	National Academy of Sciences (Washington) founded.
1864	Traube studied pathology of fever.
1864	Gray Herbarium (Harvard University) founded.
1864	Chicago Medical College incorporated.
1864	St. Louis College of Pharmacy founded.

SYDENHAM: PROPONENT
OF CLINICAL MEDICINE

Textbooks, not patients, were the basis of medical study and practice during the Middle Ages. The rebels of the Renaissance upset this comfortable, static way of medicine, so that more importance was accorded patients than philosophers. As the seventeenth century got under way, an era of discovery and rediscovery of diseases began. "Never was there a period when the medical profession underwent a more rapid change," says Dr. Joseph F. Payne, "than it did in London after the Restoration (circa 1660). Before the Civil Wars (begun in 1642), physicians in London had been a very limited and, on the whole, a very uniform class. They were guided chiefly by the Galenical tradition . . . The traditions of the classical school still bore almost undisputed sway . . . The only other school of medicine which had any distinct name, or formed a distinct school in practice, was the Chemical, or Spagyrical, constituted by the disciples of Paracelsus and van Helmont . . . Their exorbitant pretensions to infallible skill and their trafficking in secret remedies caused them to be ostracized by the College of Physicians. The very name *quack*, originally *quacksalber*, invented for them . . . meant originally nothing more than *quecksilber*, or quicksilver, the German name for mercury, a drug the use of which was one of their distinguishing marks . . . But during the Civil Wars and under the Commonwealth the upheaval of thought and disregard of traditional opinion put a sort of premium on unorthodoxy . . .

"After the Restoration the bonds of professional discipline were drawn tighter together . . . but the strife of conflicting opinions and methods of practice became keener than ever . . . The growth of physical science naturally tended to foster scepticism in regard to traditional doctrines of all kinds . . ."

The custom for young doctors from universities to spend a short time at one of the London hospitals was only just beginning and was by no means universal. Most physicians of the day, unless they had studied

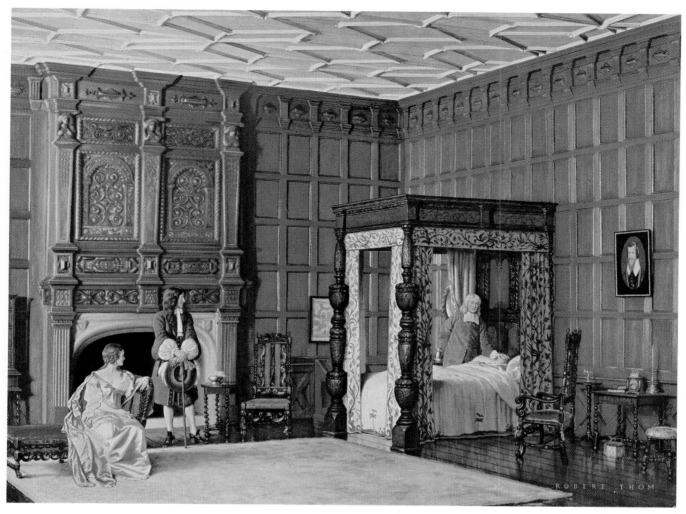

SYDENHAM: PROPONENT OF CLINICAL MEDICINE

Thomas Sydenham (1624-1689), seventeenth-century London physician, at the bedside of a patient—the only place, he believed, where doctors could learn about disease. Sydenham's plain Puritan costume contrasts markedly with high-fashion raiment worn by his lifelong friend, John Locke, physician-philosopher, who frequently accompanied him on his rounds of patients. Sydenham's honest and straightforward observations, accepted and published in many countries, earned him such posthumous titles as that of the "English Hippocrates," and also the "Father of Clinical Medicine in Britain."

117

abroad, probably had not worked in a hospital, but got their experience at the expense of their earlier patients.

Another factor that contributed greatly to change and to confusion during the second half of the century was the King himself, Charles II. On the one hand, Charles is said to have ordered medical regulation of the most conservative kind; on the other, because of an active interest in science, he gave patronage to quackery of every kind.

Besides having to compete with various kinds of spurious physicians, the regular doctors had their practice much cut into by the surgeons and apothecaries. Surgeons were not allowed to prescribe for internal maladies; nevertheless, they did so. Apothecaries, supposed to fill prescriptions of physicians for individual patients, did a large business in supplying their compoundings to any patient whose complaint seemed similar. In addition, there was a great number of others after the pennies of unwary patients—empirics, herbalists, watercasters, mountebanks, hawkers of amulets, charms, and nostrums; charlatans and imposters of every name and color. After the male quacks, says Payne, "came a great crowd of females—midwives, nurses, and 'wise women'—to sweep up the remaining crumbs of the medical feast."

It was into this melting pot of medicine that Thomas Sydenham plunged, to begin his medical career in London. It is remarkable that, out of this morass of medical practice and malpractice, he was to rise, head and shoulders above his contemporaries, as the most famous British clinician of the century.

Sydenham has been described as having a large and robust frame, reddish complexion, gray eyes, hair that was brown in early life but afterward turned gray, and which was worn long, in its natural state, without a wig. His manner was simple, as was his dress, in keeping with his Puritan background. He was essentially a man of action in a period when most physicians were men of books.

Thomas Sydenham was born in 1624 at Wynford Eagle, Dorsetshire, England, the fifth son and eighth of ten children of William Sydenham and his wife, Mary. His social background was very similar to that of Oliver Cromwell, whom he was to serve well. Sydenham came from an old family of well-to-do landowners who adhered to Puritanism. His father served as a Puritan captain in the Parliamentary army. His mother was killed by Royalist soldiers. Of his six brothers, four served in the Parliamentary cavalry, two of whom died in battle. His oldest brother, Colonel William Sydenham, became famous for military and political leadership.

In his eighteenth year, Thomas Sydenham was sent to Oxford University, where he matriculated as a Fellow Commoner, May 20, 1642, at Magdalen Hall. Hardly were his studies under way when political events began to shape his life. In the summer of 1642, conflict between King Charles I and Parliament was rapidly proceeding to final rupture. Sydenham's family connections and political feeling in his native county placed him inevitably on the side of Parliament; and some time that same summer he left Oxford to enlist in the Parliamentary cavalry, wherein he rose to rank of captain.

Back at Oxford, in 1647, Sydenham transferred to Wadham College to study medicine. Like many others of his day, as a member of the victorious party, he was granted the degree of Bachelor of Medicine by command of the Earl of Pembroke, April 14, 1648. Later that same year he was appointed a Fellow at All Souls' College to replace an expelled Royalist. Though he was a close friend of Robert Boyle, Sydenham did not participate in activities of the philosophical and scientific group known as the "invisible college," which was forerunner of the Royal Society.

Archives of All Souls' College show that, except for another brief period of military service in 1650, Sydenham continued as a Fellow there until 1655. The parish register of Wynford Eagle records the marriage of Thomas Sydenham and Mary Gee that same year. Shortly after, he took a house and started to practice medicine in Westminster.

During the years 1659 to 1661, Sydenham studied at the University of Montpellier, France. It has been conjectured that this was a very good time for Sydenham to have been absent from London: Restoration of Charles II took place in May, 1660. Because of the Act of Indemnity, however, Sydenham suffered no serious consequences; and he returned to London in 1661 to again practice medicine. At the age of 39, in 1663, he qualified as a licentiate of the Royal College of Physicians. Sydenham never attained the higher rank of Fellow, perhaps because of his earlier political affiliations, perhaps because he did not take his doctorate until 1676, at Cambridge. In view of his nature, it is likely that he cared little about academic distinctions. However, through the years, he enjoyed friendship with several eminent Fellows; and in the College's official records, Sydenham's name is frequently mentioned in terms connoting highest respect.

After settling down to practice in London a second time, Sydenham appears to have been an extremely active, successful, and respected practitioner. Though he grumbled at times that political activities of his opponents kept him from getting certain advantageous appointments, he seems to have had all the patients he could care for, considering the state of his personal health. Gout afflicted him before his thirtieth year and was a more or less constant burden throughout life.

In his medical practice, Sydenham easily gained patients' confidence with his plain honesty and strong nature. That he demanded his instructions be followed to the letter, there can be no doubt. When he deemed them necessary, he used strong measures; and he was not sparing of drugs, though at times he used no medicines at all. He repeatedly recommended use of Peruvian bark for intermittent fevers, and was one of the first to recommend the bark, sometimes "with steel," as a tonic. Sydenham's name is associated with the liquid form of laudanum; before his time, extract of opium had been used only in solid form. At times his procedures were quaint, such as directing that a puppy dog be applied to a patient's stomach, or that a small boy or girl be put in bed with a patient—forerunners of the hot-water bottle.

Fleeing London with his family during the plague of 1665, as did many of his colleagues (flight was the only effective preventive measure; and at that time such action was not looked upon as unethical), Sydenham used his enforced leisure time in the country to write his first medical book, on the subject of fevers. This volume was founded on his own observations, notes for which he had been collecting since 1661. His neighborhood was especially noted for its high incidence of febrile diseases. The first edition of the volume, in Latin, was published in 1666: it contained but 156 pages, and was dedicated to the Honourable Robert Boyle. The publication was given good notices in England; on the Continent it was received with enthusiasm; and it was reprinted in many countries. A second, somewhat enlarged edition appeared in

1668, with an introductory poem by Dr. John Locke, Sydenham's intimate friend, who, though a physician, is better remembered as a philosopher and as a politician. Dr. Locke shared many of Sydenham's unorthodox medical ideas, including depreciation of anatomy; and he frequently accompanied Sydenham on his visits to patients' bedsides.

In 1676, Sydenham's *Medical Observations* appeared. It was about four times the size of the book on fevers, and included most of that earlier work. Epidemics came in for considerable discussion; and it was that volume which became the basis for crediting Sydenham with beginning the science of epidemiology.

There followed, in 1682, Sydenham's dissertation on smallpox and hysteria; in 1683, his essay on gout and dropsy. Publication after publication came from his pen, until increasingly severe attacks of gout limited his activity.

Sydenham's works were based on his own observations; seldom did he refer to or quote other writers. The only classical man of medicine for whom he had any regard was Hippocrates. His descriptions of diseases, such as gout, hysteria, chorea minor (still called Sydenham's chorea), dysentery, scarlet fever, and measles, have become medical classics. His resolute endeavor to study natural facts by pure observation, putting aside bookish theories, facts, and fictions, and his relatively conservative methods of treatment, all are among factors that contributed to his fame. He valued knowledge only for its ethical value, as showing forth the glory of the Creator, or for its practical value, as promoting the welfare of man.

In the preface of his first book, on fevers, Sydenham displays his regard for his work as a physician. The medical practitioner, he says, should weigh the following considerations: that he will account to the Supreme Judge for the lives of sick persons committed to his care; that whatever skill or knowledge he may possess should be devoted "to the glory of God and the welfare of the human race;" that the patient is not a base or despicable creature, but one ennobled by the Creator; and finally, "that he himself is not exempt from the common lot, but is subject to the same laws of mortality and disease as others." He further states that every physician who desires to be held an honest man should not only do his best to restore health to the sick, but also to give certainty to the art which he professes (by writing and publishing his findings for the enlightenment of other medical men), so that his profession may become better and richer, and some benefit may accrue to mankind even when he himself is in his grave.

Among Sydenham's students were several physicians whose names also have come down to us: Sir Hans Sloane, Sir Richard Blackmore, and Thomas Dover, physician and buccaneer, who gave to materia medica Dover's powder. To Sloane, Sydenham epitomized his clinical philosophy: "I know an old woman in Covent Garden who understands botany better than I, and as for anatomy, my butcher can dissect a joint full as well; no, young man, you must go to the bedside, it is there alone you can learn disease." And to Blackmore's query about medical books, he recommended *Don Quixote*, implying, "Read what you like; reading books will never make a doctor."

John Locke, in addition to being a close friend who frequently accompanied Sydenham on his rounds, also was his patient, and in some ways his student. Besides Locke, and Boyle the scientist, another close friend was Apothecary Daniel Malthus.

To his eldest son, William, who also studied and practiced medicine, Sydenham left a memorandum entitled, *Complete Methods for Treating Almost All Diseases*. This volume, published posthumously, also enjoyed wide fame and large sale in many countries.

In his latter years, the torture of urinary calculus was added to Sydenham's sufferings from gout. He died December 29, 1689, at his house in Pall Mall, and was buried in St. James's Church, Westminster.

By the first quarter of the eighteenth century, Sydenham's reputation was well established in the annals of medical history abroad, and he was named with pride in Harveian orations at the Royal College of Physicians as the "English Hippocrates." He had set an example of the true clinical method. Into it went his independent and unprejudiced spirit, combined with acute powers of observation. The great Puritan, says Payne, "made his profession a part of his religion; he prosecuted his task of advancing knowledge and healing the sick with the same fervent zeal which other men have shown in what are regarded as more sacred avocations." Indeed, he well deserved the title given him posthumously: "The Father of Clinical Medicine in Britain."

WORLD EVENTS AND MEDICAL HISTORY

Dates, persons, and events of significance to the evolution of Medicine include:

1865	Joseph Lister introduced antiseptic treatment of wounds.
1865	Gregor Mendel published memoir on plant hybridity.
1865	Claude Bernard published "An Introduction to the Study of Experimental Medicine."
1865	Cornell University founded.
1865	Pasteur studied silkworm diseases.
1865	Ignaz Semmelweis died.
1865	Billings founded U. S. Army Medical Library.
1865	First International Pharmaceutical Congress convened, Brunswick, Germany.
1865-1866	Villemin demonstrated transmissibility of tuberculosis by inoculation (Klencke, 1843).
1866	J. Marion Sims published "Clinical Notes on Uterine Surgery."
1866	A. J. Ångström introduced Ångström units.
1866	Metropolitan Health Board (New York City) established.
1866	Duffield, Parke & Company formed as partnership in Detroit, Michigan. (Beginning of Parke, Davis & Company.)
1867	Lister introduced antiseptic surgery.
1867	Helmholtz published treatise on physiological optics.
1867	Bobbs performed cholecystotomy.
1867	A. W. von Hoffmann discovered formaldehyde.
1867	First International Medical Congress at Paris.
1867	Dominion of Canada established.
1867	Opening of Suez Canal and of Pacific Railway.
1867	Canadian Medical Association organized.
1867	Chicago Board of Health organized.
1868	University of Tokyo (Tokyo Teikoku Daigaku) founded.
1868	Allbutt introduced clinical thermometer.
1868	Darwin published treatise on *The Variation of Animals and Plants Under Domestication.*
1868	Hering and Breurer discovered self-regulation of respiration (rôle of vagus).
1868	Society of Czechoslovakian Physicians (Prague).
1868	Société de Médecine Légale (Paris) founded.

1869	University of Warsaw founded.
1869	Brown-Séquard introduced doctrine of internal secretions.
1869	Virchow urged medical inspection of schools.
1869	Harvey Williams Cushing born.
1869	Oscar Liebreich demonstrated hypnotic effect of chloral hydrate.
1869	Ceylon Medical College founded.
1869	American Museum of Natural History (New York City) founded.
1869	Chicago Medical College became Medical Department of Northwestern University.
1869	Massachusetts State Board of Health created.
1869	Ontario (Canada) Act for Registration of Vital Statistics.
1870	Fritsch and Hitzig investigated localization of functions of brain.
1870	Linoleum invented.
1870	Wisconsin Academy of Sciences founded.
1870	Anthropological Society of Vienna founded.
1870-71	Franco-Prussian War (test of vaccination).
1871	Establishment of German Empire and French Republic.
1871	Darwin's *Descent of Man and Selection in Relation to Sex* published.
1871	Hammarsten discovered rôle of fibrinogen in coagulation of blood.
1871	Royal Anthropological Institute (London) founded.
1871	Walter Bradford Cannon born.
1871	Joseph Lister noted antibiotic phenomena.
1871-72	First American filter for water supply at Poughkeepsie, New York.
1872	Carlos Finlay (Cuba) declared that mosquitoes transmitted yellow fever.
1872	University of Adelaide (Australia) founded.
1872	Abbé introduced oil immersion lenses.
1872	Merck introduced pyoctanin (methyl violet).
1872	American Public Health Association held first meeting.
1873	Obermeier discovered spirillum of relapsing fever.

123

JAMES LIND
CONQUEROR OF SCURVY

WORLD HISTORY and destinies of nations have been shaped on more than one occasion by alert physicians' capabilities to observe, to test, to provide solutions for health problems, and, most important of all, to convince governmental authorities that decisive remedial actions must be taken. Such a man was James Lind, naval surgeon, who pointed the way to overcome scurvy, scourge of sailing ships on the seven seas.

Scurvy was known to and described by the ancients; but it did not assume calamitous proportions until sailing ships replaced oared galleys, thereby making possible long journeys on the high seas. Prior to 1500, ships seldom ventured far from land, so frequent provisioning was not a problem. With the beginning of the sixteenth century, however, growth of nations, competition for trade with far-off places, world exploration, and colonization, set European countries to building fleets of sailing vessels and dispatching them upon journeys which ran from weeks into months and from months into years. Attendant to growth of oceanic travel came problems of provisioning, of preservation of stores, of recruitment of manpower, and of maintenance of health of crews. The latter problem, keeping crews healthy and capable of performance of duty, dependent as it was upon other factors, was of prime importance to success or failure of expeditions; yet for three centuries, it received the least official attention. Among many shipboard health hazards, scurvy was the most dangerous.

It is said that, during the three centuries from 1500 to 1800, scurvy caused more deaths among sailors than other diseases, naval engagements, marine disasters, shipwrecks, and accidents, combined. From 1600 to 1800, it is estimated that not less than one million lives were taken by this dreaded form of avitaminosis, even though naval surgeons had published reports of observations relative both to means of remedy and to prevention!

The world has been thrilled and entertained by countless tales of men who went to sea in sailing ships and of the romance of faraway

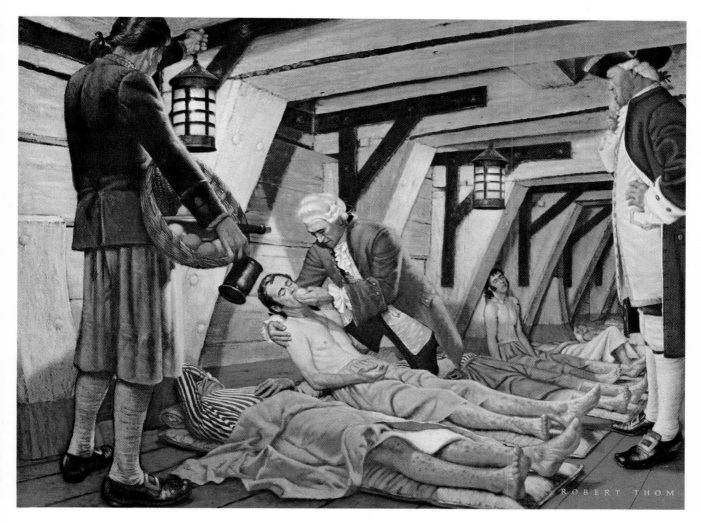

JAMES LIND: CONQUEROR OF SCURVY

Surgeon of Britain's Royal Navy aboard H.M.S. *Salisbury, in the English Channel in 1747, James Lind conducted a series of clinical experiments that definitely proved citrus fruits or their juices would cure scurvy, dread dietary-deficiency disease that killed a million seamen between 1600 and 1800. Dr. Lind's work, at sea, in Edinburgh, and at Haslar Naval Hospital, plus his three books, on scurvy, on care of sailors' health, and on tropical diseases, had much to do with reforming naval health practices, saving lives both on sea and land, and shaping destinies of nations, as world commerce increased.*

places. Few readers, however, realize the hardships and privations men had to endure on such voyages; or the "hell that no poet's imagination ever was able to invent" that made up the daily life of sailors. But medical men were obliged to report in their journals the bleak facts: the wood from which these picturesque, full-rigged sailing vessels were built never dried and slowly rotted. Materials and stores, including food, were subject to mold, to putrefaction, and to infestation with vermin. Rats infested ships; and men had to live in "a terrible odor of bilge water, stale cooking, dry rot, dead rats, and unwashed humanity." What drinking water they had soon became foul and, frequently coming from contaminated sources, brought aboard causative factors of dysenteries and of enteric fever. Food rations, consisting mainly of salt pork, salt beef, and ship's biscuit, were as insufficient as they were disgustingly full of maggots and of beetles. Sailors' few clothes soon became ragged and were nearly always wet. There was almost total absence of ventilation inside crowded ships' crews' quarters. Only in the eighteenth century did each man have his own hammock; before that, he shared a hammock and, frequently, disease-bearing vermin, with a man on the opposite shift. Allowed barely 14 inches each in which to swing their hammocks in stifling quarters, seamen readily transmitted causative factors of such other contagious diseases as the exanthemata and respiratory infections to their fellows. This condition was further aggravated by prevailing custom: Replacements to ships' personnel sometimes were made by emptying jails, and by impressment. The untrained, the unfit, and the unwary, from waterfront bars in port towns, were driven or carried aboard just before sailing. After a few weeks at sea, overcrowded crews such as these readily succumbed to scurvy. Of the crews of five ships that started Magellan's famed round-the-world cruise (1519-1522), only 18 returned. Of 961 officers and men who, in 1740, began a round-the-world voyage under England's Lord Anson, only 200 returned in 1744. More naval objectives were lost as a result of incapacitation of crews by scurvy than were lost from shot and sword. Only in the last years of the eighteenth century was this situation changed by top administrative action, and then only by enforcement of measures based upon principles laid down by Dr. Lind, who has been called the father of naval hygiene in England.

Born in Edinburgh, Scotland, October 4, 1716, into a substantial upper middle-class family, James Lind, at 15 years of age, was apprenticed to a well-known Edinburgh physician, George Langlands. This city offered favorable environment for medical students, for the University of Edinburgh had become a famous medical center.

As did many young Scottish medical students of the period, Lind entered service in the Royal Navy as a Surgeon's Mate in 1739, the same year that war began between England and Spain. Duties of a naval surgeon in Lind's day were to visit the sick twice daily, to keep the commander informed as to the health of the crew, to recommend ways of improving health conditions, to keep records, to conduct examinations, and, of course, to take care of those men wounded in battle.

During his ten years of service, Lind saw many men ill with scurvy. Because their rations were supplemented with fresh foods, by custom and by their own purchases, officers were less likely to develop scurvy; but ordinary seamen's diet was almost vitamin-free, so that after a few weeks at sea, beset by fatigue, by wetness, by cold, by loss of sleep, and by homesickness, symptoms and signs of scurvy and of other diseases appeared with appalling frequency.

Lind clearly describes the clinical picture of patients with scurvy: lassitude, weakness, swelling of legs and arms, softening and hemorrhages of gums, and hemorrhages under the skin, producing purplish or black patches. In patients in advanced stages teeth became loose and sometimes fell out; the breath became foul; strength failed to the point where the victim was unable to stand or to be up and about; and the slightest touch or movement was excruciatingly painful. If no relief could be provided, death resulted from exhaustion, from heart failure, or from acute infection such as pneumonia.

Value of the juice of citrus fruits, of sauerkraut, of fresh vegetables, and of greens, in treatment for scurvy had been recognized, and reports on success therewith published, more than a century before Lind's time; but such confusion of recommendations of useless measures and drugs also had grown out of ignorance of the cause of scurvy that true remedies failed to impress most medical men. It remained for Lind, on

May 20, 1747, to inaugurate a simple, straightforward series of tests, in the best clinical tradition, in order to determine relative effectiveness of a half dozen of the more popular measures. He reports: "I took twelve patients in the scurvy, on board the *Salisbury* at sea. Their cases were as similar as I could have them . . . They lay together in one place in the forehold; and had one common diet, water-gruel sweetened with sugar in the morning, fresh mutton-broth often times for dinner; and for supper, barley and raisins, rice and currants, sago and wine, or the like. Two of these were ordered each a quart of cyder a-day. Two others took twenty-five gutts (drops) of *elixir vitriol* three times a-day, upon an empty stomach; using a gargle strongly acidulated with it for their mouths. Two others took two spoonfuls of vinegar three times a-day, upon an empty stomach; having their gruels well acidulated with it, and also the gargle for their mouth. Two of the worst patients, with the tendons in the hams rigid, were put under a course of sea-water. Of this they drank half a pint every day, and sometimes more or less as it operated as a gentle physic. Two others had each two oranges and one lemon given them every day. These they ate with greediness, at different times, upon an empty stomach. They continued but six days under this course, having consumed the quantity that could be spared. The two remaining patients took the bigness of a nutmeg three times a-day, of an electuary recommended by a hospital surgeon, made of garlic, mustard-seed, horse-radish, balsam of Peru, and gum myrrh using for common drink, barley-water well acidulated with tamarinds; by a decoction of which, with the addition of cream of tartar, they were gently purged three or four times during the course.

"The consequence was, that the most sudden and visible good effects were perceived from the use of the oranges and lemons; one of those who had taken them, being at the end of six days fit for duty . . . The other was the best recovered of any in his condition; and being now deemed pretty well, was appointed nurse to the rest of the sick."

Cider, Lind reported, had the next best effect. There was no remarkable alteration of the course of the disease in any of the other patients at the end of the two weeks' tests.

Lind retired from the Royal Navy in 1748, and returned to Edinburgh to obtain his doctorate in medicine from the University and his license from the Royal College of Physicians of the city. In 1750, he was elected a Fellow of the College; and, in 1757, its treasurer. In 1753, his classic, *A Treatise on the Scurvy*, was published in Edinburgh. Three more editions were to be published in the next twenty years.

Appointment of Dr. Lind to the post of Chief Physician at the new Royal Naval Hospital—Haslar Hospital, near Portsmouth—came in 1758, probably due to the interest and admiration of Lord Anson, then First Lord of the Admiralty. At the time, Haslar was the largest hospital in Europe, capable of providing care for more than 2,200 patients. Lind served in this post for 25 years and had the satisfaction of seeing his son, Dr. John Lind, serve, first as his assistant, and later as his successor, when he retired, in 1783.

Just prior to his appointment to Haslar, Lind's second great volume on nautical medicine was published. First edition of *An Essay on the Most Effectual Means of Preserving the Health of Seamen in the Royal Navy* was published in 1757. It was to go through two later editions, in 1762, and 1779. During his years at Haslar, Lind not only observed patients with scurvy and with many other diseases common to seamen in European waters, but patients sick with a variety of diseases acquired all over the world—the Orient, India, Africa, North America, South America, and the Pacific islands. From this experience came the third book in his remarkable series, *An Essay on Diseases Incidental to Europeans in Hot Climates*, published in 1768, which was to go through six editions. These volumes formed a trilogy comprising observations relating to problems in most of the fields included in nautical medicine.

Readers of Lind's works are impressed with the soundness of his reasoning, the accuracy of his observations, and the logic he reveals in dealing with problems of diagnosis, of treatment, and of prevention of disease. In summing up achievements in improved naval medicine which may be credited to Lind, Louis H. Roddis cites these points:

1. The classic experiment proving the importance of citrus fruits or their juices in prevention of and in treatment for scurvy. Application of these principles late in the eighteenth century and early in the nineteenth century led to virtual elimination of scurvy in men of the Royal Navy.

2. Recommendation that new recruits be brought first to receiving

ships for quarantine, and that they be bathed and issued clean clothing. This did more to eliminate shipboard typhus fever than any other measure.

3. The suggestion that special ships be run between England and naval blockading squadrons to supply fighting ships with fresh provisions, fruits, and green vegetables. Adoption of this suggestion for maintaining ships' crews in fighting trim is believed to have been a definite deciding factor in favor of the British in their wars with Napoleon.

4. Demonstration of a practical method of obtaining fresh water from sea water by simple distillation, adapting utensils normally found on shipboard.

5. Recommendations for physical examination of naval recruits with maintenance of records thereof.

6. Suggestion of issuance of naval uniforms to seamen, a measure favorably affecting both health and morale of these men.

7. Insistence on physical exercise and on cold baths as "toughening-up" processes.

8. Use of cinchona bark for prevention of malaria.

9. Recommendations that, in the tropics, ships be anchored well off shore, and that crews not be given work details or liberty ashore at night. This did much to reduce incidence of malaria.

Dr. Lind did not live to see the Admiralty make use of lemon juice obligatory as a prophylactic against scurvy (this came at the insistence of Lind's pupils, Blane and Trotter, in 1795), but he did see his recommendation for receiving ships, to which recruits were sent to be examined, clothed, outfitted, and quarantined for an indoctrination period, put into effect, in 1781.

On July 18, 1794, death came to Dr. Lind, then in his seventy-eighth year. Benefits of his work, however, continued thereafter, indirectly exercising powerful influences upon the course of history of his nation and of the world, and upon successes in sea commerce and in exploration, well into the nineteenth century.

130

WORLD EVENTS AND MEDICAL HISTORY

Dates, persons, and events of significance to the evolution of Medicine include:

1874	Cholera conference in Vienna.
1874	Joseph Goldberger born.
1874	Fiedler stressed danger of morphine habit.
1874	Willy Kühne discovered trypsin.
1875	Faculté de Médecine et Pharmacie (Lille) founded.
1875	Landois discovered hemolysis from transfusion of alien blood.
1875	Hardy and Gerard introduced pilocarpine.
1875	Chesebrough obtained vaseline.
1875	English Public Health Act.
1875	Boston Medical Library founded (opened October 18).
1876	Imperial Board of Health founded at Berlin (April 30).
1876	Royal Sanitary Institute founded (London).
1876	Johns Hopkins University founded.
1876	Royal Academy of Medicine founded at Rome.
1876	Kolbe isolated salicylic acid.
1876	Koch obtained pure cultures of anthrax bacilli on artificial media.
1876	Pictet invented artificial manufacture of ice.
1876	Max Nitze introduced cystoscope.
1876	American Dermatological Association (Boston) founded.
1876	Bell telephone introduced.
1876	American Chemical Society (Washington, D. C.) founded.
1876-1909	New Cook County Hospital (Chicago) begun and completed.
1877	Pasteur discovered bacillus of malignant edema.
1877	L. Pasteur and J. Joubert observed antibiotic phenomena.
1877	Esmarch introduced aseptic bandage.
1877	Ernst von Bergmann introduced corrosive sublimate antisepsis.
1877-1878	Bollinger and Israel described actinomycosis.
1878	Koch discovered causes of traumatic infections.
1878	J. Marion Sims performed cholecystotomy.
1878	Von Basch measured blood pressure with sphygmomanometer.
1878	Claude Bernard died.
1878	Nägeli discovered that bacteria are not given off by moist surfaces.
1878	Edison invented platinum wire (incandescent) electric lamp.
1878-79	Welch, Prudden, Sternberg and Salmon introduced bacteriology in United States.
1879	Neisser discovered gonococcus.
1879	Sir William Macewen removed brain tumors.
1879	Hansen and Neisser discovered lepra bacillus.
1879	First chemically standardized pharmaceutical preparation, *Liquor Ergotae Purificatus*, introduced by Parke-Davis.
1879	Max Nitze introduced cystoscopy.
1879	Manson discovered transmission of filariasis by mosquitoes.
1879	Billings and Fletcher started *Index Medicus*.
1880	Pasteur discovered streptococcus, staphylococcus, and pneumococcus (Sternberg).
1880	Albert Ladenburg, German chemist, isolated hyoscine.
1880	Aseptic surgical techniques developed.
1880	Eberth isolated typhoid bacillus.
1880	Charcot published studies on lesions of the brain.
1880	Pasteur and Sternberg demonstrated carriage of pneumonia bacillus in healthy mouth.
1880	American Surgical Association founded.
1880-81	Laveran discovered parasite of malarial fever.
1881	Ogston discovered staphylococci in abscesses.
1881	Pasteur produced vaccine against anthrax.
1881	Medin discovered epidemic nature of poliomyelitis.
1881	Koch introduced gelatin media (solid plate cultures) and steam sterilization.
1881	Grimaux obtained codeine from morphine.
1881	Carlos Finlay surmised transmission of yellow fever by *Stegomyia fasciata* (August 14).

MORGAGNI AND
PATHOLOGIC ANATOMY

THE CONCEPT that processes of disease might originate in localized areas of the body was unfamiliar to ancient men of medicine. In their opinion, diseases acted generally throughout the body; illness either was ascribed to disturbance of the four humors, or to upset of atoms and of pores. During the Renaissance these old ideas slowly changed as medical men began to do autopsies. Systematic examination of the dead led to realization that in beginning stages disease usually affects but one organ or group of tissues, and sometimes for long periods may be localized in one area of the body. To adjust to this new concept of disease, physicians had radically to change their ideas regarding both diagnosis and treatment for ailments suffered by their patients. Yet despite the accumulating evidence, "generalistic" and "localistic" philosophies regarding illness existed side by side, peacefully and incongruously, for many years in schools, in books, and in minds of medical teachers. It was not until the end of the eighteenth century that the localistic, or anatomic, idea became dominant.

Contributing largely to this changing viewpoint in medicine was publication, in 1761, of a significant treatise entitled *On the Seats and Causes of Disease*. The author was a 79-year-old practitioner, Professor of Anatomy at Padua, Giovanni Battista Morgagni. This publication still may be considered one of the great landmarks in medical history, because tremendous progress, in medicine as well as in surgery, during the nineteenth century would have been impossible, had not the localistic image of disease become generally accepted.

Author of the books and protagonist of the idea relating pathologic anatomy to diagnosis of disease, Giovanni Battista Morgagni (or, as Anglicized, John Baptist Morgagni) was a happy, home-loving man who lived in almost patriarchal simplicity, as contrasted with the turbulent lives of many of his fellow greats in medicine's history. He raised a large family, and spent most of his days in Padua. In addition to being both a great teacher and a great writer, he was an intimate friend

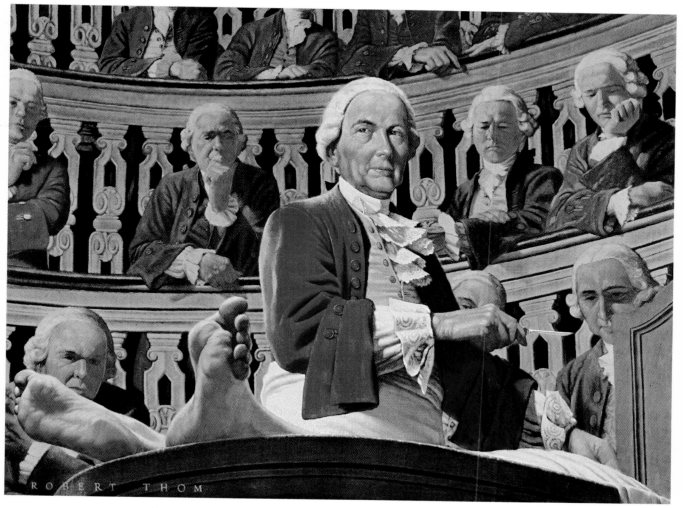

MORGAGNI AND PATHOLOGIC ANATOMY

In the famous anatomic amphitheatre built in 1590, Giovanni Battista Morgagni (1682-1771) demonstrated before medical students from many countries during the 56 years he served as Professor of Anatomy at the famed University of Padua. Although his first book was published in 1704, Morgagni's greatest contribution to medicine, On the Seats and Causes of Disease, *came out 57 years later, in 1761. This five-book work, embodying a lifetime's experience in dissection and in observation, convinced medical men that diseases were not dispersed generally throughout the body, but got their start locally in specific organs or tissues. It ranks high among 18th-century scientific works.*

of kings and princes, of popes and cardinals. He enjoyed an influence among his contemporaries seldom equaled in medical circles.

Giambatista Morgagni (as he habitually signed his writings) was born February 25, 1682, in Forli, capital of a small Papal state southeast of Bologna. His father having died while he was young, Morgagni's education was supervised by his mother. At age 15 he began the study of medicine at the university in the neighboring city of Bologna. He was fortunate to come under the influence of two celebrated professors of the period, Albertini, and Valsalva, a pupil of Malpighi. Morgagni soon attracted the attention of Valsalva, who was engaged in research on the anatomy of the ear, and became his assistant.

In 1701, Morgagni was granted doctorates in medicine and in philosophy. During graduate studies, from time to time he took over the professorial chair during Valsalva's absences. Morgagni's activities in Bolognese academic and organizational circles continued until he retired, for health reasons, to his native village to recuperate and to take up active practice of medicine. It was during this period of his life that he published, in 1704, the first volume of *Adversaria Anatomica*, a collection of essays that was to establish his position as a scientist.

Morgagni's reputation grew; and in 1711 he was offered a second professorship of medicine at the University of Padua, which he took over, March 17, 1712. Three years later, in 1715, the Senate of Venice elevated him to the chair of Professor of Anatomy at Padua. Thus, before reaching the age of 35, Morgagni occupied one of the great university professorships of the eighteenth century—one which had just been vacated by Vallisnieri, and which had been held by men of such stature as Vesalius, Colombo, Fallopius, Fabrizio d'Acquapendente, Casserius, Spigelius, and Vesling. Morgagni proved to be an enthusiastic teacher. He enjoyed nothing better than applause from his students. Furthermore, opportunities for research were ample. Popularity of his lectures and demonstrations, in the famous anatomic amphitheatre built in 1594 under the direction of Fabrizio d'Acquapendente, attracted many students to Padua from other countries, especially from those of northern Europe. The venerable amphitheatre, its steep balconies rising like an oval cone, still exists as one of the show places at the University of Padua.

In Padua Morgagni founded a new branch of medical science—pathologic anatomy. Dissection of human bodies combined with a genius for observation led him to connect external signs of disease with anatomic changes found to have taken place in organs as a result of injury or of disease. Throughout his lifetime he kept notes of these observations, setting them down in the form of letters to interested contemporaries.

In his writings, Morgagni reveals mastery in several fields, as literary scholar, as historian, and as experimental physiologist. His case histories began by setting forth signs observed in the patient during life. Then followed consideration of causes thereof. Next was an account of observations made at autopsy, and descriptions of lesions observed during dissection. Finally, Morgagni drew conclusions from facts accumulated and added various suggestions, theoretical and practical, that might serve physicians in treatment of patients exhibiting similar combinations of symptoms and signs. Morgagni's interests were not limited to rare or curious diseases; primarily, he was concerned with those ailments occurring most frequently in patients confronting physicians in daily practice.

Dissection was considered essential by the great teacher. He insisted on good clinical histories, without which autopsy results were meaningless. Furthermore, he frequently resorted to comparative anatomy, using animal dissections and experiments to obtain information useful in solving human clinical problems.

Morgagni realized that delicate interconnections between various parts of the nervous system might be related to symptoms quite remote from the site of actual disease. He paid considerable attention to the possibility of influence of mind and emotions on blood circulation and on aneurysms. He knew that apoplexy primarily resulted from changes in blood vessels and not from lesions in the brain itself; and that cerebral abscess was the result, not the cause, of a discharging ear. Also he correlated cerebral lesions on one side of the brain with affected movements of the opposite side of the body. He conducted many experiments involving pulmonary veins, jugular veins, and the pericardium. He ligated blood vessels and observed effects thereof. Morgagni also believed that weather had considerable influence on the body, especially on circulation. He paid much attention to the influence of occupation on disease. He was familiar with syphilis and its lesions in skin, in cerebral vessels, and in bone, and he described gummata of the liver and of the brain. He described cirrhosis of the liver, various calculi, and numerous tumors. Where feasible he recommended surgical operation for malignant tumors.

While Morgagni seriously considered the importance of mechanical causes associated with disease processes, he was well aware of the operation of chemical causes. He was aware of dangers of infectious and contagious diseases; this was the basis of his refusal to dissect cadavers of persons who had died of tuberculosis, of smallpox, or of other dangerous fevers.

Epilepsy, Morgagni believed, was caused by too-early closing of external sores and that syphilis was sometimes a cause. Reopening epileptics' healed ulcers to permit removal of acrid and irritating substances was recommended. Further, he advocated internal medicines and purges to augment this treatment. Prescriptions for epilepsy included combinations of such ingredients as peony root, dittany, scrapings of deer's horn, mother of pearl, amber, cinnabar, sarsaparilla, viper's flesh, chicory, primrose, mercury, and asses' milk.

While Morgagni's first publication, *Adversaria Anatomica*, in his twenty-fifth year, founded his reputation, his greatest work, the one that preserved his fame for all time, was not published until 1761, when he was in his seventy-ninth year. Entitled *De sedibus et causis morborum per anatomen indagatis libri quinque* (*On the Seats and Causes of Disease, Anatomically Studied*), this five-book opus (published in two volumes) was one of the great scientific works of the eighteenth century. After nearly 50 years of teaching, Morgagni had assembled 70 of his epistles, describing findings in some 700 autopsies, to which he added his comments, analyses, and conjectures. He quoted freely from the works of other scientists, including Valsalva, Bonetus, Wepfer, Vallisnieri, Lancisi, Haller, Boerhaave, and Mead, always giving them due credit. It is interesting to note that, though published 101 years before discovery of the famous surgical papyrus by Edwin Smith, Morgagni's essays follow virtually the same order as did that ancient Egyptian document dating from 1550 B. C.—conditions found in the head were discussed first, then in order, those of the chest, of the abdomen, and of the extremities. Additional chapters were devoted to general diseases and to surgery.

Although Morgagni's *De Sedibus* contained no single great discovery, it added innumerable important new details and observations to the body of medical knowledge of the day. From his accurate descriptions many diseases could be identified, though in his time their differentiation was not understood, even by the author. *De Sedibus* is impressive and unprecedented in its systematic arrangement, its massive quantities of carefully evaluated evidence, its contributions to understanding of gross anatomy, and its rational and extensive methods for determining sites of disease in relation to human anatomy.

Morgagni's personal life seems to have been happy and tranquil. Few controversies disturbed his professional career. It was a satisfaction to him that most members of his large family entered services of the church. Scholar, historian, stylist, anatomist, experimental physiologist, and clinician, he also was a man of cultivated tastes in art, in literature, and in languages. Patricians of Venice, who ruled Padua also, and King Emanuel III of Sardinia, were proud to consider him a personal friend. Morgagni had a close acquaintance also with five Popes. These relationships helped to spread Morgagni's ideas regarding medical education throughout the eighteenth-century world.

In addition to local honors, Morgagni received wide recognition in other countries. His work as an anatomist brought him memberships: in the Leopoldinian Academy in 1708; in the Royal Society of England in 1724; in the Academy of Sciences of Paris in 1731; in the Imperial Academy of St. Petersburg in 1735; and in the Academy of Berlin in 1754. Much later came still another honor—*Il Morgagni*, which became one of the best known of Italian medical journals for three quarters of a century, was founded in Milan in 1857, continuing until 1935.

The great anatomist of Padua was to live another ten years after publication of *De Sedibus*. He continued to teach until the very last and was nearly 90 years of age when he died, quietly, in 1771.

LAVOISIER: OXYGEN, COMBUSTION, AND RESPIRATION

Unveiling of the mystery of respiration, probably the most decisive scientific contribution to medicine in the eighteenth century, was not the work of a medical man, but of a chemist, Antoine Laurent Lavoisier. After thousands of years of unsubstantiated theories and inaccurate guesses, Lavoisier was first to demonstrate what actually happens during the process of respiration.

Lavoisier's great discoveries relating to respiration represent but one of the many facets of his extremely busy life. Though keenly interested in all natural sciences, including meteorology, mineralogy, geology, hydrometry, and illumination, Lavoisier early revealed his great talents for pure scientific research in chemistry, and for application of scientific knowledge to solution of practical problems. Thus, to medicine and to public health, he not only contributed sound advances to understanding of chemical processes, of combustion, and of gases, but he used his scientific knowledge to help improve water supplies for Paris, ventilation and sanitation in prisons, and to bring about hygienic and procedural reforms in hospitals. Similarly, he served his government on many occasions in solving economic, social, agricultural, chemical, military, and political problems. He brought about an almost complete change in eighteenth-century philosophy and theory of chemistry.

Antoine Laurent Lavoisier was born August 26, 1743, in the heart of Paris. His family was middle-class, comfortably situated financially. Lavoisier's mother died when he was quite young, so that he was reared by a maiden aunt and by his lawyer father. Following his father's guidance, young Antoine first studied law at Mazarin College, qualifying as a Bachelor of Law in 1763, and as a licentiate in 1764. However, he had already developed a compelling interest in science, having had some remarkable teachers in astronomy, mathematics, botany, chemistry, and geology. In 1765, Lavoisier published his first paper on a subject in chemistry, wherein he used the quantitative approach, one

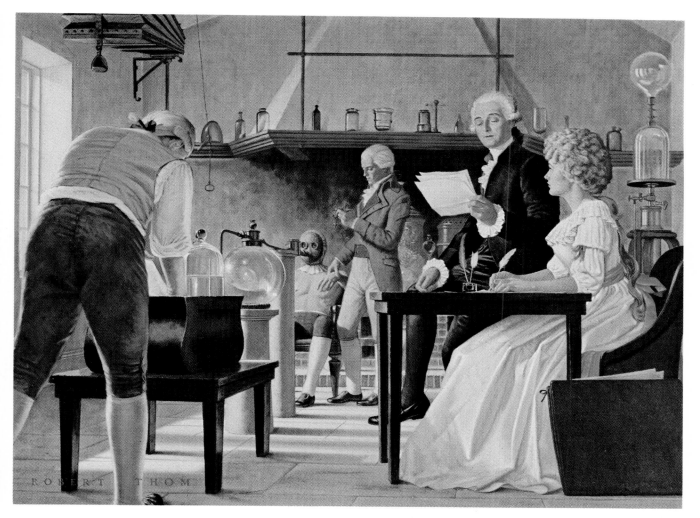

LAVOISIER: OXYGEN, COMBUSTION, AND RESPIRATION

Greatest contribution of science to Medicine during the eighteenth century came from experiments relating to the processes of respiration, conducted between 1789 and 1792 by the Parisian chemist, Antoine Laurent Lavoisier, in his laboratory at the Royal Arsenal. Mme. Lavoisier was his closest collaborator. Together with a young assistant, Séguin, Lavoisier recorded oxygen intake and carbon dioxide exhalation by a man while resting, while working, and while eating, and compared the results with statistics on combustion of carbon. Lavoisier made many scientific, social, economic, financial, and political contributions before French revolutionary radicals executed him in 1794.

which he was to make dominant in chemistry later in life. He won a medal from the king in a prize essay contest on metropolitan street lighting, in 1766; and two years later, when he was but 25 years old, Lavoisier was admitted to membership in the Royal Academy of Science. This was the beginning of a long and fruitful association with France's foremost scientists. Their regard for him is best revealed by the great number of commissions to which Lavoisier was assigned, and by the fact that in most instances, Lavoisier was asked to write reports of commissions' findings and to present these to the Academy. Because the French government relied on this scientific body to investigate a wide variety of subjects and to report its conclusions and advice to the nation's officials, Lavoisier soon was plunged deeply into service of his country. Among these activities was one that eventually was to cost him his life. In 1768, the same year that he became a member of the Academy, Lavoisier bought a part share in the *Ferme Générale*, a much-hated, privately owned organization to which the French monarchy "farmed out" a profitable tax-gathering monopoly in return for guarantees of the government's financial requirements. Lavoisier seems to have served this organization sincerely and with a fine sense of fairness toward those from whom taxes were collected. However, tax collectors seldom are objects of public admiration; and fate was to prove so to Lavoisier.

Out of his relations with the *Ferme Générale* came one of the brightest of Lavoisier's experiences. In 1771, at age 28, he married Marie Paulze, 14-year-old daughter of one of his colleagues in the *Ferme*. Though a "marriage of convenience" at the time it was solemnized, it proved to be a very happy union. Mme. Lavoisier, brilliant and talented, took a great interest in her husband's work and became a devoted collaborator. She translated papers from foreign languages into French for him; made notes of many of his experiments; drew sketches and engraved plates to illustrate some of his publications; and was hostess to a brilliant corps of friends and internationally prominent scientists.

Lavoisier's greatest accomplishments undoubtedly are to be found in his work on oxygen, which led him to study respiration, and to completely refute long-standing theories of chemistry. Though oxygen had been discovered independently by Scheele, in Sweden, and by Priestley, in England, and had been studied by Cavendish, also of England, Lavoisier, stimulated by their reports, carried on further experiments. These enabled him, in 1776, to report on the true nature and role of the gas that was called "dephlogisticated air," or "respirable air," and to suggest that it be named "oxygen" (acid-maker). His experiments began with oxidation of metals, and reduction of metallic oxides. In the course of a few years he determined that oxygen makes up only about one fifth the volume of atmospheric air and is the only gas in air that sustains either combustion or respiration; and that, in combustion, a definite ratio exists between the amount of oxygen consumed and the amount of "fixed air" (carbon dioxide) released. He also determined that water is not an element, but a compound of oxygen and "inflammable air," to which he gave the name "hydrogen." Thus began Lavoisier's nearly complete reconstruction of the scientific bases of chemistry: overthrow of the ancient theory of four elements—air, earth, fire, and water; and of the phlogiston theory (that substances burned because of escape of an unknown substance called phlogiston). He proved that water is the end product of combining hydrogen and oxygen by combustion, and therefore, is a compound rather than an element. His many chemical experiments and logical conclusions drawn therefrom, and from work done in collaboration with other scientists, including Guyton de Morveau, Fourcroy, and Berthollet, were summed up in his *Traité Elémentaire de Chimie*, published in 1789. This volume included a new system for naming chemical substances, a system which, with only minor revisions, is still in use today.

Most prominent of assignments given Lavoisier by the French government was his appointment in 1777 as head of a committee to direct the Royal Powder Factory to remedy a shortage of gunpowder that constituted a threat to the nation's security. Rapidly, Lavoisier changed the powder factory from an inadequate and inefficient operation to one that filled the Royal Arsenal with good-quality gunpowder. This placed France in a new position with other nations: as a seller rather than a buyer of gunpowder. Significantly, this work by Lavoisier made it possible for France to supply the rebellious American colonists with powder to sustain their effort toward independence from France's traditional enemy, Great Britain. Lavoisier was to contribute, without his knowledge, in another way to the growth of the struggling young nation across the Atlantic: the training he gave a young man, Eleuthère Irénée du Pont, who assisted in the powder mill and in the research laboratories, was to become basic to founding the great chemical dynasty of E. I. du Pont de Nemours, in Delaware.

It was during his years of residence and work at the Royal Powder Factory that Lavoisier carried out his experiments relating to combustion and to respiration. Having proved that in combustion, burning substances combine with oxygen, giving off both heat and carbon dioxide, Lavoisier and Laplace developed methods of measuring heat generated by various chemical changes, and of measuring oxygen consumed and carbon dioxide formed therein. Then they devised ways of determining oxygen intake, heat output, and carbon dioxide exhalation produced by respiration in a guinea pig during a specific period. By complex comparisons, in which an ice calorimeter was used, they proved that a guinea pig produced approximately the same amount of heat, during consumption of a predetermined amount of oxygen, as was produced by burning charcoal consuming the same amount of oxygen. From these investigations, Lavoisier and Laplace concluded that: "Respiration is therefore a combustion, admittedly very slow, but otherwise exactly similar to that of charcoal; it takes place in the interior of the lungs, without the evolution of light, since the matter of fire set free is immediately absorbed by the moisture of those organs . . ." Lavoisier erred in believing that this combustion took place in the lungs, was communicated to the blood, and thereby diffused through the body. Another century was to pass before this bit of biological chemistry was to be thoroughly elucidated. Later, with the cooperation of Armand Séguin, Lavoisier measured the amounts of oxygen consumed and of carbon dioxide produced during respiration by a man while resting, while working, and while eating.

Despite time-consuming tasks at the powder factory and experiments carried out during free time, Lavoisier engaged in many other activities. He prepared for the government of France an outstanding memoir on economics including a survey of the nation's natural resources; he conducted research into a number of agricultural problems, from which came practical applications resulting in increased yields of crops and of

142

livestock; he assisted in political reorganization of the province in which his farm lands lay; and he continued to work as a member of the tax-gathering body, *Ferme Générale.*

The later years of the 1780's and earlier years of the 1790's, however, were troubled years. The French Revolution was imminent; and Lavoisier's positions as powder commissioner and as a member of the *Ferme Générale* brought him into the limelight of unpopularity as early as 1789. Among the Revolution's principal targets, after the royal family, was the tax-collecting company, members of which the people considered "blood-suckers" and "thieves."

Though he participated moderately in the Revolution, along with Lafayette, Bailly, Mirabeau, and Talleyrand, Lavoisier tried to retire from public office and devote himself entirely to scientific work; but such was not to be his destiny. In 1791, the *Ferme Générale* was abolished, and he was dropped from the powder commission. He continued to work as a member of the Commission on Weights and Measures (which established the metric system) until 1793. In that year, he saw the revolutionary movement become more radical: his beloved Academy was closed, despite his efforts in its defense; and his campaign for better educational standards came to nought. The menace to Lavoisier was so obvious that it seems strange that he did not leave France, or at least seek shelter in the provinces. Apparently having no fear for his life, he chose to remain in Paris; and in November, 1793, Lavoisier and his father-in-law, Paulze, together with their colleagues of the *Ferme Générale,* were arrested. Though Lavoisier tried to secure release on the basis of his many services to the nation, most of his powerful friends, including Fourcroy, abandoned him. Others, however, like Hallé and Saint-Hilaire, remained faithful to the end. Lavoisier accepted his fate calmly, remarking: "This probably saves me from the inconveniences of old age."

Together with 26 colleagues, Lavoisier and Paulze were tried and condemned, May 7, 1794, and executed the following day, May 8, for "plotting against the people of France."

A most befitting epitaph was spoken of Lavoisier by Joseph Lagrange, who said: "It took only a moment to sever that head, and perhaps a century will not be sufficient to produce another like it."

JOHN HUNTER: FOUNDER OF SCIENTIFIC SURGERY

"THOSE who far precede others must necessarily remain alone; and their actions often appear unaccountable, nay, even extravagant, to their distant followers, who know not the causes that give rise to them, or the effects that they were designed to produce. In such a situation stood John Hunter in relation to his contemporaries. It was a comfortless precedence, for it deprived him of sympathy and social cooperation." In these few words, John Abernethy, one of Hunter's famous pupils, appropriately epitomized the life and the work of the eighteenth century's leading surgeon, and one of its outstanding comparative anatomists. "He sought for truth, for truth's sake alone: is there a nobler aim in life?" commented George Peachey; and Stephen Paget wrote: "Paré advanced the art of surgery, but Hunter taught the science of it."

Medicine and surgery had been separated during the Middle Ages, to the detriment of both branches of the healing art. Surgery had been left in the hands of uneducated craftsmen such as barbers, bathkeepers, or sowgelders, primarily engaged in menial tasks. In the eighteenth century, surgery regained standing as an independent branch of medicine—a step toward the reunion which took place in the nineteenth century. Probably no one man contributed more to this salutary development in Great Britain than John Hunter.

The youngest of ten children, John Hunter was born February 13, 1728, at Long Calderwood, the family farm in Lanarkshire, Scotland, a few miles from Glasgow. His father died when John was thirteen years old; and his mother was overindulgent. Thus young Jock grew up to be a rough red-headed country lad who successfully evaded almost all formal education; yet whose keen mind formulated an endless variety of questions about subjects his exasperated seniors thought useless. Nature, and things mechanical, were his school; for books he had little regard.

Almost completely opposite was his brother, William, ten years

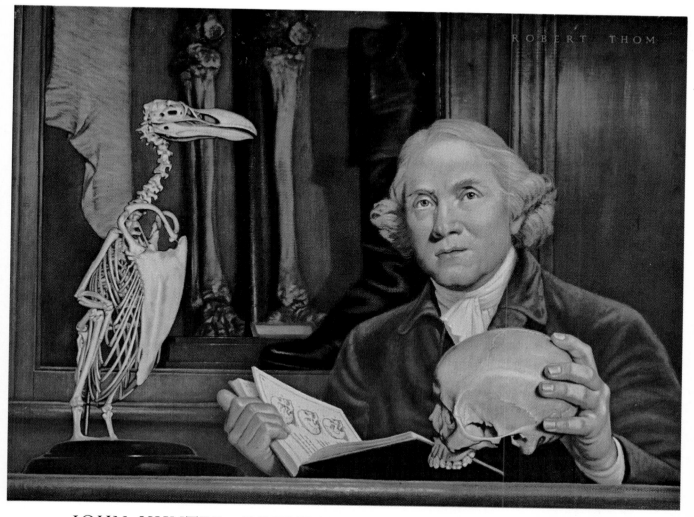

JOHN HUNTER: FOUNDER OF SCIENTIFIC SURGERY

From an untutored Scottish country boy, John Hunter (1728-1793) rose to become eighteenth-century London's foremost surgeon and medical scientist. Combining natural talent, insatiable curiosity, and keen observation, he was one of the greatest comparative anatomists of all time. The skeletons of the now-extinct Great Auk and of the Irish Giant are two of 13,682 specimens which comprised his famous collections, war-spared remnants of which still are on exhibit in London's Royal College of Surgeons. Posthumously, Dr. Hunter was honored as "The Founder of Scientific Surgery."

John's senior. Having first studied for the ministry, William soon turned to medicine. Establishing himself in London, well-educated, well-dressed, socially correct William soon earned a reputation as surgeon, anatomist, and obstetrician; later he was recognized also as a physician. By the time John Hunter reached twenty years of age, William was successfully operating a school of anatomy at Covent Garden. This was at the time when surgery, separated from barbering in 1745, was just beginning to be regarded as a respectable profession in England.

John Hunter, tired of wasting time, wrote William, asking if he might work under him. Receiving a cordial answer, John mounted his horse, rode to London, and joined his brother in September, 1748.

Skeptical at first of this untutored brother's abilities, William set John at dissections in his anatomy demonstration room. He was more than surprised at the excellent results: John revealed a natural aptitude for the work, plus an insatiable curiosity. William took John on as assistant, taught him how to make anatomical preparations, and, later, gave him teaching responsibilities. John Hunter spent eleven winters in his brother's anatomical laboratory. While there he learned not only anatomy, but also the ways of "resurrectionists," those unscrupulous characters who, in the absence of proper legal measures, provided schools of anatomy with subjects for dissection. Bodies came to the Hunters' back door by several routes: from hangmen's gibbets; from dark alleys where murder had stalked some hapless soul; from reopened fresh graves; or from caskets awaiting burial, stones having been substituted for weight of removed corpses. Furthermore, according to Robinson, John Hunter "did not pray to be delivered from the evil of the great city, but smilingly met temptation in a rollicking spirit— with a wine-bottle in his hand and a doxy on his knee. No one who saw him in the shilling gallery (of the theaters) bawling with his companions at a production of a dramatist that displeased these critics would have taken him for the brother of the cultured William Hunter . . ."

In summers, when weather made dissecting impossible, John Hunter studied surgery, first under William Cheselden, at Chelsea Hospital, in 1749 and in 1750, and under Percivall Pott, at St. Bartholomew's

Hospital, in 1751. Under these masters he walked the wards, was present at major operations, and learned simplicity of treatment and avoidance of unnecessary interference with healing processes. He was honored to receive, simultaneously with the already famous Pott, the degree of Master of Anatomy from the Surgeon's Corporation, in 1753. Early in 1754, John Hunter entered St. George's Hospital as a surgeon's pupil. The following year, upon his brother's insistence, John was persuaded to enter St. Mary's Hall at Oxford as a gentleman commoner; but again aversion to formal learning asserted itself. His Oxford career over in two months, Hunter returned to the anatomy laboratory. He continued to develop his intense interest in comparative anatomy, and during these years, he conducted his well-known researches on the lymphatic system.

Strenuous and confining work affected Hunter's health. Mindful of his family's history of tuberculosis, John decided to leave the school at Covent Garden, to secure a commission as surgeon on the staff of the British Army. He participated in campaigns at Belleisle and in Portugal from 1761 to 1763, serving for a time as chief surgeon and director of the hospital at Belleisle, acquiring extensive knowledge of treatment for gunshot wounds.

Returning from Portugal in 1763, John Hunter, now 35, entered upon practice of surgery in Golden Square, in London. The early years were thin; and his passion for scientific work hindered his success as a surgeon. He started his famous collection of specimens on comparative anatomy. To make possible the study of living animals, he purchased two acres of land, in 1764, "about two miles from London, near Brompton, at a place called Earl's Court." Here he built a house and gathered an extensive menagerie both of common and of rare animals. He came here to study and to "relax" over the dissection table, where one pupil reports having found him busily at work at 4 A.M., preparing specimens of bees. It was at Earl's Court that Hunter wrote his firsthand "Observations on the Structure and Economy of the Whale;" and there, too, that he prepared the famed skeleton of the Irish Giant, Byrne, who died in 1783. Young Byrne, nearly eight feet tall, in declining health, on learning that Hunter hoped to secure his body at death, made elaborate preparations for burial at sea in a lead coffin; but one of Hunter's "resurrectionists" was able to bribe the undertaker's guards; so the magnificent skeleton may be seen today among remnants of Hunter's collection.

In 1767, John Hunter became a Fellow of the Royal Society; and, in 1768, he was elected one of the surgeons at St. George's Hospital, an office he was to hold until death a quarter century later. In this position, he was permitted to have pupils in surgery; and in his years at St. George's he instructed no less than 449 young men, many of whom became famous. Among these were: Astley Cooper; John Abernethy; Henry Cline; Hunter's brother-in-law, Sir Everard Home; his nephew, Matthew Baillie; John Thompson; Edward Coleman, who later headed a school for veterinarians; and Americans, including William Shippen; and Philip Syng Physick, who became known as the father of American surgery. Most famous of all John Hunter's pupils and one who became a lifelong friend and collaborator in study of natural sciences, was Edward Jenner, who practiced at Berkeley, and who, some years after the death of his teacher, was to give the world the method of vaccination against smallpox.

In 1771, Hunter, who as a youth had no time for the printed word, published his first book, *Treatise on the Natural History of the Human Teeth*. The proceeds he used to finance his wedding to Anne Home, daughter of surgeon Robert Boyne Home, whom Hunter had met during his army days. To the union four children were born, of whom only a son and a daughter survived. Everard Home, Anne's brother, eventually became Hunter's pupil, his protégé at St. George's, his executor, his biographer, and, finally, the man who plagiarized his notes, then destroyed them.

Hunter experienced his first attack of angina pectoris in 1773—the disease which eventually was to kill him. It slowed him but little, however, for in 1775 he began courses of private lectures on surgery and on anatomy. He became Surgeon Extraordinary to the King in 1776; brought out a second section of his *Natural History of the Human Teeth* in 1778; and entered into bitter controversy with his brother William in 1780 over who deserved credit for discovering the true structure of the placenta—an embroilment that was to estrange the brothers until William's death in 1783. In 1785, John performed a daring pioneering operation for a popliteal aneurysm, tying off the main artery above the aneurysm, allowing collateral circulation to supply blood to the lower leg, an idea he conceived from animal experiments.

With Pott's death in 1788, Hunter became the acknowledged head of his profession in London. Honors came to him, including membership in the American Philosophical Society; and, in 1790, appointment as Surgeon-General of the British Army and Inspector-General of Hospitals. His now-famous collection was approaching its total of 13,682 individual specimens, besides which there were innumerable manuscripts, notebooks, and notes scribbled on scraps of paper. His interests ranged from surgery and anatomy to dentistry, biology, and natural history. His influence on the infant profession of veterinary medicine was profound and far-reaching, and he had an important part in development of the first English school for veterinarians.

One of Hunter's tragic errors was his belief that syphilis and gonorrhea were different manifestations of the same disease. No stranger to self-experimentation, he is said to have infected himself from an individual manifesting signs of gonorrhea, believing that he could demonstrate a quick cure; but the host must have donated spirochetes, too, for Hunter's last years were complicated by syphilitic lesions in addition to angina. Nevertheless, though crippled and crotchety, he continued his rounds, his lectures, and his anatomical preparations until the end.

The eyes of his colleagues at St. George's Hospital, however, were blinded to Hunter's strides in surgery and in comparative anatomy by bitter animosities, acrimonious disagreements, and jealousies. Not given to soft answers or to diplomatic maneuvers, the blunt Hunter experienced repeated frustrations at Board meetings due to opposition from other surgeons, one of whom evaluated Hunter's collections as equivalent to "petittoes." It was in the heat of one of these Board meetings, October 16, 1793, that, with his wrath rising, Hunter died in an anginal attack, at 65 years of age. Coincidentally, his death occurred on the same day that, across the Channel in revolution-torn France, Marie Antoinette lost her head on the guillotine.

John Hunter has been described as strongly built, five feet two inches in height, broad of shoulder, with a short neck. His hair was of an auburn tint, afterward gray, and at last white. His eyes were light colored, his jaw prominent. He dressed plainly and not always neatly. He was possessed of a sharp wit and of considerable humor. In his early days he was fun-loving and boisterous; in later years, work consumed most of his time. Because of his illness he abstained from wine. He loved his family and enjoyed the rare moments he could spend with them. Not averse to social life, he collected good art as well as anatomical specimens. He was greatly admired by his pupils. Patients he regarded as a necessary source of income to support his scientific studies, though frequently he left the dissecting table with reluctance to attend them. Even so, he was likely to let a wealthy patient wait while he attended one from whom he could hardly expect pay.

Never well off financially, because of the drain of his scientific pursuits, Hunter left his family little but his real estate and his monumental collection; and it was not until 1799 that Parliament, plagued with the expenses of war, saw fit to purchase the collection for £15,000, to turn it over to the Corporation of Surgeons. Through this period, the collection was guarded by Hunter's student and secretary, William Clift, to whom medicine also is indebted for much of what is left of Hunter's notes and writings. Of many, only Clift's painstaking copies remain.

The scope of the Hunterian collection taxes imagination. It comprised thousands upon thousands of specimens—wet, dry, stuffed, mounted. There were plants and animals; monsters and mummies; skulls of the five great divisions of the human race; the skeleton of the Irish Giant; and that of the now-extinct Great Auk. But of special interest were his many series showing comparative anatomy. In demonstrating the organs of taste, of smell, of hearing, of sight, and of reproduction, Hunter started, not with organs of human subjects, but with those from the simplest forms of life, progressing to next higher species, through insects, birds, fishes, lower and higher mammals, and finally to perfectly prepared and demonstrated human specimens. This collection constituted one of the irreplaceable losses of World War II, having been nearly destroyed by a direct bomb hit in the blitz of London in 1940. However, the Royal College of Surgeons takes pride in exhibiting some 1,100 of Hunter's specimens that survived those grim days, among them, the skeleton of the Irish Giant.

Though an able surgeon, Hunter did not contribute many new operations to the field, apart from that for popliteal aneurysm. His experimental pathology and comparative anatomy stand out, as does his work on inflammation. His two treatises on teeth laid the foundation for scientific dentistry. His book on blood, inflammation, and gunshot wounds, written late in life, contains some of his best work. Perhaps his greatest contribution to surgery, apart from his collections, came through having imparted to his pupils reliance on scientific observation and courage to try new ideas. Through them he transformed the craft of surgery to an experimental science.

The body of John Hunter was first buried, October 22, 1793, in the vaults of St. Martin-in-the-Fields. There the casket remained, forgotten, until 1859. On March 28 of that year, John Hunter's remains were reburied with great honors in the North Aisle of Westminster Abbey. Thus, sixty-six years after the controversy that precipitated his death, the great Scotsman received his just dues: the brass plaque over his grave is inscribed with the words, "The Founder of Scientific Surgery."

BENJAMIN RUSH
PHYSICIAN, PEDANT, PATRIOT

For LEADERSHIP in medicine, as well as in most other daily activities, mid-eighteenth century British colonists in North America looked overseas to the homeland. Physicians of the New World, like their brethren in the Old World, practiced medicine under confusing philosophies in transition between medieval and modern; while reluctant to relinquish adherence to traditions and systems centuries old, they had to grapple with new problems posed by the raw new land. Without anyone to fall back upon, physicians had to compare new experiences with old teachings; pioneer new therapeutic regimens based on quick bedside decisions.

The man who contributed most to systematization and progress of medicine in the American states, and who led the way in founding a body of medicine independent from that of Europe, was Benjamin Rush. Without question Dr. Rush was the most striking, the most impressive, and the most controversial figure in North American medicine of his day. Brilliant and well educated, he was a restless soul, impatient and impulsive, quick to make decisions and to defend them against all disagreement. Though domineering as a teacher, his magnetic personality profoundly influenced students. Though bitter and acrimonious in attacks upon contemporary physicians, or in defense of his own methods, he had a way of gaining the confidence of his patients and of comforting them. In times of great danger, when other physicians fled, Rush had the courage to remain with his patients; he was never too tired or too busy to try to care for them. Nor did he confine his attention solely to medicine: he was interested in every phase of life about him; and he wrote and published on many subjects. A natural reformer, he advocated abolition of slavery, penal reform, better general education, and better sanitary systems. One of the first to advocate preventive medicine, he was an ardent proponent of inoculation, and later, of vaccination, against smallpox. His work on mental illnesses was the standard for a half century. Rush wrote illuminatingly on causes and treatment

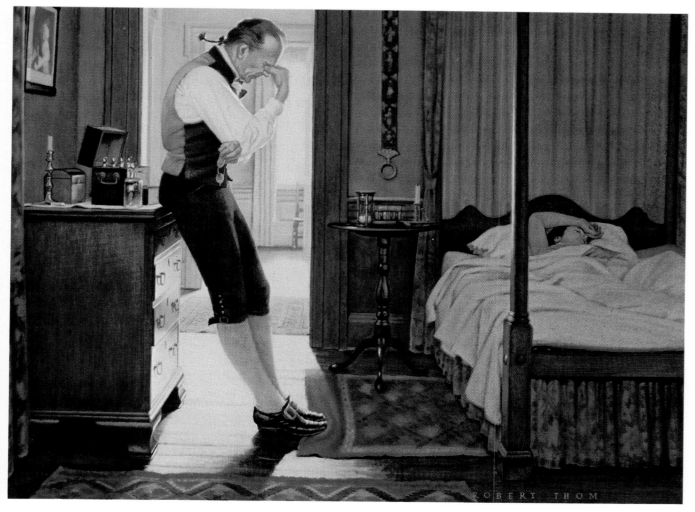

BENJAMIN RUSH: PHYSICIAN, PEDANT, PATRIOT

Professional, moral, and physical courage of Dr. Benjamin Rush (1745-1813) was taxed to exhaustion during the 1793 yellow fever epidemic in Philadelphia, capital of the new United States of America. Those residents who could, fled; those who could not were decimated by disease. Horror and hysteria reigned. Hundreds died daily. Dr. Rush stayed, cared for patients, personally survived two attacks of fever. Though his heroic treatments were severely criticized, Rush was unswerving. Patriot, signer of the Declaration of Independence, leader in the country's first medical school, Dr. Rush came to be called the first great physician in the United States of America.

153

of many diseases, and he pleaded for simplification of medical nomenclature and for elimination of all but a few key drugs. He urged medical students to acquire practical knowledge of veterinary medicine. Chief exponent, in his time, of bloodletting as a therapeutic measure, Rush, wrote Flexner, "shed more blood than any general in history." Goodman credits him with many ideas a century in advance of his time, and with dedication of his life sincerely and unselfishly to a profession which did not always use him kindly. Intensely human, often a victim of self-deception, many times tragically and disastrously wrong, Dr. Rush nevertheless stuck to his job, sick or well, with rare heroism. During the tragic epidemics of yellow fever, according to Powell, "there was only one doctor who would enter a fetid chamber, scorn all protections, sit on the edge of a vomit-soiled bed, smile cheerfully to the frightened patient, say blandly, 'you have nothing but a yellow fever'." Despite his faults, errors, and controversial career, Rush's influence on North American medicine was profound, lasting until well past the middle of the nineteenth century.

Dr. Rush has been described as above medium height, his slender body erect, and his manner dignified. His face was long and thin with forehead high and rounded, high cheekbones, and firm jaw. Bright piercing eyes under heavy brows, an aquiline nose, long upper lip, and resolute mouth gave evidence of his stubborn determination and indomitable will. In youth he wore a powdered wig, but he discarded this in middle age, his own long, rather thin graying locks softening his sharp features. Meticulous about appearance, he wore clothes with an air of elegance. Strong, well-shaped hands and long, slim fingers were indicative of sensitivity of touch and skill.

Benjamin Rush was born on Christmas Eve, 1745 (old calendar), or January 4, 1746 (new calendar—England did not adopt the Gregorian calendar until 1752). His birthplace was the Rush farm at Byberry, Pennsylvania. He was the fourth child in a family of seven. An early ancestor had been one of Cromwell's men before migrating to the colonies. Benjamin's father died when he was but 6 years old. His preliminary education was supervised by an uncle, Rev. Samuel Finley. He received his Bachelor of Arts degree from the College of New Jersey (now Princeton) in 1760. The 15-year-old graduate then apprenticed himself to a busy Philadelphia physician, Dr. John Redman. During more than five years in this association, he was permitted to observe physicians at work in Pennsylvania Hospital and to attend lectures by Dr. John Morgan (who in 1755 had served as pharmacist at the hospital), and by Dr. William Shippen, Jr. Upon his preceptors' advice, Rush enrolled in the University of Edinburgh, Scotland, in 1766, studying under the famed Dr. William Cullen. After receiving the degree of Doctor of Medicine in June, 1768, with letters of introduction from Benjamin Franklin, Rush visited Paris and London, where he studied for a time under Dr. William Hunter. He returned to Philadelphia in 1769 to enter practice and to receive appointment as Professor of Chemistry at the College of Philadelphia. His was the first formal chair of chemistry in America; and there he joined Drs. Shippen, Morgan, Adam Kuhn, and Thomas Bond, on the faculty of the medical department. This appointment gave his career a good start, and Rush added prestige in 1770 by publishing a *Syllabus of A Course of Lectures on Chemistry.*

When Dr. Rush opened his office in Philadelphia, most of his older colleagues practiced according to the teachings of Hermann Boerhaave, the great master of Leyden, Holland. Rush adhered to the system of Dr. Cullen of Edinburgh. Always hot-headed and stubborn, the tactless Rush could not resist publicly attacking his colleagues, thereby alienating most of them, with the consequence that they refused to refer patients to him. Rush struggled on with the poor patients who flocked to his door.

Always an individualist, the cocksure young man became further embroiled in controversy as he revealed his traits as a crusader and reformer. In 1772, he published a pamphlet against slavery, and another on temperance.

On January 11, 1776, Dr. Rush was married to Julia Stockton. To this union thirteen children were born, nine of whom survived. Two sons followed their father's profession. Most distinguished son was Richard, born in 1780, who became an attorney. At various times Richard held offices as Attorney General of his state and of the nation,

Comptroller of the United States Treasury, Secretary of State, Minister to England, Secretary of the Treasury, and Minister to France.

The decade, 1774-1783, was one of great significance to the embryo nation; to its largest city, Philadelphia; and to Dr. Rush. When the First Continental Congress met in 1774, Dr. Rush entertained many of its members, including John and Samuel Adams, Patrick Henry, George Washington, Thomas Jefferson, and Benjamin Franklin. After blood was shed in 1775, Rush headed companies formed to manufacture needed items for the Colonies, introduced the first spinning jenny for manufacture of cotton cloth, and superintended a saltpeter factory. Rush is credited with supplying notes for and bringing about publication of Thomas Paine's *Common Sense*, which, more than any other pamphlet, led Americans to embrace the cause of independence. Elected to Congress in 1776, Rush and his father-in-law, Richard Stockton, were among signers of the Declaration of Independence. (Four other physicians attached their signatures to this famous document: Josiah Bartlett and Matthew Thornton, of New Hampshire; Lyman Hall, of Georgia; and Oliver Wolcott, of Connecticut.) Later, in 1787, Rush was to be influential among framers of the Constitution of the United States.

In April, 1777, his congressional term having expired, Dr. Rush accepted a commission in the Medical Department of the Continental Army. True to his independent nature, he became embroiled both in medical and in military controversies: at one time he quarreled with General Washington; and on another occasion he took part in the bitter battle between Dr. Shippen and Dr. Morgan over direction of the Army's Medical Department. Despite wartime differences, Rush and Washington later renewed friendship; and Rush rejoined Shippen on the faculty of the Medical School of the University of Pennsylvania, successor to the College of Philadelphia.

As the new nation and Philadelphia, its capital, settled back to postwar living, Dr. Rush returned to practice and to teaching. As a teacher, he exerted more influence on the medical profession in America during the quarter century following the Revolution than any other person. His students were in practice from Massachusetts to Georgia; and Rush carried on heavy correspondence as their consultant. By 1786, his lectures at the university embraced medicine and chemistry. When Dr. Morgan died in 1789, Rush was elected to the chair of theory and practice of medicine. In 1792, Rush was elected professor of the institutes of medicine and of clinical medicine at the University; and in 1796, he received the additional appointment of professor of the practice of physic. He continued to teach throughout his life, advised his students to be guided both by observation and by experience, propounded codes of ethics for them, coached them on patient-physician relations, and cautioned young doctors to write prescriptions legibly, lest deaths be caused by mistaken interpretations.

During 43 years (1769-1812), over 3,000 students were registered in his classes; in addition, he tutored, privately, a number of apprentices and assistants.

Greatest test of Dr. Rush's ability as physician and as medical leader, and certainly of his physical and moral courage, came with Philadelphia's tragic epidemic of yellow fever in 1793. At the time, Dr. Rush was extremely busy with a large private practice, with lectures at the Medical School of the University of Pennsylvania, with clinics at Pennsylvania Hospital and at Philadelphia Dispensary, and with his voluminous writing. This devastating epidemic, and those of following years, were to plunge Rush so deeply into controversy that his practice never fully recovered economically; and to this day his detractors attach a stigma to his name.

The first patients began to show symptoms of "a serious bilious fever," and to die, in August, 1793. Dr. Rush, who had seen patients with yellow fever twenty years before while an apprentice, recognized the disease. At first, his conclusions were treated contemptuously by his fellow physicians. Before long, they were to change their minds.

Some patients first exhibited violent chills and fever; others, nausea and languor. Other symptoms included slow pulse, bloodshot eyes, vomiting, stupor, and delirium. Yellowness nearly always followed. Vivid spots on the body, "that resembled mosquito bites" were reported; and Rush wrote in his voluminous notes that "a bleeding at the nose, from the gums and from the bowels, and a vomiting of black matter in some instances close the scenes of life."

Fearing for his children, Dr. Rush sent them to Princeton, where their mother was visiting; but, though thousands of citizens fled Philadelphia, among them physicians, Dr. Rush stayed on. As officials of the Federal Government hastily departed, city officials conferred frantically and the public gave way to hysteria resulting in near chaos; more medical controversies broke out. Dr. Rush considered the infection to be of local origin, attributed it to "noxious miasma—evil air caused by rotting matter, stagnant swamps, or the breath of infected patients." Specifically, Rush felt that the epidemic arose from offensive odors arising from a shipment of spoiled coffee rotting on the docks. Others civic-mindedly looked afar for the fever's source, believing it to have been imported by ships entering the harbor from the Caribbean. Though never suspecting the true source of the disease—infected *Aedes aegypti* mosquitoes—on several occasions Rush nearly determined the cause. He advocated that streets be cleaned; he believed puddles, ponds and marshes should be drained; and he complained, more than once, of swarms of mosquitoes that plagued the city.

By the end of August, hundreds were ill and the city's activities ground to a standstill. Few wheels turned, other than those of doctors' carts as Dr. Rush and his few remaining colleagues hurried on new and probably fruitless missions; and those of vehicles used by Negroes (at first thought to be immune) carting away the dead. Hysteria reached a new high: husbands and wives deserted sick spouses; parents abandoned sick children; and children, their ill parents. Many persons were left to starve or to die alone and unattended. Only a handful of brave citizens and doctors remained to care for yellow fever victims. All known remedies failed.

Casting about for a solution one night, Dr. Rush, too tired to sleep, recalled a paper on yellow fever written in 1744 by Dr. John Mitchell, advocating depletion of the body with severe purges. Also Rush recalled use in military hospitals of "ten and ten"—ten grains of calomel plus ten grains of jalap—as a purge. Rush experimented, adding another five grains of jalap for good measure. Along with purges, he prescribed

158

copious bloodletting, cool air, cool drinks, and light diet. Trial led Dr. Rush to believe his treatment successful. Characteristically, he told other physicians and wrote about it in newspapers, only to be bitterly attacked by Dr. William Currie. Philadelphia's remaining medical men were split widely into two groups: Rush's friends, who used heroic purges and bleeding; and Currie's followers, who employed milder measures.

By mid-October, Rush estimated that no less than 6,000 persons were ill with the fever, and "only three physicians were able to do business out of their houses." More than one hundred persons were dying daily. Rush worked day and night; patients were on his doorstep at dawn; he prescribed as he ate his meals. His sister aided his apprentices as they put up purge powders, until she, too, died of the fever. Dr. Rush himself fell victim of the disease and was seriously ill with fever on another occasion; but he survived vigorous application of his own treatments, prescribed for patients from his bed, and rose again to minister to the sick. Finally, with the advent of frost, the epidemic subsided. Philadelphia's loss was 5,000 persons, one tenth of its population. Dr. Rush recorded the experience the following year in *An Account of the Bilious Remitting Yellow Fever, As It Appeared in the City of Philadelphia, in the year 1793.*

Further epidemics occurred in 1794, 1796, and 1798. The scenes of horror and desperation were repeated. Rush doggedly stuck to his purgings and bleedings, absorbing more and more abuse and criticism from fellow physicians and citizens; but never did he run away from his responsibilities as he saw them. His practice suffered, however, to the point where he was grateful to supplement his income by accepting, in 1797, appointment as Treasurer of the United States Mint from his friend, President John Adams.

Dr. Rush was to see the turn of the century, and to teach, to write, and to practice a dozen years beyond it. Last volume of his many works was *Medical Inquiries and Observations Upon the Diseases of the Mind*, which appeared in 1812. Although out of date by today's standards, it was the first work on psychiatry published in the United States, and for a half century, the only one. It became a standard reference for physicians and medical students. Rush believed insanity to be a disease of the brain. He has been credited with anticipating Freud's "mental catharsis" theory, because Rush advised physicians to listen sympathetically and seriously to patients, who should be given every opportunity to relieve their subconscious minds by talking. Furthermore, he recommended kind treatment, good living conditions, and occupational therapy. Contrasted with these enlightened views, however, was Rush's advocacy of bloodletting, and recommendation of use of his "tranquilizer"—a rather cruel, uncomfortable chair, with headpiece, into which uncooperative patients were strapped.

Dr. Rush continued working into his sixty-eighth year, calling on patients as late as April 13, 1813. That night, a chill and general indisposition sent him to bed. His condition did not improve, and on April 19, he died, rational and composed.

Benjamin Rush's first venture into authorship was at age nineteen and he continued writing until his last days. No phase of life around him escaped his attention. Despite his controversial nature and the animosity of his local contemporaries, Rush was respected as a scientist and as a philosopher by such men of stature as Franklin, Washington, Samuel and John Adams, and Jefferson. Easily the ranking teacher of medicine of his day in the United States, he was idolized by former students and physicians outside Philadelphia. The British physician, John Coakley Lettsom, called Rush the "Sydenham of America;" and, indeed, Rush was influenced by Sydenham's rules regarding "bedside manner." Though critics hold that his treatment of patients probably did more harm than good, his methods were in keeping with medical understanding of his day, and he sincerely believed in them. Says Goodman: "His character was laid upon foundations of integrity and service, and once he was sure within himself of the soundness and morality of his stand, he resolutely refused to compromise." He has been justifiably called the first great physician in the United States of America.

WORLD EVENTS AND MEDICAL HISTORY

Dates, persons, and events of significance to the evolution of Medicine include:

1882   Koch discovered tubercle bacillus.

1882   Löffler and Schütz isolated bacillus of glanders in pure culture.

1882   Max Sänger improved cesarean section.

1882   Liebreich introduced lanolin.

1882   Langenbuch excised the gall-bladder.

1882   Public Health Act (Canada) passed.

1882   Royal Academy of Medicine in Ireland (Dublin) founded.

1882   Royal Society of Canada (Ottawa) founded.

1882   Frank invented process for purifying water by filtration through infusorial silica.

1883   Edwin Klebs discovered diphtheria bacillus.

1883   J. Marion Sims died.

1883   Kjeldahl introduced method of estimating nitrogen.

1883   Golgi introduced silver stain for nerve cells.

1883   Pasteur vaccinated against anthrax.

1883   Metchnikoff stated phagocytic theory of immunity.

1883   Unna introduced ichthyol.

1883   Koch discovered bacilli of cholera and infectious conjunctivitis.

1883   Adolf von Baeyer obtained formula of indigo.

1883   Kühne and Chittenden demonstrated role of trypsin in digestion.

1883   Conner (Cincinnati) performed gastrectomy.

1883   A. F. A. King propounded theory of malarial transmission by mosquitoes.

1883-85   Gustav Neuber (Kiel) introduced aseptic hospital.

1884   Nicolaier discovered tetanus bacillus.

1884   Credé introduced silver nitrate instillations for infantile conjunctivitis.

1884   Ludwig Knorr discovered antipyrine.

1884   Baumann discovered sulphonal (Kast, 1888).

1884   Gaffky obtained pure culture of typhoid bacillus (Eberth, 1880).

1884   Loeffler obtained pure culture of diphtheria bacillus (Klebs, 1883).

1884   Emmerich isolated colon bacillus (Escherich, 1886).

1884   Hueppe investigated lactic acid bacilli in sour milk.

1884   Chamberland invented porcelain bacterial filter.

1884   Mergenthaler introduced linotyping.

1884   United States Bureau of Labor established.

1884   Carl Koller employed cocaine in eye surgery.

1885   Golgi discovered glia cells.

1885   Pasteur developed vaccine against rabies.

1885   Yamanashi isolated ephedrine (Nagai, 1887).

1885   H. H. Rusby made extensive trip through South America, seeking new botanical drugs.

1885   Oscar Loewi discovered bactericidal property of formaldehyde (formalin).

1885   Fraser introduced strophanthus.

1885   Bumm obtained pure cultures of gonococcus.

1885   Halsted introduced conduction anesthesia.

1885-86   Sigmund Freud studied under Charcot at the Salpêtrière.

1886   Von Bergmann introduced steam sterilization in surgery.

1886   Moissan discovered fluorine.

1886   Limousin developed glass ampoules for hypodermic solutions.

1886   Escherich investigated bacteria of intestines in infants.

1886   Fitz described pathology of appendicitis.

1886   Marie connected acromegaly with the pituitary body.

1886   Marcel von Nencki introduced salol.

1886   Soxhlet introduced sterilized milk for nutrition of infants.

1886   Kopp, Cahn, and Hepp introduced acetanilide as antifebrin (Gerhardt, 1843).

1887   Weichselbaum discovered meningococcus.

1887   Gram introduced diuretin.

1887   Kast and Hinsberg introduced phenacetin.

PINEL UNCHAINS THE INSANE

COMMON DENOMINATORS of those men who have significantly contributed to the progress of Medicine seem to have been: imagination to conceive a regimen contrary to tradition; courage to effect nonconformist procedures; and skill to carry these to a conclusion sufficiently successful to convince doubters and to confound detractors. Possessed of such qualities was Philippe Pinel, eighteenth century French physician, to whom insane patients seemed not freaks or subhuman creatures but ordinary people badly in need of compassion, care, and medical treatment. Pinel felt that treatment must include large measures of patience and of understanding rather than punishment and cruelty.

Mental disease seldom kills; but the burdens it places upon the patient, both psychological and economical, are perhaps worse than those of any other affliction. Not only is the patient's life disturbed— in more serious manifestations mental disease is more frightening than any other to those with whom the patient comes in contact; and, further, the patient's condition is less known and less understood. This is due in part to the unnatural and sometimes disgusting aspects of mental maladies; and in part because, as a branch of Medicine, psychiatry had such a late beginning.

Medicine in general had its renaissance in the sixteenth century; but at this period progress in psychiatry was abortive. Well into the eighteenth century the insane were burned as witches; well into the nineteenth century they were treated, not as sick patients, but like animals or criminals. Restriction by chains and manacles, while customary, perhaps was among the more humane methods of treatment. Incarceration in dank, sunless dungeons was the lot of many patients. Cruel beatings, cold duckings, violent purges, emetics, and physical humiliations were routine. Seldom visited by physicians, the insane were subject to the whims, caprices, and sadisms of ignorant keepers;

162

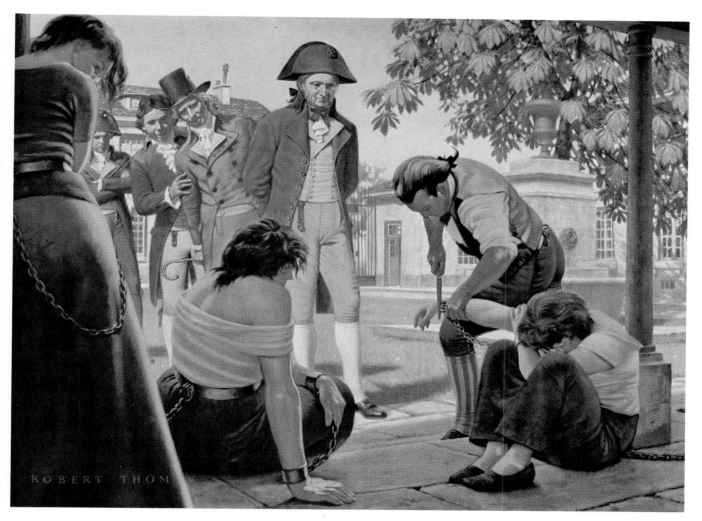

PINEL UNCHAINS THE INSANE

The Father of Psychiatry, French physician Philippe Pinel, in 1795 ordered chains and fetters removed from insane women in the Salpêtrière, large Parisian hospital. Two years earlier, he had similarly unchained insane men in the Bicêtre. Despite political and medical opposition and uncertainties of life during the hectic period of the French Revolution, Pinel persisted in replacing cruelty and inhumanity with kindness, understanding, and rational therapy. His success in curing and relieving patients suffering from mental diseases opened new perspectives for psychiatric research and practice.

163

frequently they were nursed by hardened criminals or outlaws impressed from nearby jails.

The latter years of the eighteenth century witnessed a great philosophical movement called the Enlightenment. The true birth of psychiatry paralleled this movement. It was then that a limited number of humanitarian physicians removed chains from the insane. Among them were: Abraham Joly of Geneva, in 1787; Vincenzo Chiarugi of Toscana, in 1788; Pinel of Paris, in 1793; and the Quaker, William Tuke, of York, in 1796. Of these, Pinel was the most influential; his action became most widely known, and his philanthropic and humanitarian gestures, resulting from an advanced understanding of mental disease, were further developed by his pupils and by his pupils' pupils. From Pinel's leadership there grew the great French school of psychiatry, which included such physicians as Esquirol, Ferrus, Bayle, Calmeil, Falret, Baillarger, Moreau, and others.

Philippe Pinel was born April 20, 1745, in St. André d'Alayrac, a small village in southern France. Originally studying to be a priest, he switched to medicine to become a physician, like his father and his grandfather. At Toulouse, he took an exceptional interest in mathematics, in which subject he earned his degree of Master of Arts. He received his medical degree in 1773. Continuing his studies, he spent five years at the University of Montpellier.

Coming to Paris in 1778, Pinel did not begin the practice of medicine for some years, but found himself a modest place in the Latin Quarter, where he earned his living by tutoring in mathematics and by doing medical literary work. He abstracted and edited the first three volumes of the *Philosophical Transactions* of the Royal Society, and translated William Cullen's *Institutions of Medicine* into French. He was a frequent visitor to the private hospital of Dr. Belhomme, where mental patients were treated. Having established a minor literary reputation, he was invited to edit the *Gazette de Santé*. He continued to write and to contribute articles to publications, therein revealing a growing interest in problems of mental disease. (This interest, it is said, became more intense after 1783, when a close friend became insane and died as a result). At one time Pinel came close to emigrating to the United

164

States, influenced by friendships with Benjamin Franklin and Thomas Jefferson, whom he met at the salon of Mme. Helvétius.

Philippe Pinel has been described as shy, modest, studious, and intellectual; and as moral, moderately pious, and conservative. The rational, the scientific, the orderly, and the logical, appealed to him. He was polite, composed, matter-of-fact; yet quick-witted and forceful when occasion demanded.

To have lived in Paris during the last quarter of the eighteenth century and the first quarter of the nineteenth century meant to have lived in the very center of a cauldron seething with politics, intrigue, violence, and history. Many of Pinel's colleagues and contemporaries lost their lives in the rapid changes in power during those revolutionary years. Yet Pinel served under all these changing governments and received plaudits from each. Pinel had to be present, in line of duty, at the execution of Louis XVI; he served in medical positions of trust during the Revolution and through the Terror; he saw Napoleon come and go, and served equally well under the restored Bourbons. He was honored and decorated for excellence of service by each of these conflicting governments; yet he remained true to his convictions and steadfast in his efforts to obtain better care for the mentally ill and to relieve them of their afflictions.

As the French Revolution increased in intensity, some of Pinel's friends became politically influential. These officials united in requesting the studious physician to assume charge of the Bicêtre, a combination of prison and insane asylum for men. The decree appointing Pinel was published August 25, 1793. The conditions he found there were almost beyond imagination. Disorder, irresponsibility, and pandemonium reigned. Desiring at once to remove chains from poor, mistreated patients, Pinel was informed that he could not carry out his plan without permission of the Bureau Central and authorization of the Commune. Pinel personally made his plea to these authorities. However, almost everyone in power was suspicious of his fellow officers; and there was fear that political enemies might be hidden among Pinel's patients. After personal investigation, Couthon, president of the Commune, granted permission for Pinel's experiment but with an implied question as to Pinel's own sanity in attempting to release "these animals." Pinel quietly replied, "It is my conviction that these mentally ill are intractable only because they are deprived of fresh air and of their liberty."

Chains were removed first from a small number of patients. The favorable results justified Pinel's beliefs. Release; treatment like human beings; fresh air and exercise; baths and good food; and above all, patience, kindness, firm authority, and an understanding search for the roots of the problems that disturbed these patients, resulted in recoveries of many who once were considered hopeless.

Among the first to be freed from chains was an English officer who had been kept in a dungeon for 40 years. When he saw the sun, he exclaimed, "Oh, how good it is!" Two years later he was released. Another, a writer, started running until he fell exhausted. Dismissed as cured a few weeks later, he was soon to die under the guillotine. Another man, chained 34 years, died shortly after release. A priest, chained for 12 years, recovered after ten months of patient treatment. An athletic ex-soldier, who had worn fetters for ten years, became Pinel's servant, once saved the doctor's life when menaced by a mob.

In addition to supervising the Bicêtre, Pinel was appointed Professor of Medicine, December 4, 1794, in the new medical school created by the government. This post he retained until he was "purged" as a liberal in 1822.

His work only well under way after two years at the Bicêtre, Dr. Pinel was called upon in 1795 to become administrator of the Salpêtrière. This institution, today a hospital community of some 6,000 patients and attendants, originally was called the Petit-Arsenal, or Salpêtrière, because saltpeter for the Royal Army's gunpowder was made there; but by command of Louis XIV in 1656 it was converted into a hospital for indigents. In 1660, it was made an asylum for madwomen.

Working with women patients at the Salpêtrière, Pinel again put his ideas into effect—again in the face of considerable opposition. Chains and fetters were removed from patients. Pinel had to reorganize and to train nurses, guards, and medical personnel. Added to these difficulties, politically the times were growing no less turbulent. Disturbances, bloodshed, social and personal uncertainty, all kept pace with revolutionary upheavals, the chaos of rapid changes of the

166

government, and the rise of Napoleon. Despite difficulties, Pinel persisted, developing his psychiatric techniques to meet new situations.

His mathematically trained mind was of great advantage to Pinel in his work at the Bicêtre and at the Salpêtrière. He began first to keep notes for his own use, then developed and introduced permanent, systematic case records—setting the pattern for what is now the measure of good mental hospital administration. He was first to demonstrate by personal example the value of research within the hospital.

Pinel's assistant at the Bicêtre was a man named Jean-Baptiste Pussin, who had an unusual ability to handle mentally ill patients and who has been referred to as the first psychiatric nurse. Pinel put great trust in him, and left him in charge as supervisor at the Bicêtre. Later, Pussin was to rejoin Pinel in the same capacity at the Salpêtrière.

Philippe Pinel continued to work, and to receive honors, until 1823, when he suffered an incapacitating cerebral hemorrhage. On October 25, 1826, another such attack ended his life.

Though Pinel's writings on classification of disease (*Nosographie philosophique*) and his publications on psychiatry (*Traité médico-philosophique sur la manie*, which, in second edition, was titled *Traité médico-philosophique sur l'aliénation mentale*) were well known, their importance pales in comparison with Pinel's work in development of hospital reform and of reorganization. These forward steps, made in such uncertain times, established new traditions and opened new perspectives for practical psychiatric treatment and for research in psychiatry. In addition to illustrious students who carried on his work, Pinel's son, Scipion Pinel, followed in the footsteps of his father and became a prominent psychiatrist in his own right. A nephew, Casimir Pinel, was a leading psychiatrist in the middle of the nineteenth century. Armand Semelaigne, the first psychiatric historian, was married to Casimir's daughter; and their son, René Semelaigne, devoted thirty-five years to psychiatric history before his death in 1934.

Perhaps Philippe Pinel's philosophy of handling mental patients is best summed up in a statement of his own in the introduction to the first edition of his *Traité:*

"The habit of living constantly in the midst of the insane, of studying their habits, their different personalities, the objects of their pleasures or their dislikes, the advantage of following the course of their alienation day and night during the various seasons of the year, the art of directing them without effort and sparing them excitement and grumbling, the gift of being able to assume at the right time a tone of kindness or of authority, of being able to subdue them by force if methods of kindness fail, the constant picture of all the phenomena of mental alienation, and finally the functions of supervision itself—the combination of all of these must give an intelligent and zealous man an immense number of facts and minute details usually lacking in a narrow-minded physician unless he has taken a special interest during fleeting visits to asylums . . . I abandoned the dogmatic tone of the physician; frequent visits, sometimes lasting several hours a day, helped me to familiarize myself with the deviations, shouting, and madness of the most violent maniacs . . . I take careful notes on the facts observed."

Pinel was best known to his contemporaries as the professor of internal medicine whose *Nosographie philosophique* was the bible in Parisian medical circles for twenty years. Today, however, he is remembered first of all as a great psychiatrist: a man who not only loved his patients and believed that they might be cured, but who replaced vain theories and classifications with exact observations, and who, acting upon the basis of these observations, was better able to help mental patients than anyone before him. He transformed insane asylums from ignominious dungeons into instruments of therapy. He abolished not only chains but many other violent and deleterious forms of treatment, such as severe bleeding, submersion in water, and heroic dosage with medicines. These illogical methods he replaced with: proper physical care; classification and separation of patients for specialized treatment; psychological measures; and work therapy. His deep insight into the psychological causes of insanity; his employment of statistics as a means of objectively evaluating procedures; his courage to record failures as well as successes; his devotion to observation; his conservatism regarding medications; his ethical stature—these all combined to make Pinel a worthy successor to the ancient master of medicine whom he greatly admired—Hippocrates.

WORLD EVENTS AND MEDICAL HISTORY

Dates, persons, and events of significance to the evolution of Medicine include:

1888	Institut Pasteur founded.
1888	Roux and Yersin isolated toxin of diphtheria.
1888	Chantemesse and Widal introduced vaccines against typhoid fever.
1888	Celli demonstrated fly transmission of typhoid fever.
1889	Johns Hopkins Hospital (Baltimore) and Hamburg-Eppendorf Hospital opened.
1889	Von Mering and Minkowski produced experimental pancreatic diabetes.
1889	Ramón y Cajal (Spain) demonstrated neurohistological studies at German meeting.
1889	Behring discovered antitoxins.
1889	Vuillemin coined name, "antibiotic."
1889	Kitasato obtained pure cultures of tetanus bacillus.
1889	Pasteur, Chamberland, and Roux employed attenuated cultures in preventive inoculation.
1889	Roux and Yersin pointed out danger of diphtheria convalescents as carriers.
1890	Koch introduced tuberculin and noted that tuberculous animals resist reinoculation.
1890	Schmidt isolated scopolamine.
1890	Behring treated diphtheria with antitoxin.
1890	Schleich introduced infiltration anesthesia.
1890	Ritsert prepared benzocaine.
1890	Jahns synthesized arecoline.
1890	German Pharmaceutical Society (Berlin) founded.
1890-93	Behring and Kitasato developed antitoxin treatment of diphtheria.
1891	Institute for Infectious Diseases (Berlin) opened under Koch.
1891	Frederick G. Banting born.
1891	Lister Institute for Preventive Medicine (London) opened.
1891	Halsted introduced rubber gloves in operative surgery.
1891	Von Bergmann standardized general aseptic ritual in surgery (Koch, 1881; G. Neuber, 1882-5).
1891	Gabriel Lippmann introduced color photography.
1891	S. M. Copeman introduced glycerinated lymph for smallpox vaccination.

1891	Stanford University (California) founded.
1891	Association of American Medical Colleges (Chicago) founded.
1891-93	S. P. Langley experimented with aëroplanes.
1892	Smith and Kilbourne demonstrated tick transmission of bovine piroplasmosis (Texas fever).
1892	Welch and Nuttall identified gas bacillus (*Bacillus aerogenes*).
1892	Sedgwick emphasized necessity of fly control in prevention of typhoid fever.
1893	The Johns Hopkins University School of Medicine opened.
1893	Jean-Martin Charcot died.
1894	Wellcome Physiological Research Laboratories (London) founded.
1894	Field Museum of Natural History (Chicago) founded.
1895	Röntgen discovered x-rays.
1895	Louis Pasteur died.
1895	Ronald Ross demonstrated development of malarial parasite in mosquito.
1895	First pharmaceutical research laboratory established by Parke-Davis.
1895	Calmette introduced serum against snake venoms.
1895	Marconi introduced wireless telegraphy.
1895	Cameron introduced septic tanks for purifying sewage sludge.
1895	Nobel Prize Foundation established at Stockholm.
1895	Friedrich Wilhelms Institut (Berlin) became Kaiser-Wilhelms Akademie.
1896	Max Gruber discovered bacterial agglutination.
1896	Röntgen demonstrated x-rays to public.
1896	Wright, Pfeiffer, and Kolle vaccinated against typhoid fever.
1896	Widal and Sicard introduced agglutination test for typhoid fever.
1896	Leo Arons (Berlin) invented mercury vapor lamp (elimination of red or orange rays).
1896	Friedrich Bezold devised tuning-fork method of testing and training deaf-mutes.
1896	W. J. Dibden and Schweder invented method for bacteriological purification of sewage.

JENNER: SMALLPOX IS STEMMED

"MAY I NOT with perfect confidence congratulate my country and society at large on their beholding . . . an antidote that is capable of extirpating from the earth a disease which is every hour devouring its victims; a disease that has ever been considered as the severest scourge of the human race!"

With these mild, modest phrases did Edward Jenner, in the year 1800, close his third publication, *A Continuation of Facts and Observations Relative to the Variolae Vaccinae, or Cowpox*. The statement was typical of this homeloving English country doctor of Berkeley, whose keen sense of observation and persistence in experimentation had given to Medicine and to the world an entirely new principle with which to combat disease: vaccination.

Smallpox had been a scourge upon humanity for untold centuries. Described accurately by the Persian, Rhazes (865-925), smallpox evidently had been known in China and in India long before; and for centuries Orientals had sought to protect themselves against the disease by inoculation: by snuffing dried crusts of smallpox pustules into the nose; inserting pustular material from an infected person into a vein of a healthy person; or by binding a bit of such material over a scratch in the skin. By one of these methods, practitioners sought to confer immunity to smallpox upon healthy persons, particularly children, by producing in them a mild form of smallpox. If the procedure was successful, the patient was unlikely to be affected during subsequent inevitable epidemics of smallpox in his community; and hazards of severe scarring and of crippling from infection were lessened. If unsuccessful—well, the patient probably would have succumbed to smallpox later on, anyway. The risk was considered worthwhile, even though the procedure carried the further risk that inoculated persons might convey active infection to others in the community.

Inoculation, though long practiced in the Far East, in Greece, and in the Ottoman Empire, did not find acceptance in Europe until 1717, after the idea was advocated by Lady Mary Wortley Montagu, wife of

170

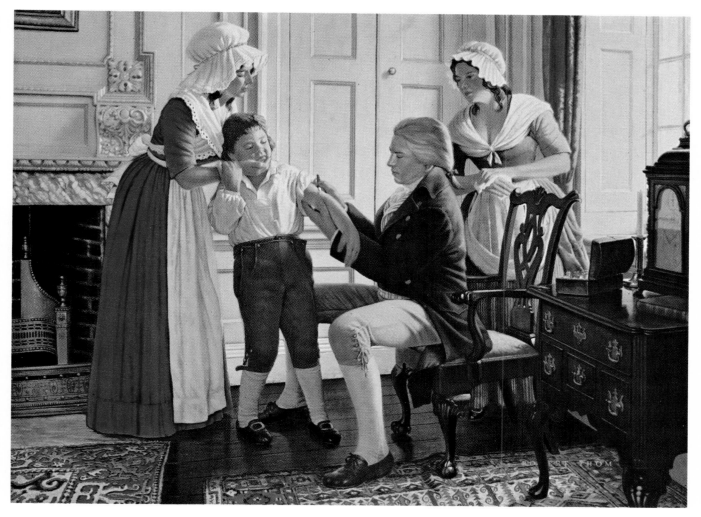

JENNER: SMALLPOX IS STEMMED

The first vaccination against smallpox was performed by Edward Jenner, English rural physician, in his apartment in the Chantry House, Berkeley, Gloucestershire. Exudate from a cowpox pustule on the hand of dairymaid, Sarah Nelmes, was inserted into scratches on the arm of eight-year-old James Phipps, May 14, 1796. The vaccination was effective, for two later attempts to induce infection with smallpox were unsuccessful. Proving and reproving his discovery, Jenner published his vaccination findings in 1798. Despite opposition, vaccination became accepted practice during Jenner's lifetime.

the British Ambassador to Turkey. Lady Montagu had her three-year-old son successfully inoculated by the Embassy physician; her daughter inoculated upon their return to Europe. Lady Mary's efforts were at first violently denounced; but when, through her influence, King George I permitted his two granddaughters to be inoculated, the practice was at first accepted, and then became the current fashion in Europe. Concurrently, the Reverend Cotton Mather, in Boston, was pressing the cause for inoculation in the American colonies, with the cooperation of Dr. Zabdiel Boylston. On June 26, 1721, Boylston inoculated his six-year-old son and two Negro slaves. His experiment was successful—but his acts and Mather's publications touched off near-riotous reactions.

Such was the status of the medical profession's and of the public's attitudes toward smallpox when Edward Jenner came into the world. As prevalent as measles, but far more deadly, smallpox during the latter half of the eighteenth century accounted for 10 per cent of all deaths. Often smallpox disfigured faces of those whom it did not kill, and caused much of the blindness of that time.

The impact of Jenner's work was not limited to his victory over smallpox: extension of his principle, of vaccination as a means of prevention of disease, in the next 160 years was to enable the medical profession to score almost total victory over several other infectious diseases.

Edward Jenner was born May 17, 1749, the son of the Reverend Stephen Jenner, vicar of Berkeley, in Gloucestershire, England. When he was five, his father died, and he was looked after by his elder clergyman brother. Early in life he exhibited an extraordinary interest in nature. At age thirteen he was apprenticed to Daniel Ludlow, surgeon and apothecary of Sodbury. In 1770 Jenner became a student at St. George's Hospital, in London, and a house pupil of the famous London surgeon and naturalist, John Hunter. From this relationship developed a lifelong friendship, a strong interest in comparative anatomy, and collaboration in research and observation of natural phenomena. Young Jenner's abilities as a naturalist earned him the job of classifying and of arranging zoological specimens brought back by Joseph Banks from Captain Cook's first voyage to the Pacific, in 1771, and an offer to accompany Cook's next expedition. Jenner turned down this and other lucrative offers, for he preferred to return to his native Berkeley to engage in the practice of medicine.

Dr. Jenner is described as a rather handsome man of stocky build who liked to dress well. He was generally beloved for his congenial and kindly personality and for his readiness to go to the sick through storm or mud. He did not disdain to look at a farmer's sick cow, after having cared for his family. Not only was he a competent physician; he also was interested in music and in poetry—even to composing bits of verse from time to time. At Berkeley, where he lived in Chantry Cottage near the church, he continued his studies of natural history, goaded frequently by letters from John Hunter demanding this investigation or that specimen. From Hunter he received a famous bit of advice: "Why think? Why not try the experiment?"

Jenner was quite familiar with inoculation as a means of preventing smallpox; he carried a vivid memory of the severity of his own experience following inoculation when he was but a boy.

Early in his career, Jenner was impressed by the insistence of dairymaids, suffering from sores and from mild reactions to cowpox, that they now would be safe from smallpox. Medical men believed this to be but an old country folk saying; but the idea intrigued Jenner. He then collected examples of persons who had had cowpox and afterward had escaped smallpox; or who, having had cowpox, did not react successfully to smallpox inoculation. Of this methodical work, Underwood says: "Even at this early stage he seems to have been obsessed by the feeling that cowpox *ought* to give complete and permanent immunity to smallpox. This is indeed strange, since every practitioner knew that smallpox did not always give complete and permanent protection against itself . . . Jenner set out to show that cowpox protected against smallpox, and also that cowpox could be transmitted from one human being to another just as smallpox could . . . that cowpox, naturally acquired, could be transmitted artificially *from person to person* so that there would result an increasing reservoir of persons who had been given the opportunity of becoming . . . immune . . . to smallpox . . . That was the cardinal factor in Jenner's doctrine, and it was an idea which had probably not occurred seriously to anyone before; at least, no one had attempted to put it into practice." Jenner's progress was slow. His keen observations extended over a quarter of a century.

It was in 1796 that Jenner made his crucial experiment. He found that Sarah Nelmes, a dairymaid, had a typical cowpox lesion on her hand. On May 14, he inoculated a young friend, eight-year-old James Phipps. Jenner reported: "The matter was taken from a sore on the hand of a dairymaid, who was infected by her master's cows, and it was inserted . . . into the arm of the boy by means of two superficial incisions, barely penetrating the cutis, each about half an inch long.

"On the seventh day he complained of uneasiness in the axilla, and on the ninth he became a little chilly, lost his appetite, and had a slight headache. During the whole of this day he was perceptibly indisposed, and spent the night with some degree of restlessness, but on the day following he was perfectly well."

But Jenner wanted to be sure. Therefore, he wrote: "In order to ascertain whether the boy, after feeling so slight an affection of the system from the cowpox virus, was secure from the contagion of the smallpox, he was inoculated on the 1st of July following with variolous matter, immediately taken from a pustule. Several slight punctures were made on both his arms, and the matter was carefully inserted, but no disease followed . . . Several months afterward he was again inoculated with variolous matter, but no sensible effect was produced on the constitution."

In 1797, Jenner sent a short treatise embodying his results to the Royal Society. The paper was refused, with the admonition that he "should be cautious . . . and ought not risk his reputation by presenting to the learned body anything which appeared so much at variance with established knowledge, and withal so incredible."

By spring, 1798, Jenner had collected further evidence to substantiate his claims, and privately published his famous booklet: *An Inquiry into the Causes and Effects of the Variolae Vaccinae, a disease discovered in some of the Western counties of England, particularly in Gloucestershire, and known by the name of the Cowpox.*

Jenner's great discovery at first evoked resistance, not acceptance. Three months in London in 1798 failed to arouse interest either among physicians or among patients. His first break came when Henry Cline, a surgeon, used a quill of dried cowpox serum, which Jenner had left with him, as a counterirritant in treating another disease, and found later that his patient had become immune to smallpox inoculation. From interest created by Cline's report of this incident the practice of vaccination began to spread.

As vaccination became popular, there was no lack of detractors, nor of persons seeking spurious credit for its discovery. Jenner's work, however, was based upon sound experimental data; his results were so positive and so convincing and the need for this surer, safer, and less torturous prophylaxis was so great, that he received official recognition earlier in life than did most medical innovators. In 1800, Jenner was invited officially to London to vaccinate the 85th regiment, which assignment he took personally. In the United States, Professor Benjamin Waterhouse performed the first vaccination in July, 1800, with material received from England. After lengthy investigation of Jenner's claims, Parliament in 1802 voted him a sum of £10,000; and again, in 1806, a grant of £20,000.

Despite swirling currents of fame and of defamation, Jenner continued to make his home in Berkeley and to practice medicine. He published two additional pamphlets on vaccination: *Further Observations on the Variolae Vaccinae or Cowpox*, in 1799; and *A Continuation*, previously mentioned, in 1800. His correspondence grew in volume apace with his fame, taking up more and more of his time. In the midst of such circumstances, the life of the great benefactor of mankind ended, at Chantry Cottage, in his seventy-fourth year. A cerebral hemorrhage was fatal to Jenner on January 26, 1823.

Jenner's dedication to his cause and to singleness of purpose is well defined in his own words:

"While the vaccine discovery was progressive, the joy I felt at the prospect before me of being the instrument destined to take away from the world one of its great calamities, blended with the fond hope of enjoying independence and domestic peace and happiness, was often so excessive that, in pursuing my favorite subject among the meadows, I have sometimes found myself in a kind of reverie. It is pleasant for me to recollect that these reflections always ended in devout acknowledgments to that Being from whom this and all other mercies flow."

LAENNEC AND THE STETHOSCOPE

DURING the past century, perhaps the most characteristic symbol associated with physicians has been the stethoscope. It replaced the urine glass, the symbol which had prevailed since medieval times. Today's physician acquires his first stethoscope during his second year in medical school. From then on, employment of percussion and auscultation in his study of patients becomes as automatic as counting pulse or taking temperature. Yet it required three generations of medical men and lifelong efforts of two physicians dedicated to research to introduce these methods to medicine, to instruct physicians in their use, and to overcome resistance and prejudice of contemporaries to whom any change was offensive.

Percussion was introduced to medicine by an Austrian, Leopold Auenbrugger (1722-1809). Appointed physician to the Spanish Military Hospital, then Vienna's finest, in 1751, Auenbrugger had exceptional opportunity to observe the processes of disease, especially disease of the chest. He noted that, when the thorax of a healthy person is struck lightly, a sound resembling that of a drum muffled with a thick woolen cloth is produced. In sick persons, such sounds vary in accordance with the nature of underlying change, its location, and its extent. Auenbrugger spent seven years testing his idea, especially checking opinions formed while examining moribund patients with conditions found at autopsy. In 1761, he published his epochal contribution, *On Percussion of the Chest*, in a small volume of 95 pages. Auenbrugger's preface was prophetic. Therein he wrote:

"I here present the reader with a new sign which I have discovered for detecting diseases of the chest. This consists in the percussion of the human thorax, whereby, according to the character of the particular sounds thence elicited, an opinion is formed of the internal state of that cavity. In making public my discoveries . . . I have not been unconscious of the dangers I must encounter; since it has always been the fate of those who have illustrated or improved the arts and sciences

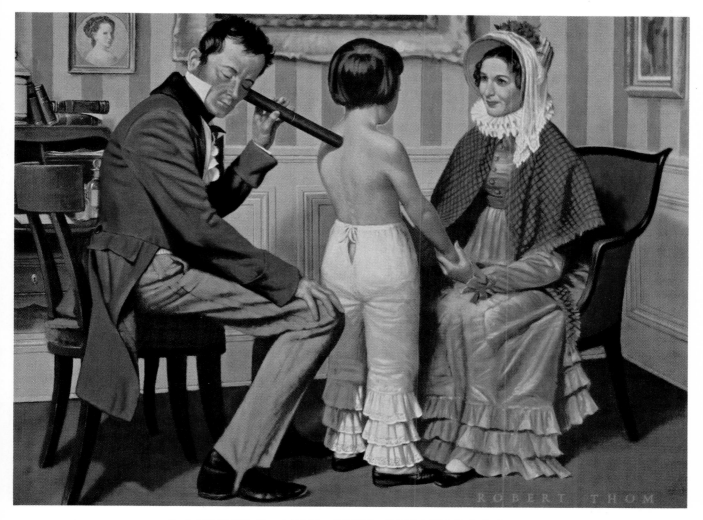

LAENNEC AND THE STETHOSCOPE

Theophile Laennec (1781-1826), young French physician, while at Necker Hospital, Paris, in 1816, devised foot-long, hollow, wooden cylinders for listening to sounds in patients' chests. These he called "stethoscopes." Comparing opinions formed during stethoscopic examinations with later findings at autopsy, Laennec learned to accurately diagnose pathologic heart and lung conditions, and to better understand many chest diseases. His instrument and his published reports on its use were among the greater contributions to nineteenth-century medicine, helping physicians to understand pulmonary diseases—especially tuberculosis, the malady that ended Laennec's own short life.

by their discoveries to be beset by envy, malice, hatred, detraction, and calumny. This, the common lot, I have chosen to undergo . . ."

Though a second edition appeared in 1775, Auenbrugger's work was unappreciated until 1808, when Jean Nicolas Corvisart, physician to Napoleon I and leader of medical thought in France, translated *On Percussion of the Chest* into French and gave unstinted praise to the discoverer of percussion, 47 years after Auenbrugger's little volume first appeared in Austria. Auenbrugger lived just long enough to see the beginning of recognition of his discovery; he died on May 17, 1809. Corvisart became one of Laennec's teachers, providing the link between Auenbrugger and percussion, and Laennec and indirect auscultation. As the career of the Austrian physician was drawing to a close, that of the young Frenchman was just beginning.

Laennec's embarkation upon a career in medicine closely coincided with recognition of Paris as world capital of medicine between 1800 and 1850. The foundations had been well laid. Morgagni of Padua and Bichat of Paris had established the importance of anatomic pathology and of autopsy. Pinel had proved the value of statistical compilations from patients' records. Corvisart, the clinician, emphasized need for adequate physical examination, including employment of Auenbrugger's methods of percussion. To these advances, Laennec was to add mediate (indirect) auscultation. This combination of clinical and diagnostic procedures revealed basic characteristics of diseases prevalent at the time, such as tuberculosis, typhoid fever, and diphtheria. Laennec's was perhaps the greatest single contribution to this half century of progress.

René Théophile Hyacinthe Laennec was born at Quimper, Lower Brittany, France, February 17, 1781. He was not quite 5 years of age when his mother died of pulmonary tuberculosis, a disease prevalent in the area. His father, an advocate with considerable education, preferred literature to law, and accepted practically no responsibility for his children. Early in life Théophile Laennec went to live with an uncle, Guillaume François Laennec, a professor on the faculty of medicine at Nantes, who had studied at Montpellier, and under Hunter, in London. This uncle saw to it that young Théophile received a sound basic and classical education, despite the turbulent times. The

178

French Revolution was under way, with its rioting and political brutalities. Théophile must have seen at least 50 heads roll into the basket under the guillotine set up in the square outside his window. Uncle Guillaume was called upon to minister to victims of the wrath of man, of war, and of the inevitable typhus which followed. In his fifteenth year, Théophile was given the title of military surgeon, third class, and set to work as an apprentice, assisting his uncle in military hospitals at Nantes.

After preliminary studies in local educational institutions, Laennec, at 19 years of age, was able to go to Paris to complete his medical education. Shortage of funds and poor living conditions did not improve his already delicate health. He immediately enrolled in the Ecole de Médecine, and attended clinics at l'Hôpital de la Charité under Corvisart and his assistant, Bayle. Corvisart's influence upon Laennec was not dissimilar from that of John Hunter upon Jenner. Corvisart stressed bedside instruction, and trained his students thoroughly in autopsy examinations. Laennec studied carefully and methodically; during his first three years at la Charité he wrote up careful histories of more than 400 patients whom he had seen. Among other favorite teachers were Bichat, and Dupuytren, at the time a pathologic anatomist, later to become a great surgeon. Driven by his inborn intensity, Laennec, advanced beyond the ordinary medical student, won two governmentally sponsored first prizes in surgery and in medicine by competitive examinations and while still an undergraduate student published papers on heart disease and on the capsule of the liver. His memoir in 1802 on peritonitis was particularly valuable in clarifying this age-old problem.

Théophile Laennec received his doctorate, June 11, 1804, at age 23. For five years after graduation he was editor-in-chief of the *Journal de Médecine*. At the same time he lectured on pathologic anatomy. Paper after paper flowed from his pen. Tuberculosis in particular attracted his attention, and percussion was one of his favorite diagnostic methods. Among his prominent patients were Chateaubriand and Madame de

Staël. During this period he held posts at the Hôpital Beaujon and at the Salpêtrière.

By 1814, Laennec was badly in need of a vacation. He returned to an estate inherited from his grandfather at Kerlouarnec, near Quimper, seeking to throw off exhaustion from his busy life, as well as persistent attacks of asthma, and to indulge his lively interests in natural history and in roots of the Celtic language spoken in his home area.

Returning to practice in Paris in 1816, at 35 years of age, Laennec was appointed visiting physician to l'Hôpital Necker. This provided him the opportunity of his lifetime. Likely his name would have found its place in history because of his publications on pathology and methods of correlating clinical observations with post-mortem findings; but the clinic at Necker Hospital, in his first year there, presented Laennec the challenge that led to his greatest discovery.

Laennec was familiar with palpation and percussion; and from his friend and former teacher, Bayle, he had learned of immediate, or direct, auscultation (listening to sounds in the thorax by placing the physician's ear directly on the patient's chest wall). Many patients were not accustomed to bathing and some even were verminous, so many physicians were reluctant to use this diagnostic method. Layers of fat that sometimes obstructed transmission of sounds, and modesty of women patients, were further deterrents.

One day, in 1816, while walking through a littered yard pondering the problem of a very obese young woman suspected to be suffering from heart disease, Laennec noted a group of children at play about a pile of beams. One would put his ears against the end of a beam, while another would scratch or tap the opposite end. To their childish amazement the sounds were conveyed from one end to the other. Laennec, grasping the physical principle involved, hurried back to Necker and his overweight patient.

"I rolled a quire of paper into a kind of cylinder," says Laennec in the introduction to his great book, "and applied one end of it to the region of the heart and the other to my ear, and was not a little surprised and pleased to find that I could thereby perceive the action of the heart in a manner much more clear and distinct than I had ever been able to by immediate application of the ear. From this moment I imagined that the circumstance might furnish means for enabling us to ascertain the character, not only of the action of the heart, but of every species of sound produced by the motion of all the thoracic viscera and consequently for the exploration of the respiration, the voice, the rhonchus (râle), and perhaps even the fluctuation of fluid extravasated in the pleura or the pericardium. With this conviction I forthwith commenced at the Hospital Necker a series of observations from which I have been able to deduce a set of new signs of diseases of the chest . . . to render the diagnosis of the diseases of the lungs, heart, and pleura, as decided and circumstantial as the indications furnished to the surgeon by the introduction of the finger or the sound, in the complaints wherein these are used."

Laennec then set about experimenting with various forms of the instrument, which he named *stethoscope*. First he tried a compact roll of paper, then a wand with no aperture. This he found would convey heart sounds, but a cylinder with a central aperture and a funnel-shaped opening at the applied end proved best suited for chest examinations. He finally settled on a cylindrical instrument made of light wood, about an inch and a half in diameter and a foot long, perforated longitudinally by a quarter-inch bore, hollowed out to funnel shape at the end for application. He fitted this end with an insertable perforated plug that would convert the device to a simple cylinder. The instrument was divided into two portions of about equal length that would slip or screw together. This had the double advantage of being more convenient for carrying in a pocket, and, when desired, of providing a shorter instrument by use of only one segment. Various adaptations of this form of instrument continued in use by physicians until the binaural stethoscope was developed by Dr. George Philip Cammann, of New York, in 1855. Cammann's instrument, which in essence was similar to those used today, afforded convenience and freedom of movement to the physician by providing aural ends which fitted into the ear, instead of just against it.

For the next three years, 1816 to 1819, Laennec intensively studied sounds heard through his stethoscopes, and like Auenbrugger, checked his impressions with autopsy findings. He presented reports to the Société de l'Ecole, and to the Academy of Sciences, describing use of his instrument in diagnosis and sounds encountered in patients with such conditions as pneumothorax, bronchial dilatation, pulmonary emphysema, edema, gangrene, and tuberculosis. He also described significant attributes of voice transmission through the chest wall, which he termed "pectoriloquy" and which he interpreted as indicative of serious tuberculous lesions. So closely did he apply himself to this work that his health broke down and he was forced to take another holiday at Quimper. He returned to Paris thereafter and set about publication of his findings in book form. In 1819, *A Treatise on the Diseases of the Chest and on Mediate Auscultation* appeared in two thick volumes.

Laennec's treatise met with cool reception and harsh criticism. However, some prominent physicians began using the stethoscope; and translations of his book were made in other languages. Laennec's ideas had better reception in other European countries and in North America than in his own country.

Laennec's health again broke down (likely he was already suffering from tuberculosis) and he retired to his farms at Kerlouarnec for two years. He returned to Paris in November, 1821, this time to be welcomed with many honors. He was appointed personal physician to the Duchess of Berry; and in 1822 he was appointed professor of practical medicine at the Collège de France, to succeed Corvisart as clinical professor one year later. Physicians from all over Europe and America came to hear lectures by the discoverer of auscultation, who had resigned his position at Necker and had taken over a clinic at la Charité. In 1824 he was made a Knight of the Legion of Honor. The emaciated, asthmatic little physician plunged again into an intensive work schedule, which included preparation of the second, enlarged edition of his treatise on auscultation. Again he was defeated by poor health. He contracted a cold, and his dry cough became more severe. At the end of May, 1826, Laennec returned once more to Brittany, hopeful for relief. One of his pupils, called to care for him, on examining him heard the telltale pectoriloquy, harbinger of death from tuberculosis. Laennec's condition worsened, and on August 13, 1826, the dread consumption that had claimed his mother and many of his patients took the life of the little physician in his forty-fifth year.

Tribute to Laennec as a man of medicine may be found in Sigerist's writings: "Laennec was something more than the discoverer of auscultation. He was a distinguished anatomist and a great clinician. The invention of the stethoscope was remarkable, but even more remarkable was what he himself did with the instrument." As a man among men, Ackerknecht described Laennec as: "Incredibly many-sided: a good philologist, musician, hunter, draftsman, woodcarver, and administrator, besides being a medical genius and a good man. But he exhibited a façade of coldness and few persons recognized his true value during his short life—so full of tribulations, so poor in joys, yet so rich in accomplishments."

WORLD EVENTS AND MEDICAL HISTORY

Dates, persons, and events of significance to the evolution of Medicine include:

1896	Casper employed ureteral cystoscopy and catheterization in diagnosis of renal diseases.
1896	University of Lyons founded (July 10).
1896	Stenbeck opened Röntgen Institute at Stockholm.
1897	First physiologically standardized pharmaceutical product, fluid-extract of ergot, introduced by Parke-Davis.
1897	Shiga discovered dysentery bacillus.
1897	Eijkman cured beriberi with rice polishings.
1897	Emil Fischer synthesized caffeine, theobromine, xanthine, guanine, and adenine.
1897	Jonnesco performed sympathectomy for glaucoma.
1897	Ogata found plague bacilli in fleas of plague-ridden rats.
1897	Nuttall demonstrated fly-transmission of plague bacilli.
1897	Ehrlich stated side-chain theory of immunity.
1897	E. Van Ermengem discovered *Bacillus botulinus*.
1897	J. V. Laborde introduced artificial respiration.

1897	Horton Smith showed danger of chronic (urinary) typhoid carriers.
1897	Germano showed that dryness is fatal to bacteria.
1897-1902	Cannon investigated movements of stomach and intestines by röntgenoscopy.
1897-1904	Ramón y Cajal published treatise on texture of the nervous system.
1898	P. and M. Curie discovered radium.
1898	Howard Florey born.
1898	Loeffler and Frosch investigated filterable viruses.
1898	Looss demonstrated mechanism of hookworm infection.
1898	Theobald Smith isolated and cultivated bovine tubercle bacilli.
1898	Dreser introduced heroin.
1898	Simonds demonstrated transmission of bubonic plague by fleas.
1898	Tschirch explained chemical mechanism of common purgatives.
1898	Affiliation of Rush Medical College with University of Chicago (January 5).
1898	Cornell University Medical College (New York City) founded.
1898-1908	Zeppelin experimented with dirigible airships.

CONQUERORS OF PAIN

PAIN associated with surgical operations had been a scourge upon mankind long before the dawn of history; and its searing, agonizing, frightening finger followed the surgeon's scalpel like a shadow until the middle of the nineteenth century. Then, within the short span of four years, means of relief were twice discovered in a new nation, the United States of America, whose medical men until then had looked to Europe for leadership in medical progress.

Nature yields her secrets to man only as his mind and his imagination expand sufficiently to cope with new ideas. Ether had been synthesized by Valerius Cordus in the middle of the sixteenth century— 300 years before its anesthetic properties were realized. Humphry Davy, experimenting with "laughing gas," hinted at the possibilities of nitrous oxide as a surgical anesthetic in 1800; but nearly half a century was to pass before surgical patients were to be relieved of fright, humiliation, agony, and shock on the operating table.

Four men played leading roles in bringing about the advent of anesthesia. Crawford Williamson Long, a physician, working independently, was first to use ether as an anesthetic in his practice in Jefferson, Georgia, March 30, 1842. Horace Wells, a dentist, of Hartford, Connecticut, who used nitrous oxide as an anesthetic in his dental practice as early as December, 1844, sought to demonstrate its possibilities for use with surgical patients before Dr. John C. Warren's class at the Harvard Medical School in January, 1845, but failed through a technicality. William Thomas Green Morton, a dentist studying medicine at the time, successfully demonstrated use of ether as an anesthetic upon a patient undergoing a surgical operation, October 16, 1846, in the operating amphitheatre of the Massachusetts General Hospital. Morton's claim to discovery was challenged by Dr. Charles Thomas Jackson, physician and chemist, whose suggestion led Morton to experiment with highly purified ether.

Conquering pain incident to surgical operation by means of an anesthetic agent probably was medicine's greatest gift to mankind up

184

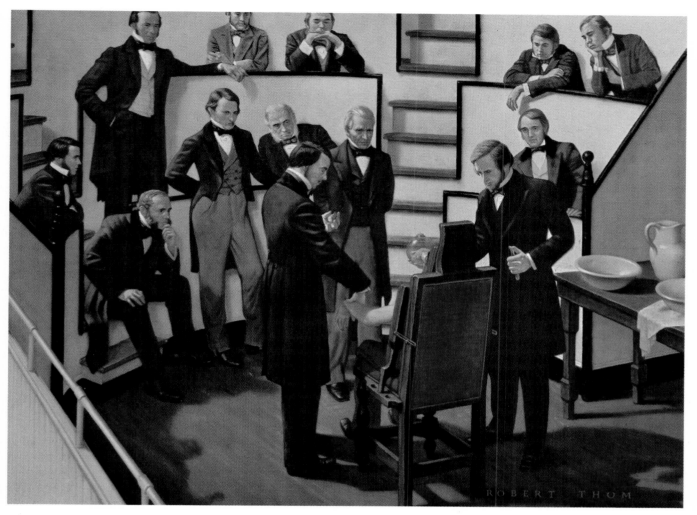

CONQUERORS OF PAIN

Before a skeptical group of surgeons in the operating amphitheatre of Massachusetts General Hospital, October 16, 1846, William T. G. Morton, Boston dentist, prepared to anesthetize Dr. John C. Warren's surgical patient, Gilbert Abbott, by causing him to inhale ether. Though Crawford W. Long, Georgia physician, had used ether for anesthesia in 1842, and Horace Wells, Connecticut dentist, tried unsuccessfully to demonstrate anesthesia with nitrous oxide in 1845, reports of painless operations resulting from Morton's methods gave practical anesthesia to mankind. Within a year, ether was being used world-widely to conquer the pain incident to surgical operations.

185

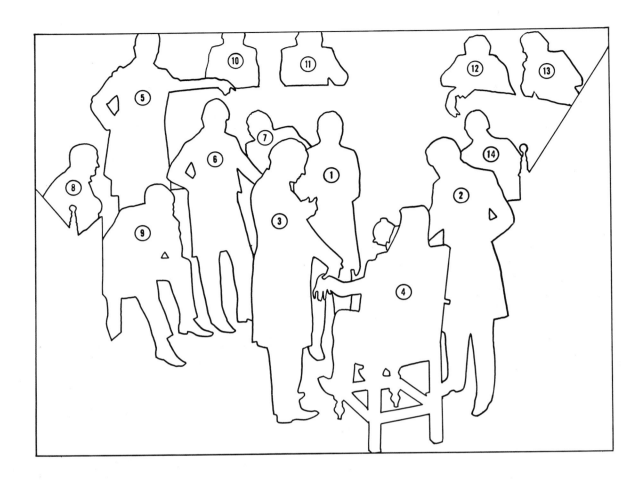

Identity of persons in the picture,
CONQUERORS OF PAIN

1. Dr. John C. Warren, operating surgeon.
2. Dr. William T. G. Morton, demonstrated
    ether anesthesia.
3. Dr. Charles F. Heywood, house surgeon.
4. Gilbert Abbott, patient.
5. Dr. Augustus A. Gould.
6. Dr. Henry J. Bigelow.
7. Dr. Solomon D. Townsend.
8, 9, 10, 11, 12, 13, 14. Medical students.

186

to that time. Ironically, none of the four men who claimed to have brought it about received the recognition he felt he deserved. As Robinson wrote: "The four men did not meet in a tavern and pledge eternal brotherhood as the world rejoiced in the Victory over Pain. Alone they drank the wine of bitterness, and tasted the lees of hatred. There was limitless glory for all, but not one would grant a share to another."

Despite tremendous advances in anesthesia during sixscore years since its world-wide adoption, we still know little about pain. Given by nature as a warning signal for the protection of life, its mechanisms can be controlled or thwarted, but these are little understood. Man early turned to his surroundings, seeking to assuage pain with herbs, leaves, cool water, or mud from the earth that bore him. When man learned to ferment wine, he created his first anodyne, physical as well as psychic. A clay tablet impressed in Babylon about 2250 B.C., proposes a remedy to relieve the pain of toothache. Theophrastus wrote of hellebore for relief of pain in the fourth century, B.C.; Herodotus the Greek and Suśruta the Hindu both discussed cannabis; Dioscorides in the first century wrote of opium, and knew about mandrake, essential ingredient of "wine of the condemned," used to ease the punishment tortures of transgressors. Dioscorides, too, was perhaps the first to use the word, *anesthesia*. Galen recommended lettuce as an anodyne. Ancient Greeks also knew that compression of carotid arteries produces insensibility. However, as Robinson stated, the term, anesthesia, was applied more often by Greek poets and dramatists than by medical men, and though sensibilities may have been blunted in various ways, there is no record that ancient Greeks performed operations under anesthesia.

Little progress was made toward relief of pain during the thousand years of the Middle Ages. Lack of standards for drugs was a primary drawback. The "spongia somnifera," a means of inhaling volatile agents, was known in the ninth century. "Sweet vitriol" was mentioned in the thirteenth century by Raymundus Lullius, and again 200 years later by Paracelsus, who distilled it from a mixture of sulfuric acid and alcohol. Cordus in 1540 described synthesis of a product that was named "ether" by Frobenius of Germany in 1730. As early as 1513, monks used alcoholic fumes to alleviate pain. Paré in 1543 used pressure to induce anesthesia—but the method was nearly as painful as the operation it masked. Seventeenth century France forbade stupefaction of patients with herbal remedies; and in the middle of that century, Severino of Naples experimented with refrigeration anesthesia—which reached limited popularity only in the twentieth century.

While ether remained a laboratory curiosity and a remedy for whooping cough, reduction of pain during operations was accomplished only as surgeons developed speed in operating. But by other routes, science was groping for the answer. Priestley and Scheele independently discovered oxygen about 1771; Lavoisier learned of oxygen's significance in respiration in 1792; and these advances gave rise to the school of pneumatic medicine—those who sought to administer medicines via inhalation. These findings also became bases for experiments in Britain: by Humphry Davy with nitrous oxide; by his student, Michael Faraday, with ether; and by Henry Hill Hickman with carbon dioxide.

Davy, in 1800, at the end of his *Researches*, wrote: "as nitrous oxide in its extensive operation appears capable of destroying physical pain, it may probably be used with advantage during surgical operations in which no great effusion of blood takes place." Faraday, in 1818, noted that: "When the vapour of ether mixed with common air is inhaled, it produces effects very similar to those occasioned by nitrous oxide." Hickman, in 1824, carried out a series of experiments on animals, proving that pain of surgical operations could be abolished by inhalation of carbon dioxide. Despite extensive publication of works of these men, in England and in France, no physicians of their day recognized the tremendous import of their experiments.

Meanwhile, experiments reported by Franz Anton Mesmer of Vienna, as early as 1776, with "animal magnetism," were enjoying a popular revival in many European countries and in the United States. First employment of mesmerism to relieve pain in surgical patients was by Jules Cloquet, a French surgeon, who removed a breast from a mesmerized patient. James Braid, surgeon of Manchester, England, was first to apply the term, *hypnotism*, to the process. Meanwhile, Samuel Guthrie, physician turned chemist in upper New York state, in 1831 was distilling "sweet whiskey" from chloride of lime and alcohol—at about the same time that Soubeiran in France and Liebig in Germany announced their independent discoveries of a heavy, sweet, volatile, "chloric ether." In 1832, Daniel Smith, one of the principal founders of the Philadelphia College of Pharmacy, wrote of its delicious flavor and intoxicating qualities, "more grateful to the taste than hydrated ether." In 1834, Dumas, a French chemist, gave the fluid the name of *chloroform*. Even though Guthrie's eight-year-old daughter once fell asleep while playing about a vat, chloroform's great promise escaped the country doctor's attention.

While it seems amazing that the idea of anesthesia did not dawn upon medical men much earlier, in view of these scientific signposts, it must be recognized that the greatest barrier to evolution of such a concept was the eighteenth century attitude toward suffering. "Behind the decent, civilized Georgian façade," wrote Cartwright, "there lies a callousness, a brutality almost unparalleled in history. Pain and suffering were held to be of no account; what mattered was not the degree of pain inflicted, but the fortitude with which it was borne. To such a mentality, anesthesia would have seemed not the greatest single boon ever vouchsafed to suffering humanity, but a matter of very minor importance . . .

"Turn over the pages for fifty years, consider the state of the world in the eighteen-forties, and we see a very different picture. During that half century . . . man's attitude to suffering had altered; instead of being an inevitable and even salutary part of life, it had become a disease to be cured radically wherever possible. In such a world, the hideous tortures inflicted by the surgeon upon the helpless sick were realized to be necessary, but were regarded with horror and disgust . . .

"The acceptance of anesthesia is not just an incidental happening, an unrelated accident . . . it is one of the outward signs of a great inward working of men's minds . . ."

Though Davy and Faraday failed to attach much importance to pain-relieving properties of nitrous oxide and of ether, revealed by their experiments, their findings led to laughing gas lectures and ether frolics of the 1840's. These popular science demonstrations, in turn, emboldened Long, Wells, and Morton to attempt what then seemed incredible—anesthesia for patients undergoing surgical procedures by inhalation of little-known chemical compounds.

The controversy over recognition and credit for practical application of the principle of anesthesia was long and bitter. The Congress of the United States investigated the claims of Morton, Wells, and Jackson, on three different occasions over an eight-year period, and, after receiving Dr. Long's belated evidence, failed to reach a conclusion. The Academy of Medicine in Paris awarded equal honors to Drs. Jackson and Morton. To this day, inconclusive arguments continue among proponents motivated for the most part by regional pride. The evidence seems clear that Crawford Williamson Long was first to use ether for surgical anesthesia for other than dental operations. It seems clear, also, that William E. Clarke, a chemist, and Elijah Pope, a dentist, used ether on a patient in Rochester, New York, for extraction of a tooth, in January, 1842. Dr. Long, having observed that he and his friends were temporarily insensible to pain following experimental inhalation of ether, administered ether on a towel held over the face of James M. Venable, and while he was anesthetized, removed an encysted tumor from the back of the patient's neck. This operation was performed March 30, 1842.

Crawford Long was born November 1, 1815, near Danielsville, Georgia. He was graduated at nineteen years of age from the University of Georgia, in 1835. After reading medicine under Dr. Grant of Jefferson, Georgia, he entered the Medical Department of the University of Pennsylvania in 1838. Among his instructors were Philip Syng Physick, once a pupil of John Hunter, and George B. Wood and Franklin Bache, who also were instrumental in development of the Philadelphia College of Pharmacy, and co-editors of the *United States Dispensatory*. After graduation in 1839, Long spent eighteen months "walking the hospitals" of New York, studying surgery, before buying Dr. Grant's practice and settling in the small Georgia town of Jefferson. After his first success, Dr. Long used ether whenever he could persuade surgical or obstetrical patients to permit it. He ran into opposition, prejudice, and rumor among country folk, however, and accumulated but few case histories. Busy with a large practice, he found no time to report his findings. It was not until he read of Morton's "Letheon" anesthetic in the *Medical Examiner* of December, 1846, that he was stimulated to write a communication for publication. Dr. Long was frequently interrupted in his writings, so that the manuscript lay unfinished until December, 1849, when the paper finally was published in the *Southern Medical and Surgical Journal*. By that time, Wells was a suicide, and Morton and Jackson were embroiled in their famous ether controversy. Crawford Long, his economic position suffering from the aftermath of the War between the States, carried on his practice, literally dying "in the harness" as he assisted a new life into the world, June 16, 1878. To the end, his most cherished treasure was evidence of his priority of use of ether for anesthesia.

Horace Wells, for a time a successful dentist in Hartford, Connecticut, was born at Hartford, Vermont, January 21, 1815. After studying dentistry in Boston, he entered practice in the Connecticut city in 1836. Ingenious and restless, he had several inventions to his credit. He had taught dentistry to several students, including William Morton, before witnessing his first laughing gas demonstration on the evening of December 10, 1844. The following day, Wells persuaded the lecturer, Dr. Gardner Q. Colton, to administer nitrous oxide to him, and induced a former dental student, Dr. John Mankey Riggs, to extract a molar. Upon regaining consciousness, he was elated to note that he had felt no pain. Wells then plunged into manufacture of nitrous oxide and administered it to fifteen patients with varying success. Full of enthusiasm, he hurried to Boston, and through efforts of another of his former dental students, Dr. Morton, secured permission to give a demonstration of painless tooth pulling before one of the classes of the famous surgeon, Dr. John Collins Warren, at the Harvard Medical School. On this occasion he failed to administer sufficient dosage of nitrous oxide: the patient cried out in pain and students jeered and called the demonstration "humbug." Wells retreated to Hartford, temporarily dropped his plans for promotion of laughing gas, and turned to selling his patented shower bath.

When, a year and a half later, Wells' former partner, Morton, successfully demonstrated use of ether for anesthesia, Wells sought to establish his claim to priority. As the Jackson-Morton battle became more heated, Wells enlisted support in his behalf in Congress, but this only added to the confusion of the issue. In New York, seeking support for use of nitrous oxide, Wells was arrested for an act suggesting derangement and committed suicide while in prison, January 24, 1848.

Though his motives might be questioned and considered anything but altruistic, William Thomas Green Morton brought the practical application of anesthesia to the attention of the world. Born on a farm near Charlton, Massachusetts, August 19, 1819, Morton early evinced a desire to study medicine, but economic circumstances led him, instead, to study dentistry, perhaps in Baltimore for a time, but not at Baltimore College of Dental Surgery, as is often claimed. In 1841, he became a student of Dr. Horace Wells; then, in 1843, he became Wells' partner for a year. Still yearning to become a physician, Morton enrolled as a medical student on March 20, 1844, under Dr. Charles T. Jackson, and in November of that same year, he enrolled in the Harvard Medical School. Morton continued to practice dentistry and established a factory for manufacture of false teeth. His method of fitting these required removal of all the "old fangs"—a none too pleasant procedure. Seeking a pain deadener as a means of popularizing his treatment with patients, Morton tried many things: champagne, laudanum, opium, and, at the suggestion of Dr. Jackson, sulfuric ether. Many of his early experiments were carried out on animals.

Having secured the ear of one of his medical instructors, Dr. Warren, Morton paved the way for Horace Wells' demonstration of nitrous oxide at the Harvard Medical School. Though Wells failed, his unsuccessful attempt fired Morton's imagination. Morton began experimenting in secret, testing ether on goldfish, on a dog, on two dental assistants, and on himself. His results were not uniform, and again he consulted Dr. Jackson. Jackson suggested that he use highly purified ether, so Morton experimented further, and his results were much better. On September 30, 1846, employing an ether-saturated handkerchief held over the face, Morton anesthetized Eben H. Frost, and extracted a molar successfully without pain. Morton now was in a frenzy of excitement and enthusiasm. His motives were not altruistic, as had been those of Horace Wells. Morton envisioned a fortune from anesthesia. Morton again approached the elderly and highly reputed surgeon, Warren, who had once experimented with mesmerism, and who had used ether in treatment for pulmonary conditions. Upon receiving word that Dr. Warren would permit his experiment, Morton hastily designed an apparatus for administering the anesthetic and sought to disguise the identity of ether with color and aromatics, giving it the name, "Letheon."

It was on the morning of October 16, 1846, that Gilbert Abbott, suffering from a tumor of the jaw, was prepared for operation in the amphitheatre of Boston's Massachusetts General Hospital. Present besides Dr. Warren were Drs. Charles F. Heywood (house surgeon), Henry J. Bigelow, Augustus A. Gould, Solomon D. Townsend, and other prominent surgeons. Morton, readying his apparatus, was late, arriving just as Dr. Warren was about to proceed. Morton saturated a sponge in the globular glass inhaler with his disguised ether preparation, spoke calmly to the patient, put the mouthpiece to his lips, and instructed him to breathe carefully in and out of the globe. Abbott at first flushed and moved spasmodically, then sank into unconsciousness. Morton turned to Dr. Warren and said: "Sir, your patient is ready."

Dr. Warren proceeded with the rather complicated task of removing the tumor, and closed the wound. The patient had only moved his legs a bit and made a few incoherent sounds. Upon emerging from the effects of the anesthetic, Morton questioned him. Abbott said he had felt no pain, only a scratching sensation. Dr. Warren is reported to have turned to his colleagues and students and said: "Gentlemen, this is no humbug."

Morton immediately applied for a patent for his discovery. Meantime, on November 7, he administered ether for the first major operation under anesthesia—amputation at thigh level performed by Dr. Hayward at Massachusetts General Hospital.

On November 12, Patent No. 4848 was issued to Charles T. Jackson and William T. G. Morton for a "new and useful improvement in surgical operations."

On November 18, there appeared an article in the *Boston Medical and Surgical Journal*, by Dr. Henry J. Bigelow. The paper had been read, November 9, before the Boston Society of Medical Improvement. In it he described the successful use of Morton's procedure. This was the article that introduced the practice of anesthesia to medical men throughout the world.

Shortly thereafter, surgeons of Massachusetts General Hospital barred Morton and declined to use his preparation "until informed what it is." Morton promptly backed away from his position of secrecy and admitted that the agent which brought about anesthesia was "sulfuric ether." From then on, there was no further opposition in the hospital to performance of operations on patients under etherization.

The medical profession, once informed, was quick to adopt the use of ether anesthesia. In Europe there was more ready acceptance of ether anesthesia than in the United States. The first successful surgical operation under anesthesia in the Old World was performed by Dr. Robert Liston, December 21, 1846, at University College Hospital of London. One observer of Liston's amputation of a patient's infected leg through the thigh that day was a young Quaker, Joseph Lister. As Flexner noted, had anesthesia not been discovered, surgical antisepsis, as developed twenty years later by Lister, could not have been achieved.

Though the medical profession generally accepted the principle of surgical anesthesia, its early course was not smooth. In December, 1846, the *Philadelphia Medical Examiner* denounced it as quackery. Both clergymen and laymen denounced it as against God and nature. Especially was there opposition to use of ether to relieve the pain of childbirth. Meantime, too, Morton was having his troubles. He had a patent, but he could not protect it. Very soon, too, it was found that ether, administered from a saturated sponge or towel, was as effective as when Morton's complicated apparatus was used. On December 9, 1846, Horace Wells published in the Hartford *Courant*, his claim as discoverer of surgical anesthesia. Dr. Jackson, who had shown little interest in Morton's work until Morton began to receive credit in the press as discoverer of anesthesia, then first advanced his claim of having suggested use of pure ether. Morton acknowledged his indebtedness to Dr. Jackson, included his name in the patent application, and made an arrangement to share with him profits expected from licensing. But, as the world became interested in anesthesia, Jackson became more selfish and more assertive. He claimed full credit, saying Morton merely was his agent. There was shadowy precedent for Jackson's actions: he had tried to take credit from Samuel F. B. Morse for invention of the telegraph; and, again, he had tried to take for himself credit due Dr. William Beaumont for his studies of gastric function made with the cooperation of Alexis St. Martin, young French-Canadian with a "window" in his stomach left by a shotgun accident.

In 1847, Morton's friends, realizing he faced financial difficulties, advised him to appeal to Congress for compensation. A petition was signed by leading Boston physicians, and filed with Congress. A representative from Connecticut objected, citing Wells' claim. The Connecticut legislature passed a resolution giving Wells credit for discovery of anesthesia. Jackson, meantime, pressed his claims in Paris with the French Academy of Sciences.

In 1847, too, Dr. James Young Simpson of Edinburgh, Scotland, began using ether in his obstetrical practice. Finding ether to have some disagreeable qualities, such as odor and tendency to irritate bronchi, Simpson searched for replacements. He tried, on himself and on his associates, such drugs as "chloride of carbon, acetone, nitric ether, benzine, vapor of iodoform, and chloroform." He found chloroform (Guthrie's "sweet whiskey") most suitable, and campaigned vigorously for its use in obstetrics and in surgery. Scottish clergymen objected to use of chloroform in women in childbirth, contending that labor was pain to be endured with patience and fortitude. This controversy was quieted only by the acceptance of chloroform by Queen Victoria during the birth of her eighth child. For a time, chloroform found considerable favor, due to its less unpleasant odor and because lower dosage was required for anesthesia; but, as use proved it to be more dangerous, ether again rose to first choice as a general anesthetic.

First to manufacture chloroform in Canada was Pharmacist J. D. B. Fraser, of Pictou, Nova Scotia, who supplied it to doctors less than four months after Simpson's first report. First Canadian physician to use chloroform in surgery was Dr. W. J. Almon of Halifax, who employed it in February, 1848. On March 22, 1848, Pharmacist Fraser supplied chloroform used during the birth of his son, Robert.

Morton's and Jackson's claims and counterclaims continued before the United States Congress, and abroad. Wells' proponents fought for his claim even after his death. Also, in 1849, Crawford Long first published his claim to priority based on having used ether in March, 1842. The French Academy, unable to reach another decision, split the *Prix Montyon* equally between Jackson and Morton.

The ether controversy continued through the period of the War between the States. United States government agencies used ether freely, ignoring Morton's patent. Crawford Long continued to present his evidences of claim. Morton's misfortunes left him in poverty. Jackson continued to publish pamphlets, making more and more extravagant claims. To one of these, written by a supposed friend, is attributed the rage followed by apoplexy that ended Morton's life in New York, July 15, 1868. Jackson was to spend the last seven years of his life in the McLean Asylum, a department within Massachusetts General Hospital, where he died, August 28, 1880.

While the world generally ignored the contenders for fame of anesthesia's discovery, progress in extending application of the principle of anesthesia, and search for newer anesthetic agents, went forward rapidly. Dr. John Snow of London was the first physician to specialize in anesthesiology. He perfected improved methods of administration of anesthetics. Benjamin Ward Richardson, another Londoner, introduced the first successful local anesthesia in the form of an ether spray, in 1867, which held its favor until the introduction of cocaine, in 1884. Dr. Isaac E. Taylor and James A. Washington of New York had begun the practice of hypodermic medicine in 1839, forcing morphine solution under the skin. Dr. Alexander Wood, of Edinburgh, devised a metallic hollow needle in 1853, and in the same year, Charles Gabriel Pravaz attached an improved hollow needle to a specially constructed syringe —now commonly referred to as a "hypodermic syringe." W. W. Greene of the United States and Claude Bernard of France in 1868 and 1869 recommended hypodermic use of morphine during inhalation anesthesia.

The alkaloid cocaine was isolated from Peruvian coca leaves in 1860 by Albert Hiemann of Germany, who also named it. Its anesthetic properties were not fully appreciated until 1873, when they were demonstrated by Alexander Bennett. In 1884, Carl Koller, house surgeon at the Allgemeines Krankenhaus (General Hospital) in Vienna, in collaboration with Sigmund Freud, studied cocaine, first as a possible agent for curing patients addicted to morphine. Freud soon turned to other interests, but Koller developed and reported the advantages of cocaine as a local anesthetic for use in eye operations. Since, research has made possible progress in anesthesia until today when there is hardly a situation for which there is not an effective anesthetic. Yet, as Keys wrote, "anesthesia remains primarily an empirical development. Our ignorance of pain is still appalling." And Robinson, pointing to the responsibility of the anesthesiologist, commented: "Since every case of anesthesia brings the patient to the gates of death, anesthesia remains the most dangerous specialty in medicine. Eternal vigilance is the price of safety in anesthesia."

To whom should final credit go? A dozen decades have not brought the answer. Long unquestionably was first to employ anesthesia in patients undergoing surgical operations; but as Robinson pointed out, "Long's first use of ether was of importance to no one except the four or five patients upon whom he used it, and for four years ether remained unknown and unavailable to the world whose pain it might have eased." Of Wells, Keys wrote: "Although Wells had failed to convince the world of the value of nitrous oxide as an anesthetic agent, he is credited with conceiving the idea of anesthesia and of publicizing the possibility of its use." Jackson, the twisted genius that sought credit for other men's ideas, no longer has proponents. Cartwright summed up the question by commenting: "By means of ether (Morton) brought about the revolution in medicine which the pneumatic physicians had looked for in vain;" and, "Of one thing there is no possible doubt: the general acceptance of anesthesia dates from Morton's successful demonstration of October 16, 1846 . . . Within a year, hardly an operation was performed throughout the civilized world without the use of ether . . ."

To Long, Wells, Morton, Simpson, and to a host of others, the world owes a great debt of gratitude. Dr. Oliver Wendell Holmes gave appropriate recognition in behalf of all mankind when he wrote: "By this priceless gift to humanity, the fierce extremity of suffering has been steeped in the waters of forgetfulness, and the deepest furrow in the knotted brow of agony has been smoothed forever."

SEMMELWEIS
DEFENDER OF MOTHERHOOD

PREGNANT WOMEN among the poor in Vienna in the 1840's feared the great lying-in wards of Vienna's General Hospital, the Allgemeines Krankenhaus. This was a charity institution, and among its rules was: in return for privileges of obstetric treatment and care of her child, the expectant mother must agree to allow herself to be used for instruction of medical students and of midwives during her labor and convalescence. But women's dread stemmed not so much from lack of privacy and modesty as from the black cloud of death that seemed to hang over the hospital—especially over the First Obstetric Clinic. No published statistics were needed for people living in the crowded streets of Austria's capital city to know that, as women in pregnancy approached term and entered the great stone hospital, there was a one-in-ten chance—sometimes one-in-five—that they might never return home alive. Childbed fever, scourge of motherhood, decimated the wards with frightful regularity, sometimes rapidly striking down all mothers in rows of a dozen beds. Often, women sought to avoid the hospital until their babies were born; other women, upon admission to the hospital, begged to be assigned to the Second Obstetric Clinic, wherein, for some unknown reason, chances for survival were much greater. In Vienna's great hospital, as in most institutions throughout Europe of that day, women in labor indeed passed through "the valley of the shadow of death." In all too many instances, newborn infants, too, suffered and died of an ailment exhibiting at necropsy pathologic changes identical with those which took the lives of their mothers.

It was in this First Obstetric Clinic that a young physician named Semmelweis began his life's work. It was to be a short career, loaded with work, brilliant in deductions and results therefrom, but fraught with frustrations, opposition, and heartache. Sinclair, a biographer, wrote: "In the whole history of medicine there is only one Semmelweis in the magnitude of his services to mankind, and in the depth of his

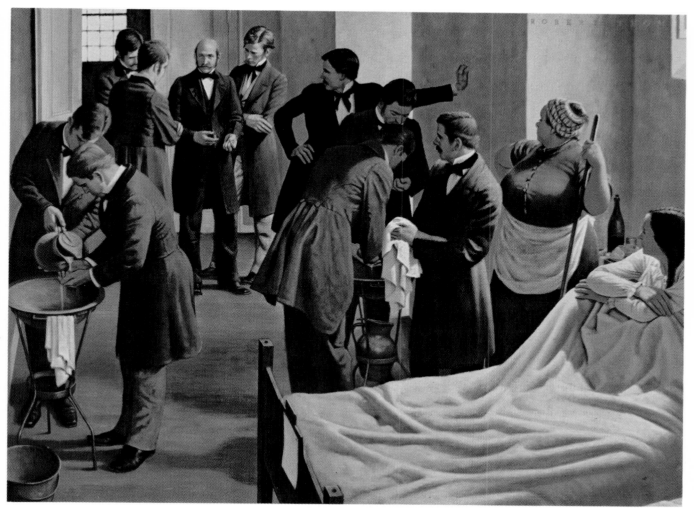

SEMMELWEIS: DEFENDER OF MOTHERHOOD

Hungarian physician Ignaz Philipp Semmelweis (1818-1865), while Assistant at the First Obstetric Clinic of Vienna's great Allgemeines Krankenhaus in 1847, discovered means of preventing puerperal fever: he insisted that physicians and medical students wash their hands in chlorinated solution before entering obstetric wards and again before examining each patient. His rule was much resented and opposed—but hundreds of mothers' lives were saved. Though his doctrine was proved repeatedly, in hospitals in Vienna and in Budapest, most of his contemporaries opposed it; and, both depressed from worry and broken-hearted from disappointment, Semmelweis died at age 47, of blood poisoning, the infection he had fought so valiantly to prevent in mothers under his care.

sufferings from contemporary jealous stupidity and ingratitude." Semmelweis found a way to save new mothers' lives, but try though he would, most of his contemporaries and not a few of his students scoffed at his ideas and mocked his methods. Worse, his superiors deliberately humiliated him and blocked his reforms. Yet he sought but to save lives, to relieve suffering, to preserve children. Analyzing Semmelweis' difficulties, Sinclair stated: "He never learned how to bow down before authorities, like so many of the unfortunate young pedants whom he had to encounter as antagonists in after years."

Ignaz Philipp Semmelweis was born July 1, 1818, in Buda, "only separated by the Danube from Pest, most populous and flourishing of all the Hungarian towns." He was fourth of seven children of a merchant. His early life seems to have been happy, but due to somewhat faulty preliminary bilingual education, he was always to have difficulty with speaking and with writing. While this was to prove a handicap in later years in conveyance of his ideas to the world of medicine, his mind was left clear to accept only what was to be seen, to discard dogmatic theories, and to reach logical deductions from experience and from independent judgment.

After beginning his medical education at the University of Pest, Semmelweis went to Vienna, capital of the Austrian empire, and in the autumn of 1837, at age 19 years, enrolled as a student of law at the University of Vienna. Shortly he discovered his true interests, and switched to the study of medicine. He returned to the University of Pest for two years, then completed his undergraduate work, receiving his doctorate in medicine from the University of Vienna, April 21, 1844. Semmelweis then took special courses in obstetrics, receiving the degree of Master of Midwifery, August 1, 1844. Previously, he had registered with the Director of the Clinic, Klein, at the Lying-in Hospital as aspirant for the post of Assistant, when a vacancy should occur. He did not receive this appointment until nearly two years later, but, as aspirant, he had access to the practice of the clinic without responsibilities of the office. During this time he became associated with leading young professors at the University—the clinician, Josef Skoda; the dermatologist, Ferdinand von Hebra; the pathologist, Carl von Rokitansky; and the professor of legal medicine, Jakob K. Kolletschka. From work in the laboratories of these men, Semmelweis learned far more about gynecology and obstetrics than he did from the stern and tedious Klein, strict adherent to past tradition who owed his position, not to professional excellence, but to political connections. In Rokitansky's autopsy room, Semmelweis studied bodies of women who died of gynecologic or obstetric disorders, laying the foundation for his superior knowledge in this field. November 30, 1845, Semmelweis passed examinations and received his doctorate in surgery.

On February 27, 1846, Semmelweis was appointed Assistant in the First Obstetric Clinic. In the great Allgemeines Krankenhaus of Vienna, the Lying-in Hospital was so large it was divided into First and Second Clinics. In the First Clinic, medical students were trained, and there they routinely examined patients; in the Second Clinic, only midwives were trained.

Well prepared for administrative and teaching responsibilities by two years' experience as aspirant, kindly and sensitive Semmelweis was deeply concerned and depressed by the high mortality from puerperal fever which devastated patients in wards of the First Clinic. In one year (1846), 459 of 4,010 women admitted to the First Clinic died. That was mortality of 11.4 per cent for the year; and in some months, deaths rose to 18 per cent. At the same time, in the Second Clinic, physically a duplicate of the First, where apparently the same conditions prevailed, except for differences in teaching midwives, only 105 of 3,754 women patients died—mortality of 2.7 per cent. Also, there were fewer deaths among women delivered at home; and even among those who, unable to reach the hospital in time, were delivered in the street. Despite unfavorable surroundings, a far higher proportion of these women, and their babies, survived than of their sisters under hospital conditions.

Semmelweis examined, again and again, traditional theories of the cause of puerperal fever—among them, seasonal influences, miasmas (poisonous air), fear, constipation, delayed lactation; but to his inquiring mind, none of these explained satisfactorily either the cause of the deadly fever, or why more women died in the First Clinic than in the Second and at home. There were no differences in patients, or in conditions, or in air, or in seasons, or in care; yet, consistently, there was a lower death rate in the Second Clinic. More and more of Semmelweis' time was spent in the necropsy room, in his search for reasons for these deaths. Always, he found the same pathologic changes, indicative of systemic "blood poisoning." Frequently, when mothers died following long and difficult labor, their babies died too—and the tiny bodies revealed pathologic changes similar to those found in their mothers. Day after day, however, professors and medical students alike habitually visited the necropsy rooms in the early mornings, proceeding directly therefrom to the obstetric clinic, and to routine examination of women in labor and in convalescence.

Semmelweis, not calloused to death's visitations, tried many measures: women's positions in labor were changed; foreign students were barred from the wards—but these measures had no effect and deaths continued to occur.

Semmelweis' activities evidently irritated Professor Klein, his superior. Suddenly, on October 20, 1846, Semmelweis was demoted, and his predecessor, Breit, was reappointed Assistant for two years. Depressed and discouraged by this humiliation, Semmelweis considered going to England or to Ireland. However, in February, 1847, Breit was appointed Professor of Midwifery at the University of Tübingen. On March 20, Semmelweis, restored to his position as Assistant, returned to the deeply disturbing and puzzling problem of deaths of so many mothers in his clinic. Semmelweis found no answer—until the sudden death of his friend, Kolletschka: a small scalpel wound, incurred during a necropsy, led to infection, fulminating into systemic blood poisoning, and to death. Necropsy performed upon Kolletschka's body revealed pathologic changes identical with those of women dying of puerperal fever. The truth came then to Semmelweis—Kolletschka died of poisons entering his body through the wound from the body of a patient who came to necropsy; Semmelweis and his students were routinely examining wounded genitalia of women patients with hands that came directly from examining bodies of patients coming to necropsy! Therefore, he, and his students, as well as hundreds of other teachers and students of obstetrics, were carrying "cadaveric poisoning" directly to their patients on their unwashed hands! Mothers sickened and died in rows because they were examined in rows! Death visited the Second Clinic less often because midwives did not attend necropsies; and they examined their patients far less frequently than did medical students.

Semmelweis checked the records. They seemed to bear out his theory. He decided to put his idea to practical test: every medical student and physician wishing to examine women in his wards was required to wash his hands—not merely in soap and water, but in chlorinated lime solution, thoroughly scrubbing with clean sand until odors of the dissecting room were removed. Only then might doctors and students examine patients.

As might be expected, such precautions were resented; protests were raised both by colleagues and by students unacquainted with reasons for such precautions (antisepsis was not to be understood for another two decades); but results were dramatic. While in April, 1847, 57 women, or 18 per cent of obstetric patients, died, the number fell, in June, 1847, after introduction of Semmelweis' procedure, to six deaths, or 2.38 per cent; and, in July, to three deaths, or 1.2 per cent.

Semmelweis felt that, at last, he had discovered the cause of puerperal fever: poison originating in cadaveric putrescence, carried to healthy patients by physicians and students themselves. Then, one week, the death count again shot up alarmingly. Of twelve women in a ward, eleven sickened and died, despite precautions. Shocked, the conscientious Assistant checked all factors and made another startling discovery: the woman patient first in line when students entered the ward had a foully discharging cancer of the uterus. Though his students had scrubbed their hands upon entering the ward, they had not done so between patients. Could it be that examiners might carry infection from live patients, as well as from cadavers, to well mothers? Semmelweis acted again: his students were required to wash in chlorine solution after *each* examination. Now, strenuous objections were raised, and these no doubt reached the ears of Director Klein—but again, the death count went down. An experience with a patient having an open wound further convinced Semmelweis that such infection could be air-borne from patient to patient. He then insisted on isolation of patients with such wounds, and further, on cleanliness of everything coming in contact with patients.

His University friends soon were convinced that Semmelweis had found the answer. They urged him to publish his findings and to speak before medical groups; but though he could be sternly positive in his teaching of students, Semmelweis refused to write, and was diffident about speaking. His medical associates, Hebra, Skoda, and others, wrote or spoke in his behalf, though, incredible as it seems, Semmelweis' fellow obstetricians failed to recognize his discovery. Instead of adopting his methods, they scorned and belittled him, and fought reforms he sought to effect. Among leaders of this opposition was his own director, Klein, who vented his resentment, March 20, 1849, by refusing to reappoint Semmelweis. As might be expected, practices in the Clinic, under his successor, reverted to Klein's methods, and again, hundreds of mothers admitted to the First Clinic died of puerperal fever.

Shocked and depressed by this poor reward for his life-saving efforts, Semmelweis tried for eight months to secure appointment as privat-dozent, or instructor, in obstetrics, only to receive, October 10, 1850, an appointment grudgingly given him, so limiting his activities as to be absurd. Without even saying good-bye to his friends, Semmelweis, five days later, fled Vienna and returned to Budapest.

His home town was none too good a place for the young physician to begin again—Hungary was suffering the consequences of defeat of the 1848 revolt against Austrian rule. However, May 20, 1851, Semmelweis received appointment as honorary senior physician, without pay, in the obstetric division of St. Rokus Hospital in Pest. Conditions were deplorable, but he began at once to put his doctrine into effect—and again, deaths from puerperal fever declined.

Despite the fact that Semmelweis' amply proved ideas were unacceptable to his Viennese colleagues, publications and letters written by his friends and students began to find acceptance elsewhere, notably in England, in Scotland, and in Ireland, where obstetricians had been conditioned to habits of cleanliness by the work of Burton, White, and Gordon, a half century before. In Hungary, Semmelweis was allowed to go on with his life-saving procedures—not, however, without occasional stubborn resistance. He was appointed Professor of Theoretical and Practical Midwifery at the University of Pest in July, 1855. The obstetric wards there were miserable and inadequate—but, despite this, Semmelweis' procedures again reduced the death toll markedly.

By this time, concern for the death of so many young mothers because obstetricians would not embrace his doctrine, preyed on Semmelweis' mind. His personality was changing. Described a few years earlier in Vienna as "of more than medium height, broad and strongly built, with round face, prominent cheek bones, high forehead and thin hair, fleshy and dextrous hands," Semmelweis in Budapest was becoming eccentric and less thoughtful of other persons, and had the appearance of an old man.

Two events changed Semmelweis' life for a time, and he was happier. Now 38 years of age, he married, June 11, 1857, 18-year-old Marie Weidenhofer; and in the same year, his friend, Markusovszky, editor of *Orvosi Hetilap*, a weekly medical journal, invited him to write. In the fall of 1857, Semmelweis at long last was persuaded, perhaps goaded by the many attacks on him, to put his doctrines and proofs into written form. In 1861, his great volume came off the press, entitled: *Die Aetiologie, der Begriff und die Prophylaxis des Kindbettfiebers* (The Cause, Concept, and Prophylaxis of Childbed Fever). This book, in spite of its being somewhat disorganized and difficult to follow, is one of the most moving, best documented, and closely reasoned books in the history of medical publications. In it, Semmelweis refuted old and silly theories regarding puerperal fever and backed his doctrine with innumerable statistics. However, if Semmelweis hoped that his book would convince his adversaries, he was sorely disappointed. Stubborn resistance continued; and mothers continued to die in obstetric clinics of the world. Semmelweis grew more impatient, excited, and violent. Added to his other perturbations, death of his first two children further depressed him. In 1862-1863, he published a series of open letters in which he accused leading obstetricians of bad faith and of murder. His friends sought to get his mind into other channels by urging him to turn to gynecologic practice—and, because he applied his ideas of antisepsis to surgical as well as obstetric patients, his practice was eminently successful. But the cries of dying mothers haunted his dreams. Colleagues whom he attacked, in return attacked him. The strain became too much. In July, 1865, Semmelweis showed signs of serious mental derangement. His wife and friends placed him in a sanatorium in Vienna, where he became even more violent. But, ironically, it was not insanity that was to defeat him. On August 13, 1865, at the age of 47, Semmelweis died of blood poisoning, the very infection he had fought so valiantly to protect parturient women from contracting. Deadly bacteria gained admission to his body through a small finger wound received during one of his last operations. Ironically too, just the day before Semmelweis died, Joseph Lister of Glasgow, acting on conclusions he had reached on reading certain publications of Louis Pasteur of Paris, for the first time used carbolic acid in treating wounds of a patient with compound fracture.

In retrospect, it appears that Dr. Semmelweis was his own worst enemy, in failing to publicize his findings earlier, in antagonizing those whom he might have convinced, and in snubbing his friends. However, Semmelweis' doctrine was about twenty years ahead of the medical world's thinking: Pasteur was to demonstrate that germs caused infection, multiplied, and spread from victim to victim, rather than generating spontaneously within the body. Further, Pasteur was to disclose the identity of the specific bacterium that caused puerperal fever. Lister's experience with surgical antisepsis was to confirm the principles Semmelweis applied to obstetric patients. Within a few years, physicians who had opposed him were to reverse themselves to declare that Semmelweis had been right. Though Oliver Wendell Holmes, of Boston, in 1843, had published a purely theoretical treatise "On the Contagiousness of Childbed Fever," he did not zealously campaign for reform, as did the Hungarian obstetrician.

Ignaz Philipp Semmelweis died at the dawn of a new age in surgery and in obstetrics. Thanks to his work, and to that of other leaders in medicine during the third quarter of the nineteenth century, pregnant women entering hospitals were no longer virtually condemned to die of puerperal fever.

WORLD EVENTS AND MEDICAL HISTORY

Dates, persons, and events of significance to the evolution of Medicine include:

1899	Reed, Carroll, Lazear, and Agramonte demonstrated mosquito transmission of yellow fever.
1899	Charles Best born.
1899	Ramón y Cajal described histology of cerebral cortex.
1899	Weichselbaum and Jaeger isolated meningococcus.
1899	Grassi and Bignami proved that *Anopheles* is sole transmitter of malaria.
1899	H. Dreser introduced aspirin.
1899	Dewar liquefied air, oxygen, and hydrogen.
1899	Beijerinck isolated filterable virus of mosaic tobacco disease.
1899	Medical Library Association (United States) founded.
1899	Ehrlich's Institute for Experimental Medicine (Frankfurt) founded.
1899-1900	Reed completed demonstration of mosquito transmission of yellow fever.
1899-1900	Stenbeck treated cancer with Röntgen rays.
1900	Bier introduced spinal (cocaine) anesthesia into general surgery.
1900	Wertheim devised radical operation for uterine cancer.
1900	A. Walkhoff showed destructive effect of radium on the tissues.
1900	Willstätter and Bode produced synthetic cocaine.
1900	Park recommended control of milk (New York City) by bacterial tests.
1900	Woodhead disinfected water supply of Maidstone (England) with chlorine after typhoid epidemic.
1900	College of Physicians and Surgeons (Chicago) became College of Medicine, University of Illinois (May 1).
1900	Conference of Pharmaceutical Faculties founded. (Became American Association of Colleges of Pharmacy in 1925.)
1900-1903	Leishman and Donovan discovered protozoön of kala azar.
1901	De Vries stated mutation theory.
1901	Dutton and Ford discovered trypanosome of sleeping sickness (*Trypanosoma gambiense*).
1901	Aschkinazi and Caspari showed that radium checked the growth of bacteria.
1901	Landsteiner discovered blood-grouping (iso-agglutination).
1901	Emil Fischer devised ester method of isolating amino acids.
1901	Takamine isolated Adrenalin.
1901	Rockefeller Institute for Medical Research (New York) opened.
1901	German Society for History of Medicine and Science (Leipzig) founded.
1901	Award of Nobel prizes begun. First recipients included Röntgen and von Behring for their contributions on x-rays and on serum therapy for diphtheria.
1902	Carrel introduced new methods of vascular anastomosis and transplantation of tissues.
1902	Walter Reed died.
1902	Bayliss and Starling discovered secretin.
1902	R. Herzog discovered site of Asclepieion at Cos.
1902	Holzknecht devised method of dosimetry for x-rays.
1902	P. C. Hewitt perfected quartz mercury vapor lamp.
1902	McClung isolated sex chromosome.
1902	Ravenel isolated bovine tubercle bacillus from a tuberculous child.
1902	Schild introduced atoxyl.
1902	Steinbuchel introduced morphine-scopolamine anesthesia in obstetrics.
1902	Finney performed gastroduodenostomy.
1902	Carnegie Institution of Washington founded.
1902	Société Française d'Histoire de Médecine (Paris) founded.
1902	Nobel prize awarded to Ronald Ross for advancing knowledge on malaria.
1902-1903	Jensen propagated cancer through several generations of mice.
1902-1906	Bayliss and Starling investigated hormones.

FOUNDING OF THE
AMERICAN MEDICAL ASSOCIATION

GUILDS were the means by which medieval craftsmen bound themselves together for mutual protection and regulation. As centuries passed, many guilds faded away. Early in the nineteenth century came a resurgence of desire, especially among professional men, to band themselves together, for solution of mutual problems and to control or to eliminate from their midst quacks, pretenders, and charlatans. From this desire grew a number of great voluntary medical organizations or associations of national scope. Growing like vines, these associations not only sprang from roots in sectional and local organizations, but, gathering strength, sent out new shoots that mothered more local societies, uniting all into vigorous, progressive corporations.

One of the first of such organizations to be formed was the British Medical Association, founded July 19, 1832. The Pharmaceutical Society of Great Britain came into being in 1841. The American Medical Association followed, in 1847; the American Pharmaceutical Association was organized in 1852; and the German Aerzteverein in 1872. Preceding all of these was the organization of the United States Pharmacopoeial Convention in 1820, a movement toward establishment of standards for medicines at first undertaken entirely by medical men.

Medical activity on the North American continent was first recorded in the sixteenth century. The first medical book in the New World was printed by Spaniards in Mexico in 1570. The first medical school was founded in Mexico in 1578. A small medical society was formed in Boston in 1735, and one in New York in 1749. Others followed in Philadelphia and in New Haven. First medical periodical to be published in the United States was the *Medical Repository*, issued in 1797.

Prior to 1800, there were several good medical schools in the United States, among them, that of King's College, New York, founded in 1764, which in 1791 became the Medical Faculty of Columbia University; that of The University of Pennsylvania, which claims to have

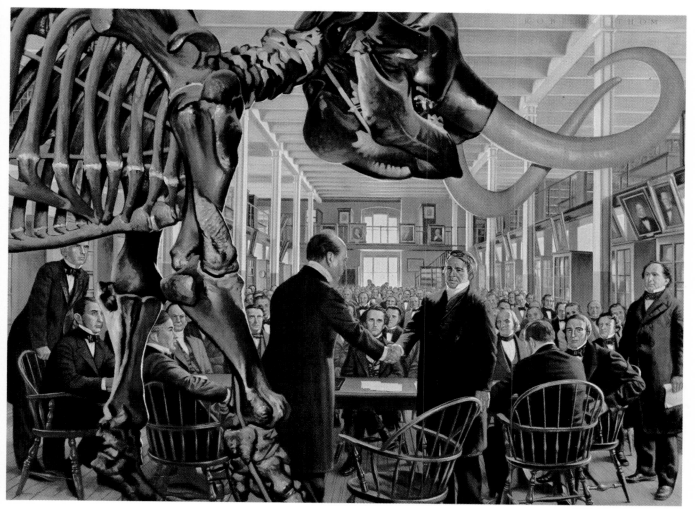

FOUNDING OF THE AMERICAN MEDICAL ASSOCIATION

Advancement of medical knowledge, improved medical education, launching of a program of medical ethics, and furtherance of public service—these were aims of The American Medical Association, organized May 7, 1847, by 250 delegates seated among exhibit cases and before ancient bones of a mastodon, Mammut americanum, *in the hall of The Academy of Natural Sciences of Philadelphia, Pennsylvania. Chairman Jonathan Knight welcomed Dr. Nathaniel Chapman, first president, and officers (foreground) as they launched what became one of the world's larger and greater medical bodies, now in its second century of service both to the public and to the profession.*

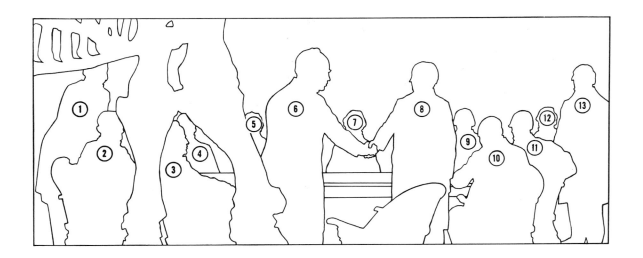

Identity of portraits in the picture,

FOUNDING OF THE AMERICAN MEDICAL ASSOCIATION

Officers and committeemen present at the time of organization of the AMA included:

1. Dr. A. H. Buchanan, Tennessee, a vice president.

2. Dr. Alexander H. Stevens, New York, a vice president; second president of the AMA.

3. Dr. J. R. W. Dunbar, Maryland, a secretary.

4. Dr. Thomas Cock, New York, committeeman.

5. Dr. John Watson, New York, chairman of the committee for organizing a permanent national organization.

6. Dr. Jonathan Knight, Connecticut, temporary chairman of the organizational meeting; a vice president of the new organization; and the AMA's seventh president.

7. Dr. Nathan Smith Davis, New York, committeeman credited with having been the "father" of the AMA; sixteenth president of the AMA; and first editor of the AMA *Journal.*

8. Dr. Nathaniel Chapman, Pennsylvania, first president of the AMA.

9. Dr. J. R. Manley, New York, committeeman.

10. Dr. Alfred Stillé, Pennsylvania, a secretary; twenty-third president of the AMA.

11. Dr. Isaac Hays, Pennsylvania, treasurer.

12. Dr. George B. Wood, Pennsylvania, ninth president of the AMA.

13. Dr. James Moultrie, South Carolina, a vice president; fifth president of the AMA.

stemmed from the College of Philadelphia, to which a medical faculty was appointed in 1765; the faculty established at Harvard University in 1783; and the Medical School of Dartmouth College, opened in 1798. Medical schools rapidly increased in number, if not in quality, in the early 1800's.

The first half of the nineteenth century was fertile insofar as medicine was concerned. Within it came acceptance of vaccination for small-pox; introduction of the stethoscope; writing of Percival's "Code of Medical Ethics"; the first ovariotomy performed by McDowell; Beaumont's experiments with gastric secretions; Holmes' essay on puerpural fever, and the work of Semmelweis in Vienna; Virchow had begun the study of cellular pathology; Helmholtz, study of the senses; and Claude Bernard was beginning to write significant essays on physiology. The greatest contribution to the advance of medical science during these fifty years was, of course, the discovery of anesthesia. Formation of strong national medical societies was to be of great significance, too; but their effect was to be demonstrated more fully within the century that followed.

While tradition and experience had developed disciplines among practitioners of medicine in the Old World, no such controls were in effect in the mushrooming communities of North America. New nations were being carved out of the wilderness; and among those men who were doing the carving were many freethinking nonconformists—rebels against older disciplines. As the Colonies rounded out their first century and new generations of pioneers carried on, few aspirants to medical careers could afford to return to Europe for education; tutoring by preceptors was the rule—but there were no laws to prevent anyone with sufficient audacity from calling himself "Doctor" and from practicing his own particular style of medicine. There developed, about the time the new nation, known as the United States of America, was created, a situation in medicine that became increasingly unsatisfactory: preceptorial training was being abandoned in favor of short courses in medical schools operated for private gain. The quality of many of these schools deteriorated as competition for students—and for their fees—became more intense. In addition to evils arising from lack of educational standards, licensure of practitioners was controlled by the very schools that produced them. Thus it became increasingly apparent to wiser and more sincere medical men of the time that some drastic action would be necessary to curb evils existing in medical education and licensure, and to restore to New World medicine dignity that would deserve public respect.

Organization of The American Medical Association was neither a spontaneous development nor the result of a moment of inspiration. According to Fishbein, "birth of the Association followed travail of many months; the pains, the jealousies, and the love associated with its conception forecast the great career to be achieved by this extraordinary progeny." It exemplified, too, courage and determination of medical men in a new world, without benefit of traditional institutions and backgrounds, to raise themselves to standards in keeping with highest professional ideals.

Rivalry among medical schools, resulting in reduced curricula and other short cuts, provided the irritant that stimulated practicing physicians of the early nineteenth century to associated action. The Faculty of the Medical College of Georgia proposed, in 1835, a convention of delegates from medical schools; but other schools of the Atlantic seaboard opposed the plan. First move toward a national medical convention was a resolution passed by the Medical Society of the State of New York, in February, 1839. However, due to lack of interest, nothing came of it. In 1844, in resolutions presented to the New York Society, Drs. Alexander Chapman and N. S. Davis attacked abuses in medical education and urged separation of licensing powers from teaching institutions. Referred to committee, these resolutions were subjected to further discussion and controversial debate at the 1845 convention of the Society. When, as the convention neared its close, it appeared that the subject of reform of medical education would be put over for still another year, Dr. Davis of Binghamton, at the urging of Dr. Alden Marsh of Albany, introduced a resolution calling for a national convention of delegates from medical societies and colleges "in the whole Union," to be held in New York City in 1846. The enthusiasm of young Dr. Davis prevailed over opposition; the resolution passed; and Drs. Davis, James McNaughton, and Peter Van Buren, were named to the committee to activate the plan.

Dr. Davis then channeled his enthusiasm into a promotional program that rivals today's best techniques. By February, 1846, medical societies and colleges of medicine, with the exception of colleges in Boston and in Philadelphia, had responded favorably. The meeting date was set for May, 1846, in the hall of the Medical Department of the University of New York. This progress was not accomplished, however, without strong opposition, stemming mainly from jealousies among medical schools. Ironically, an address severely criticizing the New York State Medical Society and referring to the proposed convention as political play, was made by Professor Martyn Paine, of the faculty of the host college. Widely published, this address had one unexpected result: it turned Philadelphians from opposition to support of the convention.

The meeting in New York convened May 5, 1846, with 80 delegates present, representing sixteen states. Dr. Edward Delafield of New York was in the chair, and Dr. William P. Buel served as secretary. A nominating committee of one delegate from each state was appointed, and, following its report, officers for the meeting were elected: president was Dr. Jonathan Knight of Connecticut; vice presidents were Dr. John Bell of Pennyslvania, and Dr. Delafield; and secretaries, Dr. Richard D. Arnold of Georgia and Dr. Alfred Stillé of Pennsylvania.

Then followed a most extraordinary move: Dr. Gunning S. Bedford, a colleague of Dr. Paine and a delegate from the host university, introduced a resolution asserting that, since the assemblage was representative of fewer than half the states and of less than a majority of the medical colleges, adjournment was in order. After a moment of stunned silence, delegates rejected the resolution by a vote of 74 to 2. The convention then settled down to work. A committee of nine, headed by Dr. Davis, was instructed to bring in recommendations regarding medical education. Reporting for the committee the following day, Dr. Davis presented four proposals:

"First. That it is expedient for the medical profession of the United States to institute a *National Medical Association*.

"Secondly. That it is desirable that a uniform and elevated standard of requirement for the degree of M.D., should be adopted by all the medical schools in the United States.

"Thirdly. That it is desirable that young men, before being received as students of medicine, should have acquired a suitable preliminary education.

"Fourthly. That it is expedient that the medical profession in the United States be governed by the same code of medical ethics."

These proposals were accompanied by a recommendation that a committee of seven be appointed to study each proposal, and to report at a meeting to be held in Philadelphia, the first Wednesday in May, 1847. Following adoption of these propositions, Dr. Davis introduced a resolution calling for separation of licensing functions from teaching institutions. Though highly controversial, Dr. Davis was able to have this proposal referred to committee. Dr. John H. Griscom requested a committee, also to report the next year, on registration of births, marriages, and deaths. The convention adjourned the evening of May 6.

The American Medical Association came into being at the convention in Philadelphia in 1847. Some 250 delegates, representing 40 medical societies and 28 colleges, and coming from 22 states and the District of Columbia, gathered in the hall of The Academy of Natural Sciences of Philadelphia, May 5, 1847. They were welcomed by Dr. Isaac Hays, chairman of the committee on arrangements. Dr. Knight was named temporary chairman. Members were named to a credentials committee and to a nominating committee. Permanent officers elected for the convention were: president, Dr. Jonathan Knight of Connecticut; vice presidents, Dr. Alexander H. Stevens of New York, Dr. George B. Wood of Pennsylvania, Dr. A. H. Buchanan of Tennessee, and Dr. John Harrison of Louisiana; and secretaries, Dr. R. D. Arnold of Georgia, Dr. Alfred Stillé of Pennsylvania, and F. Campbell Stewart of New York.

Several committee reports were disposed of and the group reaffirmed its stand on licensure. In addition, a controversial resolution, concerning requirements for preliminary education, was discussed and acted upon. These principles were to be reaffirmed, repeatedly, though many years were to pass before their aims were fully achieved.

Most important of the subjects to come before this assemblage was the report of the committee on a plan for organizing a permanent national association. The committee brought in a proposed constitution, embodying, as the basis of organization, the principle of representation. Active members of the Association were to be delegates from medical societies and medical degree-granting institutions, in accordance with a fixed numerical ratio. Purposes of the organization, set forth in the Preamble, were:

". . . for cultivating and advancing medical knowledge; for elevating the standard of medical education; for promoting the usefulness, honor, and interests of the medical profession; for enlightening and directing public opinion in regard to the duties, responsibilities, and requirements of medical men; for exciting and encouraging emulation and concert of action in the profession; and for facilitating and fostering friendly intercourse between those engaged in it."

Encouragement of formation of state and local medical associations was to be one of the organization's primary aims, and delegate membership was shaped to this end. Committees were to be established to study problems related to medical sciences, practical medicine, surgery, obstetrics, medical education, medical literature, and publications.

After considerable discussion, the proposed Constitution was adopted, May 7, 1847. The convention then resolved itself into The American Medical Association. Officers elected for the Association's first year were: president, Dr. Nathaniel Chapman of Pennsylvania; vice presidents, Drs. Jonathan Knight of Connecticut, Alexander H. Stevens of New York, James Moultrie of South Carolina, and A. H. Buchanan of Tennessee; secretaries, Drs. Alfred Stillé of Pennsylvania, and J. R. W. Dunbar of Maryland; and treasurer, Dr. Isaac Hays of Pennsylvania.

From this organizational meeting stemmed three further resolutions that helped shape the course of the Association for more than a century: one was aimed at abolition of quackery and nostrums; another, at prevention of sectional domination—no two consecutive annual meetings were to be held in the same city; and the third laid groundwork for development of the Association's Principles of Medical Ethics. The group then selected Baltimore as the city in which the 1848 meeting would be held on the first Tuesday in May.

Significant of the importance of The American Medical Association, both to the profession in this new and growing country and to its relationships with physicians of other lands, were remarks made by the

Association's second president, Dr. Alexander H. Stevens of New York, at the close of the 1848 meeting held in Baltimore:

"Our Association stands forth without a parallel in its high purposes, and its means of accomplishing them. May it prove an exemplar of similar organizations in our sister republics of the Western Hemisphere, and exhibit in a new form to our brethren in Europe, the easy adaptation of our institutions to the great end of promoting the happiness of mankind."

The man who most deserves the title of architect and founder of The American Medical Association was Nathan Smith Davis. Not only was Dr. Davis responsible in large measure for bringing about organization of the Association; he devoted a half century of his lifetime to the Association's development and to bringing to fruition the sound principles embodied in its objectives.

Dr. Davis was born in a log cabin in Chenango County, New York, January 9, 1817. Offered choice between a farm career and a term of higher education, the young man at age 16 years began attendance at Cazenovia Seminary and study of medicine under Dr. Daniel Clark. Later he continued his studies under Dr. Thomas Jackson of Binghamton, and attended three courses of lectures at the Medical College of Western New York. At 20 years of age, in 1837, he began practice in Vienna, New York, moving to Binghamton five months later. Joining the Broome County Medical Society that same year was his first step into organizational work. During the next ten years he wrote articles for various medical journals, taught medical students, and helped found Binghamton Academy. He was seated as Broome County delegate to the New York State Medical Society in 1844. His interest and activity in the state organization led to his role in formation of The American Medical Association.

In the spring of 1847, Dr. Davis moved to New York City, where, in addition to his practice, he became instructor in anatomy at the College of Physicians and Surgeons, gave lectures on medical jurisprudence, and became editor of a semimonthly medical journal, *The Annalist*.

In the summer of 1849, Dr. Davis accepted the chair of Physiology and Pathology at Rush Medical College in Chicago. Soon he was editing the *Northwestern Medical and Surgical Journal*, writing *History of the Medical Profession, from the first Settlement of the British Colonies in America to the year 1850*, and, *History of The American Medical Association from its Organization up to January, 1855*. He advocated many reforms in preliminary educational requirements and in the curriculum at Rush; but, in 1858, when these were vetoed by the Dean, Dr. Davis resigned from that faculty, joining several of his supporters to found the Medical Department of Lind College. This institution became Chicago Medical College in 1862, and Northwestern University Medical School in 1892.

Dr. Davis attended 47 of the first 50 annual meetings of The American Medical Association and was ever active in promotion of progressive projects. He served as the Association's president both at the 1864 and at the 1865 meetings. In 1882, at the age of 65 years, Dr. Davis became the first editor of *The Journal of The American Medical Association*, a position he held until 1888.

Dr. Davis' sons, Frank Howard Davis, and Nathan Smith Davis, Jr., both followed him into practice of medicine, as did two of his grandsons, John Davis Kales, and Nathan Smith Davis III. The "old doctor" was to help celebrate the fiftieth anniversary of the Association, and also of the Chicago Medical Society and of the Illinois State Medical Society, both of which he helped organize. On June 4, 1904, after walking home from a busy day at the office, Dr. Davis suffered a heart attack. The "old doctor," well past his eighty-seventh birthday, grew increasingly weaker, and died, June 16, 1904.

The weekly periodical, *The Journal of The American Medical Association*, under the editorship of Dr. Davis, first appeared in 1883. *The Journal* grew to become one of the largest and most influential publications of its kind in the world, ranking beside the *British Medical Journal* and the *Deutsche Medizinische Wochenschrift*. In 1889, English-born Dr. George H. Simmons became its second editor. For many years, Dr. Simmons also was business manager of the Association. In 1924, he was succeeded by Dr. Morris Fishbein, an able and brilliant medical journalist who had joined the staff as assistant editor in 1913. In 1949, Dr. Austin Smith, formerly Secretary of the AMA Council on Pharmacy and Chemistry, took over the editorial helm, continuing until January 1, 1959, when he resigned to become president of the Pharmaceutical

Manufacturers' Association. Dr. John H. Talbott, formerly Professor of Medicine of the School of Medicine, University of Buffalo, New York, succeeded Dr. Smith as fifth editor of *The Journal*.

The Association, which Dr. Davis was instrumental in bringing into being in 1847, was to experience many struggles and vicissitudes during the next dozen decades. Complete reorganization was effected in 1900-1901, after which growth was rapid. Chief accomplishments of The American Medical Association include:

1. *A long and determined drive for higher educational standards for medical students.* This, one of the first aims of the Association, was to make little headway until 1909, when the report of a study made by Dr. Abraham Flexner put half the medical diploma mills out of business and set new standards for the future of medical teaching in the United States.

2. *A relentless fight against quacks and charlatans.* The AMA Bureau of Investigation, founded in 1906, has been most effective in revealing facts concerning unethical and fraudulent practices and in providing regulatory bodies with evidence leading to conviction.

3. *Influence for greater scientific accuracy and for more dependable therapeutic agents.* The Council on Pharmacy and Chemistry, founded in 1905, and today known as the Council on Drugs, has been influential in developing new concepts of pharmaceutic integrity.

4. *Establishment of The Journal, which has been the lifeblood and heart of the AMA.* Exercising a powerful voice in behalf of better standards for medicine, *The Journal* today has the largest circulation of any medical periodical in a comparable field. In addition, the Association publishes 10 specialty journals and *Today's Health*, a magazine for the public.

5. *Growth*, steadily, from some 250 physicians, who attended its founding meeting, to a membership that today totals approximately 180,000 physicians. The Association owns its own headquarters at 535 North Dearborn Street, Chicago, Illinois, modernized recently at a cost of more than $2,000,000.

6. *Establishment, in 1943, of a Council on Medical Service,* "to make available facts, data and medical opinions with respect to timely and adequate rendition of medical care to the American people."

218

7. *Long, relentless, and costly efforts to prevent government encroachment into the field of medicine.* It has tried to show, forcefully and clearly, that politics and medicine do not mix.

8. *Encouragement of medical research.* As early as 1898, the AMA established annual Scientific Grants in Aid of Research. Well over one million dollars have been contributed for fundamental investigations made by selected medical institutions.

9. *Broadening of the public's knowledge and understanding of health.* In addition to *Today's Health*, addressed to the public, and *AMA News*, directed to physicians, the Association, for years, has employed every medium of communication to the people in developing interest in public health matters.

10. *Fostership of public health facilities throughout the nation.* Formation of state health departments was one of the earliest goals of the AMA; and it recommended creation of the United States Public Health Service, and, more recently, the Department of Health, Education and Welfare, within the United States government. The Association also urged use of reason and of understanding, rather than emotional blindness, in combating groups whose policies, if followed, would have prevented even discovery of antitoxins, insulin, antibiotics, and many other valuable therapeutic agents.

The American Medical Association gave birth to, and brought to maturity, many other constructive reforms and advancements, all of which are part of the printed record. Naturally, such an aggressive organization has made enemies; consequently, over the years the Association has been sued for recovery of several millions of dollars in damages. With the exception of one case, the suits brought to trial have been unsuccessful. In this one exception, damages awarded were in the amount of one cent.

The distinguished physician and teacher, Dr. William H. Welch, in his presidential address to the Association in 1910, epitomized the effectiveness of the organization, when he said:

"The Association has been from the beginning the great unifying force for the medical profession of this country, whose common interests it has been its chief endeavor to serve."

RUDOLF VIRCHOW AND
CELLULAR PATHOLOGY

FOR twenty centuries, the theory of humoral pathology, in one form or another, influenced the thinking of medical men. According to this philosophy, the body was controlled by four humors and sickness resulted from an imbalance of those humors. Effects of imbalance were thought to encompass the entire body, until Morgagni in 1761 convinced many of his contemporaries that disease usually gained foothold in one or more specific organs; and Bichat, in 1800, drew finer lines and argued that tissues which made up organs were focal points of morbid changes. It remained for Rudolf Virchow in 1855 to develop understanding that the basic units of life are self-reproducing cells of living bodies, and that pathologic conditions result primarily from changes in life processes of cells, due to external influences and irritations. The principles of "cellular pathology," based upon Virchow's scientific research, have dominated biology and pathology ever since; and they finally laid to rest remnants of the old humoral theories to which some medical men still clung in the nineteenth century.

Virchow also was to take a forward position among German medical scientists who, in the mid-nineteenth century, were to wrest leadership of world medicine from the Paris school, dominant since the turn of that century. Though men trained in Paris had advanced their profession tremendously, their methods, stressing physical examination and autopsy, were self-limiting. The future was to go with those who understood and could apply new scientific tools to clinical medicine: microscopy, experimental physiology, and chemistry. In these fields, the Germans were to excel for many decades.

Rudolf Ludwig Carl Virchow was born in the small Eastern Pomeranian city of Schivelbein, October 13, 1821, the only child of a minor city official and farmer. Virchow seems never to have forgotten his rural beginnings. Early in life he revealed an unusual aptitude for the sciences, combined with a wide range of interests, including Arabic

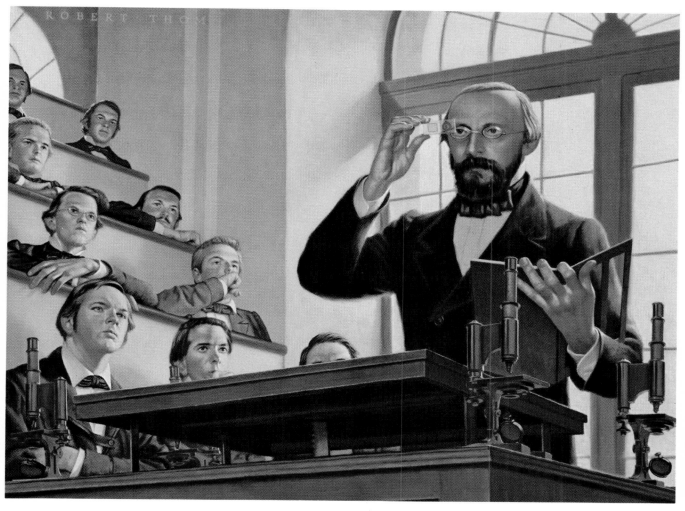

RUDOLF VIRCHOW AND CELLULAR PATHOLOGY

Just past his thirty-fourth year, in 1855, Dr. Rudolf Virchow (1821-1902) while professor at Würzburg University, Germany, propounded his theory of cellular pathology. Lecturing and demonstrating at his specially made desk in the Würzburg Krankenhaus, the slight, short, fiery professor used microscopes to convince students that cells reproduced from other cells, and taught that disease results from disturbance of cells by injury or irritants. Later, in Berlin, Virchow continued to lead international medical thought, and to teach, to engage in research, to write, to edit, to explore new fields, and to serve his community politically, until his death in 1902. The "little doctor" was a medical giant.

221

poetry, classics, and French, English, Hebrew and Italian languages. In October, 1839, Virchow entered the medical school of the Friedrich-Wilhelms-Institut, in Berlin. Primarily an instituion offering free medical education to gifted boys from the poorer classes in return for future service as military physicians, the Institute turned out other nineteenth century luminaries, including Helmholtz, Löffler, and Behring.

At the time Virchow began his studies, the position of German medicine was still at a very low level, due to the influence of romantic philosophies among physicians; but the Berlin university had two of the more magnetic teachers of the time: Johannes Müller, physiologist, comparative anatomist, embryologist, and pathologist; and Johann Lucas Schönlein, outstanding German clinician. These men influenced Virchow: he entered upon research activities while still an undergraduate, and he readily developed abilities to apply exact laboratory methods to investigation of biologic and pathologic questions. In 1843, he presented his thesis on "Rheumatic Disease, Particularly of the Cornea," and received his doctorate in medicine.

As a young student and resident physician, the man who was soon to rise to national and international prominence in several fields presented anything but an imposing figure. Short, thin, blond, dark-eyed, he was accorded the friendly nickname, *der kleine Doktor* (the little doctor). Evidently his stature was a point of personal sensitivity: in Würzburg, he had constructed a special, low desk with an adjustable center section, to deemphasize his short stature.

In 1843, Virchow was appointed "company surgeon," similar to a rotating internship, in Berlin's Charité Hospital. There he began advanced work in biochemistry and in microscopy, a field in which he was to succeed his teacher, Robert Froriep, only three years later, in 1846. From Froriep, too, he was to gain his interest in writing and in editing. In 1845, he began publishing papers on his first two discoveries: embolism, and leukemia. This marked the beginning of an almost continuous flow of papers and other publications for more than half a century. Meantime, things medical did not prevent Virchow's mind from being alert in other fields, including politics, especially as his Pomeranian homeland was involved.

In that same year, 1846, Virchow also began to give courses in pathologic anatomy, and in the following year, at the age of 26, Virchow became a *Privatdozent*, or instructor. In 1847, also, with Benno Reinhardt, Virchow launched the first volume of *Archives for Pathological Anatomy and Physiology and Clinical Medicine*, a periodical which he was to edit until 1902, and which is still being published.

Virchow in later life was to regard the year 1848 as the most decisive in his life: he was able at that time to crystallize his previous critical and constructive ideas in politics and in science into one consistent philosophy. Sent on an official mission to study an epidemic of typhus fever in famine-ridden Upper Silesia, a Prussian province occupied by a Polish minority, Virchow returned preaching political therapeutics (education, freedom, and prosperity for all). He was as audacious in criticism of his government as he was of his medical elders.

When revolution broke out in Berlin in March, 1848, Virchow was among those who fought on the barricades; and in a weekly publication of his own, *Medical Reform*, he discussed changes he believed were needed both in administrative and in medical practices.

Reactionary persecutions following the revolutionaries' defeat led to Virchow's dismissal from his academic position in Berlin, and induced him in 1849 to accept the position of Professor of Pathology at the University of Würzburg. There he entered upon seven of the most creative years of his life. His new professorship at Würzburg was the first chair in pathologic anatomy in Germany. Also, recent improvements in compound microscopes extended the field and the accuracy of the probing curiosity of "der kleine Doktor." "Learn to see microscopically!" became one of his persistent admonitions to students.

Among Virchow's discoveries while engaged in teaching, in writing, in editing, and in research during his Würzburg years, were chemical substances, such as myelin, and amyloid; demonstration that connective tissues are composed of cells; and that granulated cells are in a degenerative, not a formative, state. He continued studies related to public health and began work on physical anthropology. But of greatest significance was formulation and exposition of the basic biologic law: *Each cell stems from another cell*.

In 1838, another pupil of Johannes Müller, Theodor Schwann, had introduced his theory that the elementary unit of all animals and of all plants is the cell. This was not the first cell theory, but better microscopes had made cellular observation more accurate and convincing. Schwann, however, believed that cells were spontaneously created from an amorphous substance called "blastema." Virchow expressed doubt of the spontaneous generation theory as early as 1845; but in Würzburg he proceeded to disprove this concept by demonstrating conclusively that cells multiply by division. Disease, Virchow taught, is not located basically in organs, tissues, vessels, or nerves, but in cells; and this more specific concept became the basis of instruction in pathology. He coined the term, *cellular pathology*, in 1855, and his book on the subject was published in 1858.

Virchow was not the first man to look for pathologic changes in cells; nor was he the first to claim that cells originate only from cells. He was first, however, to systematize the theory of cellular pathology, and to give medicine again a common denominator for all diseases—something it had lost in giving up older medical philosophies. Probably the bases of Virchow's greater success than earlier observers had had lay in the soundness of his research, the prolificacy of his publishing, the crusader-like quality of his zeal, and the growth of his influence upon medicine.

Already internationally famous for his teaching in Würzburg, Virchow was called back to Berlin in 1856. Johannes Müller wanted Virchow to succeed him as teacher of pathologic anatomy. One of Virchow's conditions for return was erection of a special building for an Institute of Pathology. This building was to be used during the entire 46 years Virchow was to spend in Berlin.

The importance of "der kleine Doktor" in his field continued to grow: in Berlin, he wrote his great book on tumors; he worked on fungi; and he did important work on trichinosis. Though some writers have claimed that Virchow was an enemy of bacteriology, the facts deny the claim. He was an early participant in the trend toward knowledge of etiology through microbiology. His assistant, Obermeier, discovered the spirilla of relapsing fever; and Virchow was first to publish, in his *Archives*, the discoveries of Bravell, Hansen, and Loesch. He exercised healthy skepticism toward many "new organisms" reported to have been discovered; and frequently his skepticism was justified by later findings. He did make blunders in his views regarding tuberculosis and diphtheria; however, his basic positions were sound: that disease cause and disease process should not be confused; that bacterial toxins might exist and might be important; and that there are social and constitutional factors as well as bacteriologic factors to be considered in management of infectious diseases.

In Berlin, too, Virchow became involved in municipal and in national politics. In 1859, he was elected to the Berlin city council; and he served as a member of that body continuously thereafter until his death. His studies in public health and his growing influence permitted him to bring about construction of better sewerage for Berlin, to build new hospitals, and to bring about improved hygienic conditions in schools and in other municipal institutions. In 1861, Virchow was elected to the Prussian diet (legislative body) in which he led a desperate fight against Otto von Bismarck's internal dictatorship and external policies of "blood and iron." This was one of the few times Virchow failed to get what he wanted. Bismarck's ambition to "unify" Germany was fulfilled following three campaigns which took place during 1864, 1866, and 1870. Bismarck became so annoyed with "der kleine Doktor" that at one point he challenged Virchow to a duel, but this never came about.

Virchow now had friends, pupils, and admirers in every country. Among students who studied under him were many whose names were to become famous in medical research and in medicine's progress; who were to add impetus to the tremendous advances in world medicine during the latter half of the nineteenth century.

Once more, the center of gravity in Virchow's life shifted. While continuing his interest in medical teaching and in politics (he served in the German national Reichstag from 1880 to 1893), his main interest now turned to anthropology and to archaeology. Great interest had been developed in Darwin's theories. While Virchow recognized their merit, he warned against exaggerated claims of evolution enthusiasts, such as those of his erstwhile assistant, Ernst Haeckel. In the field of racial research, Virchow organized and directed a gigantic project involving the examination of nearly seven million German schoolchildren. Aim of the study was to determine whether or not there was a true "German type." Virchow's findings proved that less than one-third of German children were blond and that there was no evidence of a predominant skull type among them.

At an age when many men would have begun to slacken their activities, Virchow embraced his new field of interest with enthusiasm. He founded the German Anthropological Society in 1869; and in the same year, the Berlin Society of Anthropology, Ethnology, and Prehistory. He also edited the journal of the Society. His activities then spread to the Near East, where he sponsored Heinrich Schliemann in excavations on the sites of ancient Troy and of Hissarlik. In 1888, he went with Schliemann and Schweinfurth to Egypt; and in 1894 he did his own field work in the Caucasus.

Meanwhile, Virchow continued to be the dominant figure in international medicine. It is said that he could demolish an adversary in a discussion without even raising his voice. A certain coldness of character probably facilitated his ability to analyze situations and persons objectively and to get what he wanted. However, he was easily approachable; he liked, for example, to sit down with friends and students after meetings for a glass of beer and for singing. He was hospitable and could be very gay, especially in his family circle. He could be particularly warm toward the lowly and the sick. With medical men and with students, however, he could be ferocious, insisting on precise logic and order in relation to mere trifles. Still, he was tremendously popular as a teacher. Virchow continued to lecture, to write, to edit, to research, to serve in political bodies, and to influence international medicine, into his eighty-first year and until his death, September 5, 1902, caused by cardiac failure following an accident. Berliners accorded him his final honor—a public civic funeral.

While achieving many successes, Virchow's obstinacy sometimes blocked worthwhile projects. However, his record of positive accomplishments far outweighs his faults. His courage, his energy, his many-sidedness, his interest in humanity, his scientific results made him unique and unforgettable. His work on cellular pathology had far-reaching consequences, contributing to tremendous progress in medicine and in surgery, and proving to be a stimulus to modern chemotherapy.

WORLD EVENTS AND MEDICAL HISTORY

Dates, persons, and events of significance to the evolution of Medicine include:

1903   License No. 1 "for the manufacture of viruses, serums, toxins, and analogous products," issued by U. S. Treasury Dept. to Parke-Davis.

1903   Metchnikoff inoculated higher apes with syphilis.

1903   Einthoven developed the electro-cardiograph.

1903   Von Pirquet and Schick identified serum sickness with anaphylaxis.

1903   Koch stressed danger of healthy typhoid carriers as agents of infection.

1903   Emil Fischer and von Mehring introduced veronal (barbital).

1903   Albers-Schönberg noted sterilizing effect of x-rays on gonads.

1903   Bruce demonstrated transmission of sleeping sickness by tsetse fly.

1903   Dunbar discovered toxin and antitoxin (pollantin) of hay fever.

1903   Riva Rocci invented sphygmomanometer.

1903   Ramsay and Soddy demonstrated transmutation of radium into helium.

1903   Siedentopf and Zsigmondy invented ultramicroscope.

1903   Almroth Wright and Douglass investigated opsonins.

1903   Castellani discovered *Trypanosoma ugandense*.

1903   Vaccination obligatory in Spain.

1903   Nobel prize awarded to Becquerel and the Curies for their contributions on radiation.

1904   Nobel prize awarded to Pavlov for his work on physiology of digestion.

1904   Atwater invented respiration calorimeter.

1904-14   Gen. William Crawford Gorgas, U. S., headed yellow fever control making possible building of Panama Canal.

1904   Max Cloetta introduced digalen.

1904   Ehrlich discovered trypan red, effective against trypanosomes.

1904   Fourneau introduced stovaine.

1904   Ramón y Cajal published *Texture of the Nervous System of Man and of the Other Vertebrates*.

1904   F. Stolz determined composition of Adrenalin.

1905   F. R. Schaudinn and Erich Hoffmann discovered parasite of syphilis (*Treponema pallidum*).

1905   Bordet and Gengou isolated bacillus of whooping cough.

1905   Chaput employed stovaine in spinal anesthesia.

1905   Winter resuscitated the heart by Adrenalin injections.

1905   Dutton and Koch demonstrated tick transmission of African relapsing fever.

1905   E. H. Starling, English physiologist, first used the term, "hormone."

1905   Alfred Einhorn discovered novocain.

1905   Wright brothers made successful flight with aëroplane.

1905   Nobel prize awarded to Koch for his work on tuberculosis.

1906   Wassermann introduced serum diagnosis of syphilis.

1906   Ernst B. Chain born.

1906   Frederick G. Hopkins (England) predicted isolation of vitamins.

1906   Von Pirquet stated doctrine of allergy.

1906   Voelcker and von Lichtenberg examined kidney with x-ray (pyelography).

1906   Neisser demonstrated susceptibility of lower apes to syphilis.

1906   Federal Food and Drugs Act (United States) passed (June 30; effective 1907).

1906   Nobel prize awarded to Golgi and Ramón y Cajal for their work on structure of the nervous system.

1906-25   Blair Bell introduced use of pituitrin as oxytocic in lingering labor.

1907   Von Pirquet introduced cutaneous reaction in tuberculosis.

1907   Theobald Smith suggested use of toxin-antitoxin in diphtheria (Behring, 1912).

1907   Ricketts demonstrated tick transmission of Rocky Mountain fever.

1907   Adolf Schmidt employed functional test meal in diagnosing intestinal disorders.

1907   Fletcher and Hopkins demonstrated role of lactic acid formation in normal muscle contraction.

1907   Nobel prize awarded to Alphonse Laveran for discovering the etiology of protozoan diseases.

HELMHOLTZ
PHYSICIST-PHYSICIAN

Hermann Ludwig Ferdinand von Helmholtz as a youth did not want to be a physician: he wanted rather to be a physicist, or a mathematician. Later in life he became a scientific investigator who made outstanding contributions in each of these fields. Of him, Sigerist wrote: "It was a rare stroke of luck for medical science that a man with such eminent physical and mathematical gifts should be forced by circumstances to devote a considerable part of his life to medical science."

Medical men may remember Helmholtz best for his inventions: the ophthalmoscope and the ophthalmometer. However, his original research, both in physical optics and in color sensation, was much more extensive; and of almost equal importance to medicine were his studies of acoustics and of the mechanism of the middle ear. The scope of Helmholtz' interests and of his original work is amazing: in addition to the sciences of medicine, optics, and acoustics, the great German scientist made important contributions to knowledge in psychology, chemistry, physiology, physics, mechanics, hydrodynamics, electricity, color, meteorology, and mathematics. Hall comments that "It is doubtful if the world has ever produced a man who combined greater breadth of knowledge and greater depth of wisdom, with keenness of vision, persistency and patience of pursuit, and modesty of claim."

Hermann Helmholtz was born August 31, 1821, at Potsdam, near Berlin. He was the son of Ferdinand Helmholtz, teacher in the Gymnasium (high school) and a man of high culture and intelligence. The mother was a daughter of a Hanoverian artillery officer named Penne— a lineal descendant of William Penn, the great Quaker who came to North America and founded Pennsylvania. A grandmother was of French origin. Helmholtz thus had German, English, and French

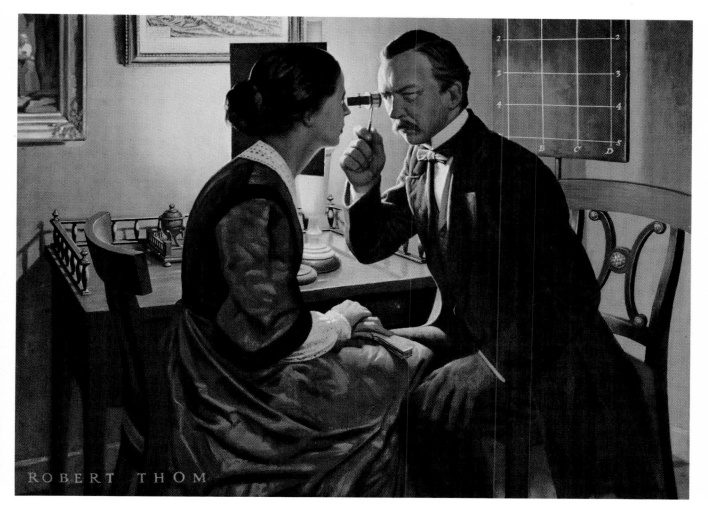

ROBERT THOM

HELMHOLTZ: PHYSICIST-PHYSICIAN

Among great contributions to medicine in the nineteenth century was the ophthalmoscope, an instrument used for inspection of the interior of the eye, invented in 1850 by Hermann Ludwig Ferdinand von Helmholtz (1821-1894), Professor of Physiology at Königsberg. Physician by training and teacher by profession, Helmholtz became Germany's foremost physicist, succeeding to the Chair of Physics at the University of Berlin. His contributions to medicine's knowledge of acoustics nearly equaled those he made to physiologic optics. His discoveries in physics advanced knowledge in a dozen scientific fields, earned him ennoblement, and brought him eminence, distinction, and world-wide recognition.

229

blood in his veins. One of four children in a family of modest means, he was sickly as a child and had poor health throughout a long life. Confined to his room by illness for long periods, the boy sought amusement through activity of mind. He read widely and whiled away time with a set of blocks, from which he gained early concepts of geometry. He grew to love nature and enjoyed hikes in the country, gaining from them an appreciation for natural laws. His early interest in physics was revealed in his construction of optical apparatus, using odd lenses; in his application of optical principles; and in his drawing diagrams illustrating passage of light through telescopes, surreptitiously while attending lectures in high school. He developed his mathematical talents without the aid of special instruction.

Young Helmholtz wanted to devote his life to the study of physics but the limited means of his father dictated otherwise. Surgeon-General Mursinna, a relative, advised the boy to study medicine, and in 1838 arranged for his admission to the Royal Medico-Chirurgical Friedrich-Wilhelms-Institut in Berlin—an appointment given freely to youths on condition that afterward they become surgeons in the Prussian army.

During his years in medical school, Helmholtz came under the influence of Johannes Müller, one of the Institute's great teachers, a circumstance which led to his association with DuBois Reymond, Brücke, Gustav Magnus, Kirchhoff, Virchow, and others who later joined with him in founding the Berlin Physical Society.

During his student years, Helmholtz suffered an attack of typhoid fever and was treated at no cost to him at Charité Hospital. With money saved from his stipend during this period, he purchased a compound microscope, an instrument rarely possessed by students in those days. In 1842, Helmholtz, at the age of 21, presented his doctoral thesis, *On the Structure of the Nervous System of the Invertebrates*, in which he contributed basic knowledge: proof that nerve fibers are branches of nerve cells, a fact therebefore unknown.

For more than 50 years thereafter, from this time (1842) on to 1894, when Helmholtz reached the age of 73, papers flowed from his pen in almost uninterrupted succession. By the end of his career, he had published 217 papers and books.

Serving for six years, after graduation in 1842, as a medical officer in the Prussian army, Helmholtz continued research in his spare time. Among subjects he investigated were fermentation (in which he preceded Pasteur), and production of heat in contracting muscle. In 1847, at the age of 26, he published in pamphlet form what perhaps was his greatest scientific accomplishment: postulation and proof of the law of conservation of energy. Though now axiomatic, Helmholtz' theses . . . that energy is indestructible and that energy may be transformed but is never lost or destroyed . . . represented the first clear and unmistakable presentation of an idea, applicable to medicine as well as to mechanics, that had been only hinted at by earlier scientific workers.

In 1848, Helmholtz was allowed to leave the army so that he might become Professor of Anatomy at the Academy of Art in Berlin. In 1849, he became Professor of Physiology in Königsberg. Continuing research there, Helmholtz measured the velocity of the nerve impulse— believed by his teacher, Johannes Müller, to be technically impossible. At this time, too, he began intensive study of the physiology of the senses.

In the course of studies relating to physiologic optics, in 1850, Helmholtz invented the ophthalmoscope. He once wrote how the discovery came about: "I was endeavoring to explain to my pupils the emission of reflected light from the eye, a discovery made by Brücke, who would have invented the ophthalmoscope had he only asked himself how an optical image is formed by the light returning from the eye. In his research it was not necessary to ask it, but had he asked it, he was just the man to answer it as quickly as I did, and to invent the instrument. I turned the problem over and over to ascertain the simplest way in which I could demonstrate the phenomenon to my students. It was also a reminiscence of my days of medical study, that ophthalmologists had great trouble in dealing with certain cases of eye disease, then known as black cataract. The first model was constructed of pasteboard, lenses and cover glasses used in the microscopic work. It was at first so difficult to use, that I doubt if I should have persevered unless I had felt that it must succeed; but in eight days I had the great joy of being the first who saw before him a living human retina."

The ophthalmoscope consists essentially of a converging or concave mirror for concentrating light through the patient's pupil thus illuminating the retina and other parts of the eye. The eye of the observer is behind a small hole in the center of the mirror. In front of this opening is a magnifying lens or combination of lenses. Invention of this instrument opened a new era, not only for ophthalmologists, but for other practitioners of medicine, as well. Ophthalmoscopic examination of the retina, which may be regarded as an outlying portion of the brain, gives information of value, not only in diagnosis of diseases of the eye, but also in assessing pathologic states in other parts of the body.

Helmholtz' interest in physiologic optics began with the ophthalmoscope and did not end until he felt he had completely mastered the whole field. Next problem to attract his attention embraced optical constants in the eye. In order to determine the curvature of refractive surfaces, Helmholtz developed the ophthalmometer, by means of which refractive powers and visual defects of the individual eye might be measured. This work he continued until he could lay down rules for guidance of practicing ophthalmologists in use of the instrument in solution of problems of ocular accommodation, and in measurement necessary for preparation of lenses for correction of visual defects.

Helmholtz next turned to problems of color sensation, which he explored intensively, including causes of color blindness. This work on optics, begun in Königsberg, was continued in Bonn, and in Heidelberg, culminating in 1867 with publication of his classic work, *Handbook of Physiologic Optics*.

In 1856, Helmholtz, then 36 years of age, accepted the Chair of Anatomy and Physiology at the University of Bonn; three years later, in 1859, he became Professor of Physiology at Heidelberg, where he remained until 1871.

Paralleling his work on optics, and of almost equal importance to medicine, was Helmholtz' work on physiologic acoustics. Begun in Königsberg, the greater part of these studies was carried out in Bonn. Before Helmholtz' research, knowledge of acoustics was rudimentary and largely empiric. He combined his advanced knowledge of physics with experimental physiology and went on, not only to define physical principles underlying transmission of sound, but followed its course through the middle ear to the brain. He accurately described, in detail, the anatomy of the middle ear, and the function of each tissue therein. Results of these studies were outlined in his book, *Sensations of Tone as the Physiological Basis of Music*, published in Heidelberg in 1863. These developments had been preceded by a number of papers over the years, including: *Vowel Tones; The Physical Basis of Harmony and Dissonance; The Theory of Organ Pipes; Musical Temperature;* and *Motions of the Strings of a Violin*. His monograph on anatomy of bones of the middle ear appeared in 1869.

After 1867, Helmholtz' work and publications were predominantly in the field of physics and mathematics, although his contributions relating to cerebral functions were of fundamental value to the field of psychology. In 1871, Helmholtz, logically, was invited to return to Berlin to take over the Chair of Physics at the University of Berlin, to succeed the great Magnus. In this position he was accorded recognition as the foremost physicist in Germany. During the next eleven years he contributed a total of 60 scientific papers on various subjects.

In 1888, Helmholtz became the first director of the Imperial Institute for Physics and Technology, at Charlottenburg, near Berlin. In addition to these new duties, he maintained his Chair at the University until his death. In his later years, instead of declining, Helmholtz seemed to increase in mental power. More and more, he devoted himself to establishment of fundamental principles related to dynamics, hydrodynamics, thermodynamics, electrodynamics, and other complex physical problems. He continued his popular science lectures, begun in Königsberg.

Despite his heavy program of scientific research, Helmholtz was a lover of art in all its forms: he was an accomplished musician; and, for recreation, he loved a climb in the mountains or a walk in a meadow. Some of the answers to his most puzzling problems, he related, came to him during his visits to nature. During his lifetime he was twice married. Two children were born to each union. His home life has been described as quiet, cultural, and pleasant. Emperor Wilhelm I ennobled Helmholtz and often received him in the imperial domestic circle. Helmholtz' seventieth birthday anniversary was celebrated as a national event, for which a gold medal was struck in his honor. The Kings of Sweden and of Italy, the Grand Duke of Baden, and the President of the French Republic each conferred special honors upon him.

Despite age, Helmholtz continued to be active: in 1892, he attended meetings of the British Association for the Advancement of Science, in Edinburgh, Scotland; and in 1893, the International Exposition in Chicago, after which he toured the United States and Canada. On his homeward journey, he fell on shipboard and suffered concussion of the brain. From this injury he only partially recovered, and in July, 1894, he suffered a stroke. Death took the great physicist and physician, September 8, 1894, just eight days after his seventy-third birthday anniversary.

Helmholtz . . . teacher, experimenter, physician, and physicist . . . left the world a great heritage of scientific advancement. There was an intimate relationship between his functions as professor and as original investigator: he investigated because he wanted to speak of matters with knowledge gained firsthand. Again and again he took up problems that he might master them himself, so that he might make clear explanations to his pupils. Students profited . . . and so did the entire world . . . for the work of the kindly, reserved professor was spread 'round the globe among practitioners of medicine and among those active in several other fields in science.

WORLD EVENTS AND MEDICAL HISTORY

Dates, persons, and events of significance to the evolution of Medicine include:

1908   Kamerlingh Onnes liquefied helium.

1908   Paul Ehrlich and Elie Metchnikoff shared Nobel prize for work in immunity.

1908   Zeppelin constructed improved airship.

1908   Cushing operated on the pituitary gland.

1908   Peking Union Medical College founded by Rockefeller Institute.

1908   American Public Health Association standardized tests for milk.

1908-10   William Pasteur described massive (postoperative) collapse of the lungs.

1909   Sorensen investigated hydrogen ion concentration.

1909   Hofmann synthesized caoutchouc (india rubber).

1909   F. F. Russell vaccinated United States Army against typhoid fever.

1909   Nobel prize awarded to Kocher for his contribution on the thyroid gland.

1909-13   Marine and Lenhart standardized iodine treatment of goiter.

1910   Flexner produced poliomyelitis experimentally.

1910   Abraham Flexner published survey of medical schools and education.

1910   Vedder demonstrated amebicidal action of emetine.

1910   Chapin, Winslow, and Robinson emphasized danger of contact infection in communicable diseases.

1910   Ehrlich and Hata introduced salvarsan (606).

1910   Nobel prize awarded to Albrecht Kossel for his work on cellular chemistry.

1910-27   A. V. Hill investigated thermodynamics of muscular contraction.

1911   Cushing described dyspituitarism.

1911   Walter Cannon published *The Mechanical Factors of Digestion*.

1911   Peyton Rous (U.S.) showed cancer in chickens caused by virus.

1911   Nobel prizes awarded to Marie Curie and A. Gullstrand for their respective works on radiation chemistry and dioptrics of the eye.

1911-14   Casimir Funk investigated vitamines.

1911-15   Van Slyke devised methods of estimating amino nitrogen and amino acids.

1911-27   Pavlov investigated conditional reflexes.

1912   Nicolle, Anderson, and Goldberger produced experimental typhus in monkey.

1912   Joseph Lister died.

1912   Weber and Lorey effected x-ray examination of abdominal viscera (pneumoperitoneum).

1912   Von Behring employed toxin-antitoxin immunization against diphtheria.

1912   Nobel prize awarded to Alexis Carrel for his work on organ transplantation and vascular suturing.

1912-13   Gustav Embden and co-workers investigated carbohydrate metabolism.

1912-14   Institut du Radium (Curie Foundation) erected at Paris.

1912-16   Cannon investigated effect of adrenal secretion on emotions.

1913   Schick introduced susceptibility test for diphtheria.

1913   Vitamin A discovered.

1913   Krönig and Gauss introduced morphine-scopolamine anesthesia in obstetrics (twilight sleep).

1913   Douglas, Haldane, Henderson, and Schneider investigated effect of acclimatization to high altitudes (Pike's Peak) on respiration.

1913   Wellcome Medical and Medico-Historical Museums (London) founded.

1913   Rockefeller Foundation (New York) chartered.

1913   Nobel prize awarded to Charles Richet for his work on anaphylaxis.

1913-16   Dochez, Gillespie, and Avery typed the pneumococci.

1913-16   McCollum, Davis, and Kennedy described vitamins A and B.

1913-27   Maude Slye experimented on hereditary susceptibility to and immunity from cancer.

J. MARION SIMS
GYNECOLOGIC SURGEON

THE IDEA that health problems peculiar to women deserve separate and distinct medical and surgical attention simply had not been conceived before the middle of the nineteenth century. Some physicians even refused to examine women or to treat them for other than ordinary afflictions. Their reasons ranged from realization of their own shortcomings to ludicrous pseudo modesty. Meanwhile, sick women suffered in silence and in seclusion.

In maintaining this attitude, New World doctors of the early 1800's followed the practice of European physicians, to whom they looked for leadership in medicine. They were importers of ideas; seldom exporters. However, there were a few, but important, exceptions. Rugged physicians, faced with the myriad medical problems of the new American frontiers, and without consultants or publications to fall back upon, were forced to improvise, to invent, to experiment, to take chances. Out of their experiences, when they could find time to write them down, came some remarkable contributions to medical knowledge; and medical communication across the Atlantic began to acquire a two-way flow.

Near the frontier village of Danville, Kentucky, Dr. Ephraim McDowell (1771-1830) performed the first of a series of ovariotomies in 1809, about which he published a report in 1816. These intra-abdominal operations, eight of thirteen of which were successful, were performed without benefit either of anesthesia or of antisepsis. Although John Light Atlee (1799-1885) of Lancaster, Pennsylvania, performed ovariotomy successfully in 1843, as did his younger brother, Washington Lemuel Atlee (1808-1878) in Philadelphia, no European physician followed McDowell's lead for several decades.

In 1833, Army Surgeon William Beaumont (1785-1853) published reports of his remarkable studies on secretion of gastric juice in his famous patient, Alexis St. Martin, which he began while stationed at a frontier fort on Mackinac Island, now a part of Michigan. On the

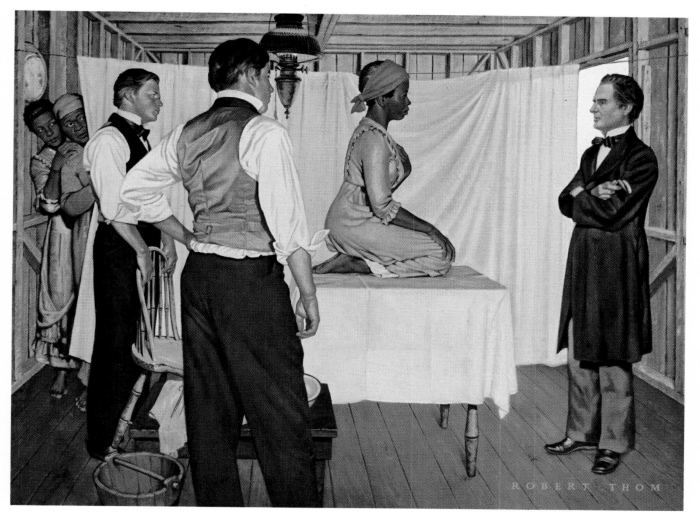

J. MARION SIMS: GYNECOLOGIC SURGEON

Little did James Marion Sims, M.D., (1813-1883) dream, that summer day in 1845, as he prepared to examine the slave girl, Lucy, that he was launching himself on an international career as a gynecologic surgeon; or that he was to raise gynecology from virtually an unknown to a respected medical specialty. Nor did he realize that his crude back-yard hospital in Montgomery, Alabama, would be the forerunner of the nation's first Woman's Hospital, which Sims helped to establish in New York in 1855. Dr. Sims, who became a leader in gynecology in Europe as well as in the United States, served as president of The American Medical Association, 1875-1876; and was honored by many nations.

237

Georgia frontier, Dr. Crawford W. Long used ether to anesthetize patients undergoing surgical procedures, as early as 1842; but reports from surgeons at Massachusetts General Hospital in Boston of demonstrations by Dr. William T. G. Morton in 1846 gave basic principles of surgical anesthesia to the world.

During early decades of the nineteenth century, a penniless South Carolina country boy was growing up. In his youth and early manhood he showed little promise beyond the ordinary—but he was destined to launch a new medical specialty, gynecology, and not only to take the lead in surgery for women in the United States, but to become an accepted leader and teacher abroad. His name was James Marion Sims.

Eldest of eight children fathered by a tavern keeper and local politician, James Marion Sims was born January 25, 1813, near Hanging Rock Creek, Lancaster County, South Carolina. He grew to manhood in Lancaster. His education began in a log cabin schoolhouse, continued at Franklin Academy, and at the College of South Carolina, in Columbia. His scholarship was not particularly distinguished. Upon receiving the degree of Bachelor of Arts in 1832, Sims was undecided as to a career. His mother wished him to become a minister; his father, a lawyer. Having no enthusiasm for either of these callings, Marion Sims decided upon medicine. Perhaps the fact that the father of Eliza Theresa Jones, the girl he loved who lived "on the other side of town," had been a physician, helped him make his decision. Sims began study in the office of Theresa's uncle, Dr. B. C. Jones, then registered for a course of lectures in the Medical College at Charleston, from which he graduated in 1834, at the age of twenty-one. The following year Sims attended Jefferson Medical College in Philadelphia, receiving his M. D. degree in 1835.

Sims has been described as a handsome though somewhat delicate young man, about five feet eight inches in height, of good figure, erect of carriage, and with a quick step. His face was oval, his nose approaching the Grecian type. He had clear, deep-set brown eyes, and dark brown hair. His smile was infectious, and his nature usually buoyant. His manner was quick and impulsive. He was brave without being aggressive, and, on proper occasions, ready to assert the courage of his convictions. He had a great capacity for sympathy, which, combined with his quickness of hand and inventiveness of mind, was to lead him into new paths and to a record of great service.

Nothing pointing to future greatness was evident either to Dr. Sims or to his home town neighbors when he returned to Lancaster, South Carolina, to practice. Of himself, Dr. Sims wrote: "When I graduated, I felt absolutely incompetent to assume the duties of a practitioner . . . I had had no clinical advantages, no hospital experience, and had seen nothing at all of sickness. I had been able to buy a full set of instruments for surgical operations, and I laid in a full stock of medicines in Philadelphia. My father rented me an office on Main Street. I had a sign painted on tin . . ." To detract further from the young physician's confidence, his first two patients, infants, died under his care. Had he not been completely without means, Sims would have given up medicine then and there; he did decide to leave Lancaster, and proceeded by horseback to the frontier town of Mount Meigs, Alabama, a trip requiring three weeks of difficult travel. In Mount Meigs, his fortune changed: most of his surgical patients recovered; most of his medical patients got well; his practice thrived.

Dr. Sims married Theresa Jones in 1836, and entered into a partnership in Mount Meigs with Dr. Boling A. Blakey. This introduced Dr. Sims to a large practice, and he soon bought out Dr. Blakey. For the next three years Dr. Sims practiced successfully—then he and his family were struck down by a series of attacks of malarial fever. These so reduced Sims' ability to practice that his savings were exhausted. He determined to seek a healthier climate and relocated in Montgomery, Alabama.

In addition to regaining his health, Sims, who previously had had little interest in medicine except as a means of making a living, began to mature professionally. He developed a successful general practice, and increased his reputation as a skillful surgeon. At the rear of his home he built a one-story frame building that would accommodate eight beds, to serve as a hospital. He also began training young men in medicine and surgery.

In Montgomery, too, Dr. Sims performed a clever, difficult operation for harelip and missing upper jaw, the report of which became his first paper published in a major journal. There, too, he believed he had discovered the cause of *trismus nascentium,* a condition of tetanus in infants. Sims ordered infants showing signs of this condition removed from their strait-jacket-like cradles, where they lay on their backs virtually immobilized, and saw to it that they were placed on their sides and their positions changed frequently to relieve pressure on the point where the spine joins the skull.

Until 1845, Dr. Sims had taken little interest in women patients beyond caring for ordinary ailments. Until June of that year, he had never encountered a patient suffering with vesicovaginal fistula—an opening resulting from tears in tissues between vagina and bladder, or rectum, from difficult childbirth, permitting drainage either from the bladder or from the rectum, or sometimes from both, into the vagina. Continuous uncontrollable leakage of urine or feces from the vagina caused both physical and mental agony to unfortunate victims, who not only were shunned by family and by friends, but hated themselves while doomed to an almost intolerable lifetime of discomfort and of seclusion. However, in the course of two months, Dr. Sims was called upon by owners of three young female slaves, Anarcha, Betsey, and Lucy, who suffered from such fistulas, and he was requested to do something to relieve them. Sims, finding no published report of successful surgical treatment for vesicovaginal fistula, pronounced them incurable. However, the owner of Lucy insisted upon sending her to Dr. Sims' office for examination. The doctor was regretfully about to send Lucy back home when a set of circumstances altered the young surgeon's life—and Lucy's life, as well.

Dr. Sims was called that morning from his routine rounds to care for a woman who, thrown from a horse, had injured her pelvis and was in great pain. Sims, having determined that there were no fractures, was faced with the problem of relieving her intense pain. According to his own report: "If there was anything I hated, it was investigating the organs of the female pelvis. But this poor woman was in such a condition that I was obliged to find out what was the matter with her. It was by a digital examination, and I had sense enough to discover that there was retroversion of the uterus . . ." A long-forgotten aphorism of one of his former teachers came to mind: he placed the patient in the knee-chest position, and with further digital manipulation, air was admitted to the

240

vagina, pressure restored the uterus to its normal position, and the patient was relieved of her pain almost instantly.

The thought flashed through Dr. Sims' mind: could he not put Lucy in a similar position and see the relationship of the fistula to surrounding tissues? "Fired with this idea," wrote Sims, "I forgot that I had twenty patients waiting to see me . . . I jumped into my buggy and hurried home. Passing by the . . . store, I bought a pewter spoon . . ."

Calling his two assistants, Dr. Sims went to the hospital and told his patient he wished to re-examine her. Placing her on a table, he directed her to assume the knee-chest position. As Sims inserted the bent handle of the spoon into the patient's vagina, he reported: "I saw everything, as no man had ever seen before. The fistula was as plain as the nose on a man's face . . . I said at once, 'Why can not these things be cured?' I immediately went to work to invent instruments for performing the operation . . ." He was so confident that he not only kept Lucy at the hospital, but he sent also for Anarcha and Betsey, telling their masters he would put them up at his own expense until they were well.

Dr. Sims' confidence that he could cure vesicovaginal fistula surgically was to be sorely tried. His first operations proved failures: while the fistulas might be greatly reduced, infections resulted around silk sutures, and small openings remained—small openings that leaked as much as large ones. Three years of trial and error and discouragement followed. Finally, in 1849, Dr. Sims determined to use thin pure silver wires as sutures, securing them with pieces of lead. Anarcha became subject of the experiment: it was her thirtieth operation. The operation was successful; there was no infection about the silver wire sutures; the fistula was closed. In the next two weeks, Lucy and Betsey were cured by similar operations.

Dr. Sims was amazed at the number of women suffering from vesicovaginal fistula who came out of seclusion to seek his help, when word of his success got around. The Sims position, a more comfortable adaptation of the knee-chest position, and the Sims speculum, bear the doctor's name even today. Dr. Sims also set about training an assistant —an act he was to regret later when the student attempted to take credit for development of Sims' techniques. Just when Sims seemed to be on the road to success, fate dealt him more blows. His second son died; and Sims himself became victim of a chronic intestinal infection —a disease that was proving fatal to many persons in the Southern states. After trying for three years to regain his health, the discouraged doctor, believing death was near, decided to publish his manuscript on operations for vesicovaginal fistula. It appeared in the January, 1852, issue of the *American Journal of the Medical Sciences*. Needless to say, it met with more skepticism than enthusiasm.

In a desperate effort to regain his health, Dr. Sims finally decided in 1853 to move permanently to New York City. This was quite an undertaking for a family rooted for generations in the South. He struggled to gain a foothold; but poor health, irritability, poverty, and jealousy on the part of his colleagues in the city, held him back. Though he had opportunities to demonstrate his operation, surgeons frequently adopted his techniques and sent no more referrals to Sims.

Out of meditation during idle time came his conviction that women deserved greater consideration by the medical profession. Gradually in Sims' mind a new idea developed: a special hospital for care of women and for performance of the operation at which he had become so adept. Dr. Sims gained little support or interest until by chance he struck up a friendship with Henri Luther Stuart, former newspaperman and freelance writer with many contacts. With Stuart's aid and introductions, Dr. Sims met a number of New York's wealthy philanthropic leaders. With the help of an active group of influential women, Dr. Sims was able to overcome almost insuperable obstacles of finance, of prejudice, and of opposition from medical men. On May 4, 1855, Woman's Hospital—the first gynecologic hospital in the United States—opened its doors. At first it had but 30 beds and Dr. Sims was its only surgeon. Constant charitable activity and much ingenuity on the part of the Lady Managers' committee were required to keep its doors open. Gradually, however, the hospital grew. Other gynecologic operations were undertaken; the staff was increased; doctors from near and far were welcome to visit the operating room to observe Dr. Sims' methods. Eventually, land for expansion was secured between Forty-ninth and Fiftieth streets (now the site of the Waldorf-Astoria Hotel) and foundations were laid in 1863 for a new and expanded state-chartered hospital

242

—The Woman's Hospital in the State of New York. Dr. Sims continued as titular head of its surgical staff.

Meantime, however, other events were developing that were to influence Dr. Sims' life. The War Between the States put him in an embarrassing position: he and his family could not put out of mind their Southern ties, and such beliefs were highly unpopular in New York. Sims decided to take a vacation trip to Europe—a sort of "postman's holiday"—for European surgeons had heard of him, and he was invited to demonstrate his vesicovaginal fistula operations in leading continental medical centers. Dr. Sims then became an international commuter; he moved his family to Paris for the duration of the war. He became physician to queens and empresses, as well as to charity patients. In 1870 and 1871, he served as military surgeon in the Anglo-American Ambulance Corps during the Franco-Prussian war. For his impartial services to wounded soldiers, he was decorated both by French and by German governments.

Dr. Sims returned to New York in 1872, and again took part in activities of the expanding Woman's Hospital. Its staff and patient load had grown rapidly. In 1874, however, the Board of Lady Supervisors passed bylaws limiting the number of visitors who could witness operations and refusing admission to cancer patients. Dr. Sims' ire was aroused: he arose and vehemently, perhaps undiplomatically, voiced his opposition. He announced that unless the two rules were repealed at the next meeting, he would leave the hospital. Dr. Sims' resignation was accepted, December 22, 1874. This was a great blow to the aging surgeon; but if his popularity was at a low ebb in New York, the condition did not prevail elsewhere. The following year, 1875, he was elected president of The American Medical Association.

Dr. Sims' work was not limited to gynecologic surgery; he also did basic work on control of dysmenorrhea, on overcoming sterility, and on artificial insemination. In 1878, he initiated an operation for removal of gallstones and gave it the name cholecystotomy. In 1880, Dr. Sims was named president of The American Gynecological Society, an organization which he had helped to found. In the same year, he was reinstated as consulting surgeon to Woman's Hospital. Dr. Sims, by then, however, was spending much of his time in Europe, where his reputation was as great as it was in the United States. In 1881, he was made honorary president of the International Medical Congress at Geneva.

About to return to Rome, where he had built a successful practice, Dr. Sims, in his seventy-first year, seemingly in good health, while sitting in bed working on his autobiography early in the morning of November 13, 1883, had a seizure of dyspnea. His son, Dr. Harry Marion Sims, rushed to his side, but the father died without a word.

Dr. Marion Sims, to whom so many women owed lifelong debts of gratitude, indeed had a fruitful, inspiring career. His first operations on suffering women were performed without benefit either of anesthesia or of antisepsis; yet, within his lifetime he was to add both these boons to mankind—and to womankind—to his operating techniques. Not only are the surgical feats he performed still outstanding; he led pioneers in gynecology to respectability and to recognition on a high plane. He invented new instruments to meet new requirements. He brought to medicine a new concept: hospitals devoted to the special surgical and medical needs of women. Equally important, he carried these bold, brilliant ideas, pioneered in America, back to Europe, and taught Old World physicians how to use them for relief of countless thousands of women world-wide.

WORLD EVENTS AND MEDICAL HISTORY

Dates, persons, and events of significance to the evolution of Medicine include:

1914	Christiansen, Douglas, and Haldane investigated CO_2 carriage by the blood.
1914	Panama Canal opened.
1914	St. Petersburg became Petrograd.
1914	Nobel prize awarded to Robert Bárány for his work on the vestibular apparatus.
1914-18	World War I.
1914-19	E. C. Kendall discovered and investigated thyroxin.
1915	Carrel-Dakin treatment of infected (gunshot) wounds.
1915	Walter Cannon published *Bodily Changes in Pain, Hunger, Fear, and Rage.*
1915	Delousing of troops organized.
1915	Paul Ehrlich died.
1915	Twort reported on bacteriophages.
1915	Preventive inoculation against tetanus in gunshot wounds.
1915	Simmonds described pituitary dwarfism.
1915	Joseph Goldberger demonstrated that pellagra results from nutritional deficiency.
1915-16	Mott *et al.* investigated shell shock.
1916	Bull introduced antitoxin for gas gangrene.
1916	Vitamin B (complex) discovered.
1916	The Johns Hopkins School of Hygiene and Public Health opened.
1917	Ruth Tunnicliff discovered diplococcus in measles.
1917	Wagner von Jauregg treated paresis by superinfection with malarial fever.
1917	Windaus extracted cholesterin (vitamin D) from cod liver oil and formulated it.
1917	Vitamin D reported.
1917-18	American commission investigated trench fever.
1918	Fahraeus introduced erythrocyte sedimentation test.
1918	Ellerman established transmission of leukemia in chickens by virus.
1918-19	Spanish influenza pandemic.
1918-24	Flexner, Amoss, and Webster investigated experimental epidemiology.
1919	Mellanby produced experimental rickets.
1919	Huldschinsky demonstrated antirachitic effect of ultraviolet light.
1919	Huldschinsky demonstrated curative effect of sunlight (quartz lamp) on rickets.
1919	Kolle and Ritz treated experimental (rabbit) syphilis with bismuth.
1919	Dale and Laidlaw investigated histamine shock.
1919	E. Mellanby treated experimental rickets with cod liver oil.
1919	Nobel prize awarded to Bordet for his contributions on immunity.
1920	E. C. Cutler (U.S.) and P. W. Souttar (England) performed heart surgery.
1920	Paul Saxl (Austria) introduced mercurial diuretics for treatment of cardiac edema.
1920	Nobel prize awarded to August Krogh for his discovery of the capillary motor regulator mechanism.
1921	Banting and Best isolated insulin.
1921	A. F. Hess treated rickets by exposure to sunlight.
1921	General use of iodine as an antiseptic (Pregl's solution).
1921	Institut Behring (for Experimental Therapy) at Marburg.
1921-26	R. L. Kahn introduced serum test for syphilis.
1922	Petrograd became Leningrad.
1922	McCollum and Steenbock discovered vitamin D.
1922	Nobel prize awarded to Hill and Meyerhof for discoveries on heat production and metabolism of lactic acid in muscle tissue.
1923	George and Gladys Dick discovered hemolytic streptococcus of scarlatina and devised susceptibility test.
1923	Wilhelm Conrad Röntgen died.
1923	Graham and Cole introduced cholecystography (examination of gallbladder by x-rays).
1923	Nobel prize awarded to Banting and Macleod for insulin research.
1923	Gwathmey introduced synergistic anesthesia.
1924	History of Science Society (United States) founded at Boston.
1924	Nobel prize awarded to Einthoven for his discovery of the mechanism of the electrocardiogram.
1925	Whipple and Robschat-Robbins treated experimental anemia with raw liver.
1925	Sir Henry S. Soutar operated for mitral stenosis.

CLAUDE BERNARD: EXPLORER OF PHYSIOLOGIC FRONTIERS

THE LEADING drama critic of Paris, Sorbonne Professor Saint-Marc Girardin, sighed. He shuffled the neatly written sheets; glanced again at a sentence, long and labored of rhetoric. Slowly he turned, looked up at the tall, slim, handsome Burgundian youth, and said firmly: "You have done some pharmacy. Now, study medicine. You have not the temperament of a dramatist."

In that simple act, Professor Girardin served his country and society far better than he knew. The disappointed literary aspirant heeded his advice: France lost a potential playwright; she gained her greatest nineteenth-century physiologist, Claude Bernard.

Laboratory sciences, and in particlular, experimental physiology, had made little progress before the middle of the nineteenth century. Then they began to flourish, particularly in Germany. Chemistry, physics, and physiology advanced and began to have decisive influence upon the practice of medicine. Up to that time, at best, treatment of the sick was based upon the practitioner's experience. At worst, it was based upon his theories and philosophic imagining.

Among the great contributions to the advance of clinical medicine of the nineteenth century was the brilliant information that came welling out of Bernard's laboratories. Alexis Carrel said of Bernard: "Before him, medicine was purely empirical. He is responsible for the introduction of the scientific method in the art of healing." Bernard's pupil, Paul Bert, wrote: "In twenty years, Claude Bernard found more dominating facts, not only than the few French physiologists working beside him, but than all the physiologists in the world." L. J. Henderson summed up Bernard's philosophy in one sentence: "His life was spent in putting questions to nature."

Claude Bernard's immortality is based upon four major contributions: studies of digestion and of the functions of pancreatic secretion;

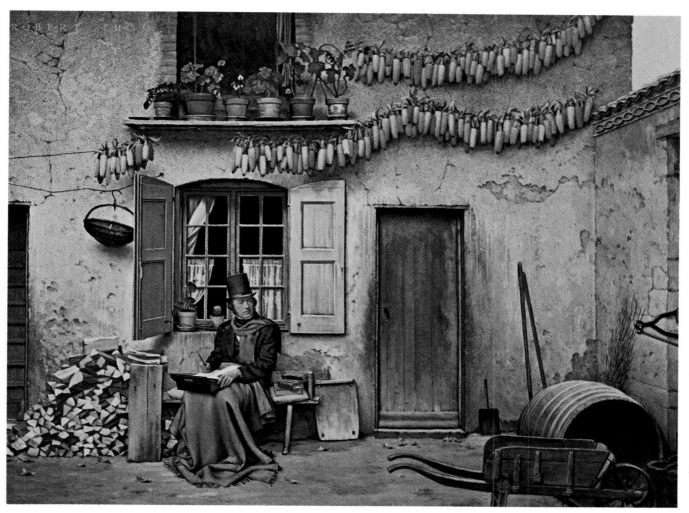

BERNARD: EXPLORER OF PHYSIOLOGIC FRONTIERS

The only place where Claude Bernard (1813-1878) felt at home, outside experimental laboratories, was at the provincial farm near Saint-Julien (Rhône), France, where he was born. Bernard's great skill at dissection and at observation gave medical science benefit of outstanding physiologic discoveries concerning pancreatic secretions, animal sugar, poisons, and vasomotor nerves. He held professorships in physiology at leading Paris schools; he was awarded national and international scientific honors; but his great book, An Introduction to the Study of Experimental Medicine, *was written at his old farm home while he recuperated from recurrent attacks of illness.*

247

discovery of glycogen, and of the glycogenic function of the liver; discovery of the vasomotor nerves and their control of bodily functions; and basic work on poisons (curare in particular) and on their pharmacodynamics. His monumental publication, *An Introduction to the Study of Experimental Medicine*, described many of his important studies. In this book, Bernard defined the relationship between theory and experiment in scientific research; roles of doubt and of intuition; of proof and of counterproof; of statistics and of individualism. His concept of existence of an "internal environment"—those mechanisms by which the several organs within the body are coordinated to permit higher animals to enjoy functional stability—served Bernard well, and still serves researchers, though today more modern terminology is used. Bernard defended the necessity of vivisection and discussed in detail the technicalities of animal experimentation. Clarity and precision in Bernard's descriptions of experimental methods and controls are of such quality that the *Introduction* still is reprinted.

Claude Bernard was born July 12, 1813, in the village of Saint-Julien, near Villefranche, Department of the Rhône, France. His father, Pierre Jean François Bernard, owned a small estate, chiefly planted with grapevines, and derived his income from making wine and from teaching. Educated locally until his eighteenth year, young Claude Bernard then obtained employment in the pharmacy of M. Millet, in Lyons. There his menial duties of sweeping floors and washing bottles were occasionally interrupted by deliveries of drugs to a nearby school of veterinary medicine. His observations there evidently made a profound impression upon the young man and helped to guide him toward his life's work.

His one night off each month, the pharmacist's apprentice spent at the theatre. Young Bernard was inspired to try his own hand at playwriting. The result was a comedy, *La Rose du Rhône*, which is said to have earned its author one hundred francs.

Bernard now began a serious work, a play in five acts, called *Arthur de Bretagne*. Pharmacist Millet decided that the boy had lost interest in his drug store duties and was a dreamer. Bernard's career in pharmacy ended after eighteen months. The play finished, the young man set out in 1834 for "the big city," Paris, to seek recognition and fortune. Gaining an introduction to Professor Girardin, then at the height of his fame as a critic, Bernard presented his play. It was at this time that Girardin gave him discouraging but kindly advice to study medicine—advice which, fortunately, Bernard accepted.

Then twenty-one years of age, Claude Bernard enrolled in the medical school in Paris in the fall of 1834. He achieved no great success as a student; some of his instructors even regarded him as lazy. Anatomy and dissection appealed to him. To add to his meager funds, he entered into partnership with another student, to open a laboratory for animal experimentation. Unfortunately, the laboratory failed; but Bernard's remarkable manual skill became more evident. He taught natural history at a girls' school, and tutored, as means of financing his studies; he passed his examinations to become an *externe* in 1836, and an *interne* in 1839. He followed the services of leading teaching physicians at hospitals in Paris—La Salpêtrière, La Charité, and L'Hôtel-Dieu. At the latter hospital, Bernard came into the service of François Magendie, then France's leading physiologist, Physician at L'Hôtel-Dieu, and Professor of Medicine at the Collège de France. Magendie had a reputation for being gruff, abrupt, and difficult. Before long Bernard's dexterity caught the old professor's attention, and in 1841 he became Magendie's *préparateur*, or laboratory assistant. At first, Bernard's relationship with Magendie was difficult, but once the old professor was convinced of his assistant's ability, their association became cordial, almost filial, and Bernard progressed rapidly along the line for which he was best fitted: experimental physiology. His first paper, published early in 1843, concerned the anatomy of the *chorda tympani* nerve. Later that same year, Bernard undertook investigation of what happens to foodstuffs during digestion. In December, 1843, he presented as his thesis for the doctorate, *The Gastric Juice and its Role in Nutrition*, concerned primarily with digestion of cane sugar.

Completion of work necessary to earn the medical degree did not greatly change Claude Bernard's way of life, except that he abandoned hospitals for the laboratory. He was never to engage in practice. Free to devote himself to his investigations, beginning in 1844, his publications appeared in rapid succession.

The next two decades of Bernard's life were busy productive years. Experimentation continued to hold his greatest interest; he pursued it throughout his life, in private laboratories and in teaching institutions.

Bernard continued to teach; yet teaching was a burden to him. He was appointed Magendie's deputy at the Collège de France in 1847. In this capacity he was required to lecture, in addition to laboratory work; but he was not accorded the rank of Professor of Physiology until after Magendie's death in 1855. Then he was appointed Magendie's successor, in the chair held before him by Laennec. In 1854, Bernard had been named Professor of Physiology at the Sorbonne. He continued to hold both posts until 1868, when, following a favorable interview with Napoleon III, there was created for Bernard a new Chair of General Physiology, and a new laboratory, at the Museum of Natural History. Upon accepting this professorship, Bernard relinquished his chair at the Sorbonne to his former pupil and assistant, Paul Bert.

While Bernard earned respect and admiration for his teaching, results of his experiments and publication of progressive reports of his findings earned for him world-wide distinction. While carrying further his early studies on nutrition and digestion, Bernard explored differences of digestive processes in herbivorous and in carnivorous animals. During these experiments, he observed that ingested fats remained unchanged until they reached the openings of the pancreatic ducts; then they were emulsified and absorbed. This led him to intensive study of pancreatic secretions and their effects. His findings were published in 1846. He was the first scientist to appreciate the importance of internal glandular secretions, and to understand interrelations of organic function.

Another idea current among physiologists of the day was that only plants synthesized sugar, and that animals only broke down sugars to basic elements in metabolism. To study these concepts, Bernard, beginning in 1846, sought to discover in which bodily organ sugars disappeared. His attention was attracted to the liver. Always open-minded, always ready to overthrow theory for fact, Bernard was astounded to realize that, even though animals were fed no sweets, their livers synthesized sugar in a form which he named glycogen. To prove his discovery, in 1848 he demonstrated that alcohol could be formed as a result of fermentation of glycogen. During the next few years, Bernard's progressive series of papers, read before the Académie des Sciences and the Société de Biologie, radically changed the medical world's concepts of organic function.

Concurrently with his studies of the pancreas and of the liver, Bernard began in 1844 to search for mechanisms by which poisons exerted killing power. He was attracted to the South American arrow poison, curare. It was he who gave the world the answer: curare causes death by destroying all motor function without affecting sensation. His description of how the victim, though retaining full consciousness and sensory powers, slowly dies, completely immobile, is chillingly vivid. Bernard published an extensive report on these studies in 1850.

Study of poisons led Bernard also to investigate how carbon monoxide kills; and it was he who found that carbon monoxide combines with hemoglobin more readily than oxygen to lower, even to destroy, the oxygen-carrying power of the blood. This observation also led to development of a method of employing carbon monoxide in measurement of various components of blood.

Another of Bernard's brilliant discoveries was that of existence and function of vasomotor nerves. The whole story of this discovery did not come to light at once. Bernard had started out, in 1851, to study the influence of sympathetic nerves on blood vessels. Results of his experiments were not what he had expected. "Thereupon," he reported, "I did as I always do; that is to say, I at once abandoned theories and hypotheses in order to observe and study the fact itself . . ." In the course of a series of carefully controlled experiments, on which Bernard reported to scientific societies from time to time over a five-year period, he established that two sets of nerves affected blood vessels. One set constricted the vessels; the other set dilated them. By 1858, Bernard had demonstrated positively the existence of the vasomotor nervous system, and importance of its functioning to other physiologic processes.

In 1860, an unidentified chronic illness began to take its toll, handicapping Bernard's efforts. His friends attributed this in part to the miserable conditions in the laboratory provided for him—a dark, damp, cold, ill-ventilated basement room with crude sanitary facilities. By 1862, sickness forced him to leave Paris and to spend two years recuperating at his birthplace near Saint-Julien. His father's vineyards had become his property; and it was to this quiet, rural setting, overlooking the Saône River and the hills beyond, that Bernard returned. Though experimentation could be but rudimentary there, Bernard found time to do something he had been planning for a long time: he began to write the *Introduction* to what he envisioned as a multivolumed work on experimental medicine. Unfortunately, the first volume was the only one he ever wrote; but the impact of *An Introduction to the Study of Experimental Medicine*, when the first edition came off the presses in 1865, was phenomenal. While many of Bernard's reports, lectures, and papers were published, it is the *Introduction* which has kept his name known throughout a century bristling with medical advances. Bernard's younger contemporary and good personal friend, Louis Pasteur, commented thus on the *Introduction:* "Nothing so complete, nothing so profound and so luminous has ever been written on the true principles of the difficult art of experimentation. This book will exert an immense influence on medical science, its teaching, its progress, its language even. I seek in vain for a weak point in M. Bernard. It is not to be found . . ."

Bernard returned to work in Paris late in 1863, but by 1865, he was forced again to return to Saint-Julien, where he remained until 1867. In his later years, Bernard did not launch many entirely new investigations, devoting his attention rather to enlarging upon and further pursuing investigations begun in his earlier years. Results of these he duly reported, in lectures at Collège de France or at the Museum of Natural History, or in papers before various learned societies. More and more of his time in later years was taken up with responsibilities to these societies.

Though Bernard had his opponents and detractors, there was no lack of honors accruing to him in his lifetime. France honored him three times with advancing degrees in the Legion of Honor. In 1854 he was elected to the Académie des Sciences, which he served as president in 1869. He helped form the Société de Biologie in 1848, and became its president for life in 1867. In 1861 he was elected to the Académie de Médecine, and in 1868 to the exclusive French Académie. He also was a founder, in 1872, and the first president of the French

Association for Advancement of Science. Nor was recognition limited to his native land (outside which he never set foot): in 1860 he received the Order of the Polar Star from Sweden and Norway; in 1864 he was named an honorary member in the Royal Society of London, England; in the Academy of Sciences in Berlin; and in the corresponding society in St. Petersburg.

At home, the impression Bernard made upon the Emperor was reflected not only in creation of the chair of physiology at the Museum of Natural History, but also, in 1869, in his elevation to membership in the Senate. This high political honor was to be short-lived, however: the Franco-Prussian War broke out in 1870, and the Senate ended when Napoleon III was captured and the new Republic proclaimed. Bernard retired to Saint-Julien for the balance of the war.

Despite a reserved demeanor, Bernard possessed great personal magnetism. His students loved him, though he had no great gift of oratory. Bernard's close friend, Georges Barral, once described the physiologist thus: "Of solemn aspect, somewhat cold as a professor, somewhat wan in his chair, Claude Bernard showed himself incomparable in the laboratory, before the dissecting table. Standing, his head covered with a large hat under which were escaping long grey locks, his neck wrapped around with an immense muffler, grey and black, which he discarded only during the intense summer heat, he could be seen stooping a little, calmly plunging his fingers into the open abdomen of a dog, explaining the object of his research . . ." Bernard's worth was recognized early in his life by his elders, such as Rayer and Magendie. Friends of his youth, Davaine, Lasègue, and Morel, remained faithful to him after they themselves became famous. Great scientists of his generation, Renan, Berthelot, and Pasteur, admired him. He trained a number of very able and devoted pupils who became great in their own right, including Paul Bert, who succeeded Bernard to the Chair of Physiology at the Sorbonne, and Arsène d'Arsonval, who followed Bernard at Collège de France. Bernard and the younger Pasteur not only were good friends, but at times collaborated; sometimes they worked separately on the same problems—and not always were they in agreement on results. Bernard, however, was chairman of the committee of Académie des Sciences that in 1860 presented the prize for experimental physiology to Pasteur for his work on fermentation. Pasteur's regard for Bernard has already been mentioned. Over the years, the spectacular nature of the younger chemist's work has tended to capture more public interest than the less dramatic but no less important findings of the great physiologist.

The honor in which Bernard was held in scientific circles was not reflected in his home life. He married in 1845; but from the beginning the marriage apparently was doomed by extreme incompatibility. Madame Bernard continually called upon her husband to quit the smelly laboratories and to build up a profitable medical practice: not only was she uninterested in his laboratory pursuits, but she had a horror of vivisection; she sought to make up for her husband's "sins" by contributions to antivivisection societies. Added deep sorrow came to Bernard in that both his sons died in infancy. His daughters were turned against him by their mother. The couple parted in 1869—the year the Emperor named Bernard to the Senate. Formal separation came in 1870. Bernard's last years were lonely, with only his "scientific family" for company in Paris; his sister and his niece, to whom he transferred his affections, frequently visited him at Saint-Julien, where he spent a part of each year tending homely agrarian pursuits.

In 1877, Bernard began his course at Collège de France as usual, He gave his last lecture December 28, after which he had to be helped to his home. On New Year's Day, 1878, he caught cold while making calls, and developed severe pyelonephritis. He died the morning of February 10, 1878, after several weeks of severe pain.

Upon notification of Bernard's death, the Chamber of Deputies of France voted that he be given a state funeral. Bernard thus became, on February 16, 1878, the first scientist to have been accorded such an honor in France.

Bernard's simple but strong feeling about his life's work is reflected in his writings. For example, he opened his course of lectures in 1847 with the remark: "Scientific medicine, gentlemen, which it ought to be my duty to teach here, does not exist." From close to his heart came the observation: "Those who do not know the torment of the unknown cannot have the joy of discovery . . . Even in science itself, the known loses its attraction, while the unknown is always full of charm." For theoretical concept, Bernard had little respect, although he recognized that: "Science goes forward only through new ideas and through creative or original power of thought," and, "Even mistaken hypotheses and theories are of use in leading to discoveries . . . The alchemists founded chemistry by pursuing chimerical problems and theories which are false . . . It seems, indeed, a necessary weakness of our mind to be able to reach truth only across a multitude of errors and obstacles." Yet he was careful to guard against temptations of the speculative method, commenting: "Our ideas are only intellectual instruments which help us to penetrate phenomena. We should drop them when they have served their turn, even as one scraps a bistoury grown rusty from long usage;" and his courage is revealed in the admonition: "When we meet a fact which contradicts a prevailing theory, we must accept the fact and abandon the theory, even when the theory is supported by great names and generally accepted." To his favorite student, Paul Bert, he is said to have remarked: "Put off your imagination as you take off your overcoat, when you enter the laboratory; but put it on again, as you put on your overcoat, when you leave the laboratory."

Research men and women, even today, find solace and comfort in Bernard's philosophy: "One must be brought up in laboratories and live in them," he wrote in his *Introduction*, "to appreciate the full importance of all the details of procedure in investigation, which are so often neglected or despised by the false men of science calling themselves generalizers . . ." and "The whole future of experimental medicine depends on creating a method of research which may be applied fruitfully to the study of vital phenomena, whether in a normal or abnormal state." Perhaps reflecting some less pleasant aspects of his work, he also commented: "If a comparison were required to express my idea of the science of life, I should say that it is a superb and dazzlingly lighted hall which may be reached only by passing through a long and ghastly kitchen."

PASTEUR: THE CHEMIST WHO TRANSFORMED MEDICINE

THE LIFE WORKS of some men seem to have been specially destined as vehicles by which bits of wisdom of the Infinite may be conveyed to waiting mankind. Among those so selected must have been Louis Pasteur. "By the design of his life," wrote Stephen Paget, "he was always being led straight . . . from each discovery to the next . . . he taught the whole world a new way of thinking of the infective diseases, and a new way of dealing with them."

Not only had Pasteur the ability to discover new facts: he knew how to adapt his findings to practical applications, and how to teach and to inspire others. His discoveries live on in the works of men who came after him.

By the middle of the nineteenth century, medical men knew but little more than had their Greek forebears about actual causes of the great scourges of the race—the plagues, the fevers, and the pestilences. At the close of the century, at the end of Pasteur's career, the germ theory had been proved and no longer was seriously contested; the patterns of many infective diseases were understood; methods had been devised for preventing or for combating some of the most serious infections; conditions under which surgical procedures were carried out had been revolutionized; and the sciences of bacteriology and of preventive medicine had been launched. Indeed, within few life spans have such revolutions taken place in medicine; and he who had brought them about was not a physician, but a chemist. His laboratories were not spacious expanses of glass and steel, but miserable garrets; he had not a background of wealth and means, but was the son of a poor tanner.

Louis Pasteur was born December 27, 1822, to Jean-Joseph Pasteur and his wife, Jeanne-Etiennette, in a very modest home adjacent to a tannery, in Dole, Department of Jura, France. He grew up in nearby Arbois, in which city his father set up a tannery in 1827. Louis' preliminary education was in schools in Arbois, and his early inclinations

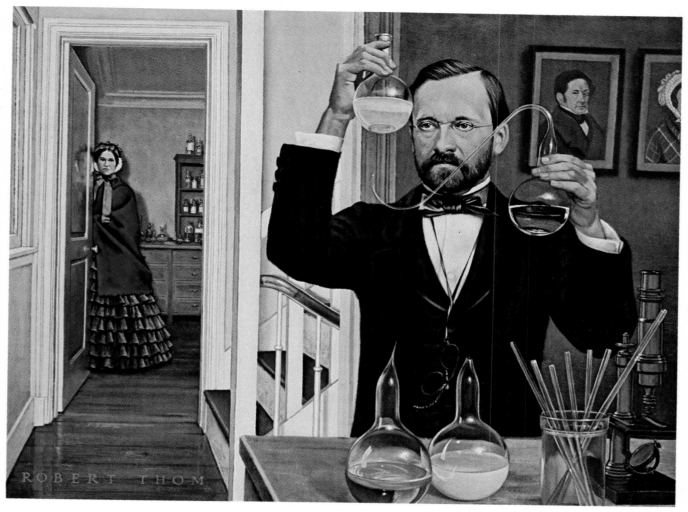

PASTEUR: THE CHEMIST WHO TRANSFORMED MEDICINE

Proof that microbes are reproduced from parent organisms, and do not result from spontaneous generation, came from careful experiments in makeshift laboratories of France's famed chemist and biologist, Louis Pasteur (1822-1895), at the Ecole Normale, Paris. Behind him are portraits of his father and mother, which he painted during his youth. Mme. Pasteur waits patiently for him to complete an observation. From basic work begun in these laboratories came proof of the germ theory of disease, which transformed medical practice; vaccines for virulent diseases, including anthrax and rabies; solution of many industrial biochemical problems; and founding of the Pasteur Institute.

257

were toward art—as is borne out by his youthful paintings of his mother, of his father, and of neighbors. Louis attended the Royal College of Besançon, from which he received his baccalaureate in science in 1842, ironically with a grade of "mediocre" in chemistry. His eyes set upon the goal of the Ecole Normale, Pasteur went to Paris in the fall of 1842, where he tutored to finance his studies until he passed examinations admitting him to the Ecole Normale in October, 1843. Pasteur was appointed assistant to the chemist A. J. Balard at the Ecole Normale, in 1846, and attended courses given by Jean-Baptiste Dumas, then France's most celebrated chemist, at the Sorbonne. In 1847, Pasteur passed his tests in chemistry and in physics, and developed interest in crystallography.

The year 1848 proved to be fateful for Louis Pasteur: he participated in the revolution of that year. Peace restored, he returned to his study of crystals, and, in his twenty-sixth year, achieved his first claim to scientific fame by presenting to the Academy of Sciences his *Report on the Relationship between the Crystalline Form, the Chemical Composition, and the Direction of Rotatory Polarization.* Therein he reported having found that tartaric acid crystallizes in two chemically identical but physically different forms, and that these right-faceted and left-faceted crystals in solution consistently rotate rays passing through a polarimeter to the right, or to the left, in accordance with their physical character. Met with skepticism, Pasteur won attention and friendship from leading French scientists, including Jean-Baptiste Biot, when at their insistence he presented them with carefully worked-out proof. The joy of this initial triumph was marred for Pasteur by the sudden death of his mother, May 21, 1848.

In September, 1848, Pasteur was appointed Professor of Physics at the lyceum (high school) in Dijon, but in December he was offered a collegiate position as Assistant Professor of Chemistry at the Faculty of Sciences in Strasbourg. There he could continue his researches on crystals. There, too, he married, May 29, 1849, Marie Laurent, daughter of the Rector of the college. Marie Pasteur proved to be just the type of wife the scientist needed—she was tolerant of his devotion to research, assisted him with his notes and his records, and looked after his physical well being during an active and hectic career.

Pasteur's teaching career progressed. He was made full Professor of Chemistry at Strasbourg in 1852, and in 1854 he was appointed to the Chair of Chemistry of the Faculty of Sciences in Lille, as well as Dean of the University. His work on crystals had launched a new branch of science, stereochemistry; and in Lille, in the heart of the sugar beet country, Pasteur began his studies on fermentation of sugar to form alcohol. Thus did Pasteur, the chemist, begin transformation to Pasteur, the microbiologist. With the help of his microscope Pasteur found that microorganisms were responsible for alcoholic fermentation; and that faulty fermentation resulted from contamination by unwanted types of organisms.

In October, 1857, Pasteur returned to Paris, having accepted appointments as Administrator of the Ecole Normale and as Director of the Scientific Department of the college. There he sought a place for a laboratory. The only space available was two small rooms in an attic, dark, unsuitable, hot in summer, cold in winter. Nevertheless, Pasteur made the best of them and was able to continue his research. A year later, he moved to a slightly better suite of five narrow rooms. His incubator, installed under a stairway, could be approached only on his knees. Finances for laboratory operation came largely from Pasteur's own pocket. However, as his associate, Emile Duclaux, said in later years, "From this wretched garret, which nowadays would hardly be considered fit for a rabbit's cage, radiated the movement that has revolutionized all aspects of science." In these laboratories Pasteur continued his studies on fermentation, culminating in a paper before the Academy of Sciences in 1859. From alcoholic fermentation Pasteur proceeded to study lactic fermentation; then to butyric fermentation, discovering the difference between aerobic and anaerobic microorganisms. Fermentation studies in these laboratories at the Ecole Normale led to Pasteur's greatest and most revolutionary contributions to science—study and refutation of the theory of spontaneous generation, undisputable proof of the existence of germs, of their modes of reproduction, and of their specificity in causing disease. These studies began in 1860.

Controversy over whether life could form spontaneously out of suitable media, or whether it could only arise from parent organisms, was more than 2,000 years old. Aristotle and Virgil embraced the idea of spontaneous generation, as did Ovid and Pliny. Alchemist Van Helmont in the sixteenth century gave a "formula" for spontaneous production of mice. The Italian, Redi, proved that maggots hatched from flies' eggs and could not arise spontaneously from putrid meat. About the middle of the eighteenth century, two priests, the Italian Spallanzani, and the Englishman Needham, entered into acrimonious and inconclusive controversy on the subject.

Of not so ancient origin, but no less controversial, was the related "germ theory"—the idea that diseases were caused by outside infective organisms, rather than by humors, miasmas, and other vague factors. Paracelsus (1493-1541) had conjectured that disease might arise from "seeds" in the air. Girolamo Fracastoro (Fracastorius) in 1546 published *De Contagione*, concluding that epidemic diseases were produced by imperceptible "seminaria" or seeds, which had the power to multiply in the body of the patient. Carl von Linné (Linnaeus) in his doctoral thesis at Hardewyck, Holland, in 1753, mentioned "argillaceous particles" as possible explanation for certain recurrent fevers.

Pasteur's contemporary and adversary, F. A. Pouchet, Director of the Natural History Museum in Rouen, and a highly vocal advocate of spontaneous generation, perhaps furnished the spark that ignited Pasteur's interest in the subject when, in 1858, he sent to the Academy of Sciences a *Note on Vegetable and Animal Proto-organisms Spontaneously Generated in Artificial Air and in Oxygen Gas*. Pasteur's copy of this paper bears underlining of passages he likely intended to submit to experimentation.

Pasteur began with study of atmospheric air. His microscope confirmed his belief that germs floated in it. The next question was: Do germs enter putrescible substances due to exposure to air, or are they generated within the substance? Pasteur conducted exhaustive experiments, in the laboratory, on mountain tops, and under every conceivable condition. When his flasks were heated to boiling and sealed to air, no growths appeared. When opened in the laboratory, contamination followed. Flasks opened, exposed, and resealed in comparatively pure air of mountain heights remained clear. When reopened at lower levels, growths appeared. But Pouchet and other supporters of spontaneous generation dogged Pasteur with denunciation, with derision, and with purported contrary evidence.

Pasteur's most spectacular demonstrations were made with his swan's neck flasks. Broth was placed in the flask, the neck of which was heated and drawn out to form a lazy ∽, the swan's neck shape. When the broth in the flask was heated to boiling, air was forced out; on cooling, air pressure outside forced air to re-enter the flask. Due to the lazy ∽ shape of the small tubular neck, if entering air were permitted to flow into the flask slowly, air-borne particles would fall by gravity to the surface of the lower curve of the neck, and, as long as the flask was not tipped or agitated, no microbial growth occurred. If, however, the flask were tilted until broth touched the lower curve of the neck, or, if air were drawn in rapidly by violent agitation, growth appeared.

Pasteur summed up his findings in a treatise entitled: *Organized Corpuscles Existing in Atmosphere*, for which the Academy of Sciences awarded him a prize. But, to clarify his position and to confound his opponents, Pasteur requested that a commission be appointed to settle the debates. Interest in the dispute had reached far beyond the walls of the Academy, however; and on April 7, 1864, Pasteur held a symposium on spontaneous generation, at the Sorbonne, before a large audience which included leading scientists of the day. After describing his experiments in detail, Pasteur summed up his findings with these words:

"There is now no circumstance known in which it can be confirmed that microscopic beings have come into the world without germs, without parents similar to themselves. Those who maintain this view are the victims of illusions, of ill-conducted experiments, blighted with errors that they have either been unable to perceive or unable to avoid."

Thus was spontaneous generation laid to rest and the "germ theory" officially introduced to science. A year later, in 1865, medicine was to receive its first dividend from Pasteur's work: Joseph Lister, surgeon of Glasgow, Scotland, seeking to apply in practice Pasteur's findings, used carbolic acid to disinfect the wound of a compound fracture in a patient at the Glasgow Infirmary, and introduced the era of antisepsis in surgery. Detractors were long-lived, however, in Pasteur's own country and elsewhere. As late as 1886, Morris Longstreth, M.D., of Philadelphia, Pennsylvania, published a serious, 16-page dissertation "Against the Germ Theory of Disease," in *The Therapeutic Gazette*.

Important as they were, Pasteur's experiments concerning spontaneous generation and controversies with Pouchet did not occupy all of his time: he introduced the autoclave to kill hardy germs and spores; he applied his growing knowledge of microbes to problems of fermentation; in 1861, he showed Orleans vinegar manufacturers how to improve their yield. From vinegar, he turned to the study of wines. He demonstrated that proper fermentation resulted from action of airborne wild yeasts deposited on ripening fruit; and that "diseases" of wines, affecting both their flavor and their keeping qualities, resulted from other parasitic germs either having fallen on the fruit, or having been introduced into the vats or presses. From these studies arose Pasteur's suggestion that vintners might protect their product, without injury, by heating bottled wine for several minutes at 55 C. (131 F.). Thus was the process, now called pasteurization, introduced. Importance of its subsequent application, in fields of public health and of food preservation, are well known. Pasteur's wine studies were summed up in his book, *Wine and Its Maladies*, published in 1866.

In 1862, Pasteur won coveted election to membership in the Academy of Sciences. In 1863, he read to that society another paper of major importance, wherein he dealt with the mechanism of the cycle of life and of death. He proved that when organic matter decomposes, aerobic microorganisms on the surface cause oxidation or combustion, while anaerobic germs, inside, produce putrefaction. Thus, "life presides at the labor of death," death itself being a manifestation of life. Dead things, he pointed out, would remain indestructible without work done by microbes; yet life would no longer be possible were not elements of biologic forms which have ceased to live returned to the air and to the earth.

Pasteur accepted a professorship at the School of Fine Arts in 1863, in addition to his work at Ecole Normale. The triumphs of this active period of his life were marred by deaths of his father, in 1865, and of three of his daughters: Jeanne, in 1859; Camille, in 1865; and Cécile, in 1866. Only his son, Jean-Baptiste, born in 1851, and his daughter, Marie-Louise, born in 1858, survived. In later years, the son entered government service; and Marie married a young secretary, René Vallery-Radot, who became his confidant and biographer, and, in Pasteur's old age, his constant attendant. A grandson, Pasteur Vallery-Radot, became Professor of Medicine at the University of Paris in 1929, and continued biographic work on his famed grandfather.

In 1865, at the insistence of the French Senate, Pasteur undertook studies of two diseases that were responsible for devastation of the nation's silk industry: silkworms were affected, sometimes by *pébrine*, sometimes by *flacherie*, sometimes by both. Silkworm farmers were threatened with economic ruin. Pasteur, who until then had never handled a silkworm, set to work with his microscope. He soon discovered the causative agents, devised means of detecting them, and measures for eliminating passage of these parasitic diseases from one generation of worms to the next. Again, Pasteur's work met with great resistance and opposition—but he persisted; and acceptance of his methods saved the silk industry, not only in France, but also in Austria, in Italy, and in Asia Minor.

More troubles were in store for Pasteur. In 1867, a series of disturbing incidents at the Ecole Normale resulted in Pasteur's being relieved of administrative duties. He accepted a chair at the Sorbonne, and a laboratory for physiologic chemistry was built for him at the direction of Napoleon III. In 1868, Pasteur suffered a stroke, which seriously threatened his life and resulted in partial paralysis of his left arm and leg. About the time his work on silkworms was completed, in 1870, the Franco-Prussian War broke out. Not only was Pasteur's work disrupted; he faced dual concern for the welfare of his country and for that of his only son, then serving in the military.

Pasteur always sought to test on a large scale those phenomena which he had observed in the laboratory. "Pure science, on its highest level," he wrote, "cannot advance one step without sooner or later bringing profit to industry from the application of its precious results." He had demonstrated this in his work with problems of the vinegar, the wine, and the silk industries. He demonstrated it again when, called upon for help by the brewing industry, he convinced brewers of the value of the microscope as a working tool; of the necessity for assuring purity of yeast cultures; and of the feasibility of applying heat (pasteurization) to preserve the quality of beer. Another book, *Studies on Beer. Its Diseases and their Causes. Method of Making it Unchangeable*, summed up these studies.

Election of Pasteur (by a margin of one vote) to membership in the Academy of Medicine, in 1873, was a great tribute to the chemist. It brought him into close contact with his friend, Claude Bernard. It also precipitated an almost endless fight with official medicine. Having in mind Lister's work, stemming from his own, Pasteur, in 1874, startled his medical colleagues by stating: "If I had the honor of being a surgeon, I would never introduce into the human body an instrument without having passed it through boiling water or, better still, through a flame and rapidly cooled right before the operation."

In 1874, too, Pasteur was forced by health to give up his chair at the Sorbonne. He also received from the National Assembly an award in the form of a life pension.

Though Pasteur already had made many important and basic discoveries, the years 1877 to 1886 were filled with new discoveries of great significance to medicine and to science. Studies on anthrax in livestock proved both that an aerobic spore-forming bacterium is its cause, and that germs cause disease. Further work demonstrated that other germs cause furunculosis (boils) and puerperal (childbed) fever in new mothers. These findings demonstrated—despite constant attacks from opponents—the importance of measures to prevent infection and to avoid contagion. However, it was during his work on chicken cholera, in 1879, that a laboratory "accident" led Pasteur to discover methods of attenuating bacterial cultures, of decreasing and of increasing their toxic attributes, at will, and of taming dangerous microbes so that they might be changed from killers to benefactors—thereby to pave the way for development of vaccines and of antitoxins. In 1881, in the face of opposition from Professor Colin of the Veterinary School at

Alfort, Pasteur conducted a field trial at Melun: 25 sheep were vaccinated against anthrax, and 25 were used as controls. One month later, each of the 50 sheep was inoculated with material from a culture of a strain of potent anthrax bacilli. Two days thereafter, all 25 unvaccinated sheep were dead or dying; all 25 vaccinated animals were alive and healthy. These results had tremendous repercussions in the scientific world; and, generally, Pasteur's authority was now firmly established. Election to membership in the Académie Française followed, in 1882.

With the collaboration of his former pupil, Emile Roux, Pasteur in 1880 began the study of rabies (hydrophobia), a dreaded infection that was always fatal to man and to animals. Terror reigned when rabid dogs or other animals were discovered, for it was well known that prolonged, agonized illness leading to death frequently followed vicious bites characteristic of these animals' attacks. Pasteur set out to see what could be done to combat rabies.

By 1884, Pasteur had not only developed a method of vaccinating dogs to render them immune to rabies; he had also developed a vaccine against swine erysipelas, and had supervised an expedition to Egypt to study a local outbreak of cholera.

Pasteur did not consider the rabies problem solved by vaccine alone. Inability to discover the causative microbe (later found to be a submicroscopic virus) handicapped him; however, he did discover the most virulent source of infective material: the medulla oblongata, or lowermost portion of the brain. Also, Pasteur found that by drying the cord aseptically, the virulence of the causative factor of rabies decreased to the point of avirulence in 14 days. Since the incubation period (from time of the bite to onset of disease) for rabies was several weeks, Pasteur found that he could successfully treat an animal, already bitten by a rabid animal, if treatment were begun within a few days after the injury. Treatment consisted of injecting daily an emulsion of cord, beginning with the least virulent material (dried for 14 days) and progressing to the most virulent (dried for 1 or 2 days). Thus, rabies could be prevented and lives saved. These experiments on animals were repeated and repeated; but Pasteur hesitated to try his method on humans.

Fate precipitated the crucial experiment: a provincial mother appeared at the laboratories with her nine-year-old son, Joseph Meister. The boy had been bitten fourteen times, two days before, by a dog declared rabid. The age of the child, plus the severity of his wounds, made it seem inevitable that he would develop rabies and die. The mother's imploring, the family doctor's urging, and the favorable consensus of his scientific colleagues persuaded Pasteur to try his vaccine on the boy. A physician began treatment, July 7, 1885—first, administering a dose of the weakest, then, progressively, doses of more virulent emulsions of infected cord. Pasteur anxiously watched for signs of reaction; but the boy stood the test, far better than the scientist. (In later years, Joseph Meister was to join the staff of the Pasteur Institute.) A few weeks later, Pasteur presented to the Academy of Sciences his famous report: *Method of Preventing Rabies After a Bite*. Publication of this report brought pilgrims to his laboratory for rabies treatment— some patients coming from as far away as New York. On March 1, 1886, Pasteur submitted to the Academy of Sciences his further report: Of 350 persons who had received treatment following bites of rabid animals, there had been but one death—a girl brought to him thirty-seven days after she had been bitten by a rabid animal.

Physicians and scientists from all over the world now flocked to Pasteur's laboratories to learn firsthand about prophylactic treatment against rabies, and about other Pasteurian doctrines which were rapidly revolutionizing the practice of medicine. Along with these ovations came waves of criticism from die-hard opponents and from sensational journalists. At the same time, a movement was launched to finance construction and operation of a Pasteur Institute, in which the scientist's work and that of his associates could be furthered.

The excitement and labor of this period proved too much for the ageing man: in November, 1886, he developed symptoms of coronary insufficiency. However, with the help of Madame Pasteur and his loyal son-in-law, René Vallery-Radot, Pasteur was enabled to supervise the ever-widening scope of work of his associates. On November 14, 1888, the Institute that bears his name was dedicated. The good work went forward: Roux and Yersin developed diphtheria toxin from filtrates of cultures of the bacillus, and this led to discovery of diphtheria antitoxin by Behring in Germany. Roux then developed serotherapy for tetanus; Calmette, serotherapy for snake bites, and Metchnikoff established existence and action of phagocytes in the blood, and carried out basic studies on syphilis.

Pasteur's seventieth birthday, December 27, 1892, was occasion for an ovation at the Sorbonne, attended by scientists and political figures from all over the world. Lister paid the tribute: "Pasteur has lifted the veil that for centuries has hidden the infectious diseases." At the end of the ceremonies, Pasteur, too moved to speak, asked his son to read his acknowledgment.

The great scientist's health steadily declined, limiting him to occasional observance of work in the laboratories and to visits from members of his devoted staff. After a series of cerebrovascular accidents, death came to Pasteur, September 28, 1895.

The government of France arranged an imposing state funeral for its great citizen, and Pasteur's body was interred in a marble crypt in a small chapel within the Institute. On its walls may be seen mosaics and plaques alluding to his work; and most impressive is the imposing list of the areas in which Pasteur's principal discoveries were made: *1848, Molecular Asymmetry; 1857, Fermentations; 1862, Spontaneous Generation; 1863, Studies On Wine; 1865, Diseases of Silkworms; 1871, Studies on Beer; 1877, Virulent Diseases; 1880, Virus Vaccines;* and, *1885, Prophylaxis of Rabies.*

LISTER INTRODUCES ANTISEPSIS

Surgery, at the beginning of the nineteenth century, had progressed scientifically little beyond the point at which Ambroise Paré had left it two centuries before. A good surgeon was he who could operate fast, could be oblivious to the patient's agonized screams of pain, and could retain hope that the patient might survive inevitable postsurgical "hospitalism." This term applied to a variety of septic infections virtually endemic in patients in hospital wards. "Hospitalism" was fatal to about one of three surgical patients. To commit surgical patients to hospitals came to be regarded as almost tantamount to signing their death certificates in advance.

Discovery of the principle of anesthesia in 1846 effected the first great change in surgical procedure. Anesthesia removed blind fear and invoked blessed insensibility for patients during operations. Anesthesia did away with the necessity for utmost speed, making possible more careful, finished surgical techniques; and making feasible surgical procedures that previously had been regarded as beyond physical endurance. Anesthesia quieted the unnerving, heart-rending screams associated with the operating theatre, relieving surgical practice of one of its least attractive aspects.

As anesthesia encouraged surgeons to widen application of their ministrations to human ills, deaths from infectious diseases, especially in crowded and none too clean hospital wards, increased apace. Suppuration in wounds was so common that it became accepted as normal: medical men discoursed learnedly about "laudable pus" and its absence was looked upon with alarm. Pyemia, septicemia, tetanus, erysipelas, puerperal fever, and hospital gangrene were the great hazards faced by surgical and obstetric patients. The situation became so alarming that some hospitals were closed; some were torn down and rebuilt on the theory that these affections arose from something unknown that emanated from the physical structures. For surgeons to operate on the surface of the body, or to amputate, though within range of surgical ability and of patients' endurance, was to court great postoperative danger to life. To treat patients for compound fractures by

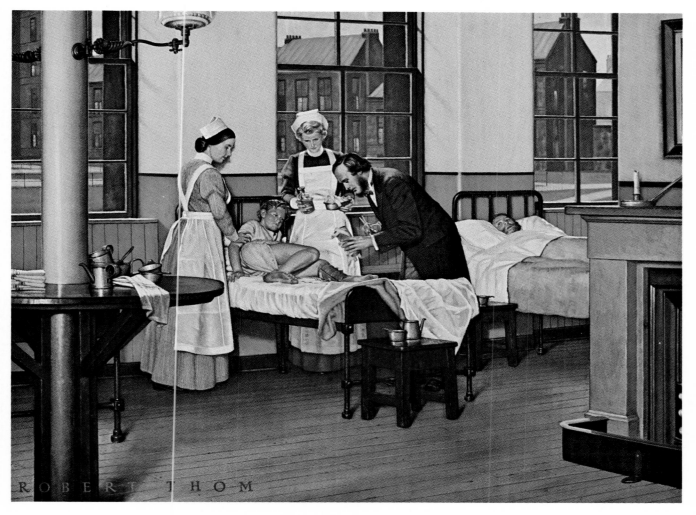

ROBERT THOM

LISTER INTRODUCES ANTISEPSIS

When Surgeon Joseph Lister (1827-1912) of Glasgow Royal Infirmary removed dress-ings from James Greenlees' compound fracture, he found the wound had healed without infection—something unheard of before. For six weeks, beginning August 12, 1865, Lister had treated the boy's wound with carbolic acid. Now, Lister had proof of success of his principle of antisepsis—which was to revolutionize methods of treatment and to open new vistas in practice of surgery, of medicine, and of environmental sanitation. Hospitals were turned from "houses of torture and death" to "houses of healing and cure." In 1897, Lister became the first British surgeon to be elevated to peerage.

269

methods other than amputation was negligence; to amputate was to take a fifty-fifty chance with patients' lives. To open the abdomen, or the chest, or the skull, was unthinkable. Ovariotomy was the one exception.

Such was the course of surgical practice until Joseph Lister introduced antiseptics in treatment of wounds and in operations. Though Lister's methods were slow to be accepted, surgery began to embrace this second great change in the final quarter of the nineteenth century. Risks to patients' lives were reduced markedly. By combining advantages of anesthesia with antisepsis, and, later, with asepsis, surgeons were able to carry out operative procedures far beyond the realm of pre-Listerian imagination. That pioneering, that pushing into new areas of surgical practices for relief of human disorders, has continued to accelerate during the decades that have elapsed.

To Joseph Lister, surgery and medicine owe a great debt of gratitude for having patiently and scientifically introduced the age of antisepsis. In turn, Lister freely acknowledged his indebtedness to earlier workers, and especially to Louis Pasteur. Douglas Guthrie summed it up well: "Standing on the shoulders of his predecessors, he beheld something that was invisible to them."

Joseph Lister was born April 5, 1827, at Upton, Essex, England, the fourth child and second son of Joseph Jackson Lister. The family had a comfortable income from the wine business, and the elder Lister had time to pursue his favorite hobby, microscopy. His discoveries for improving the microscope gained for him a Fellowship in the Royal Society in 1832. Joseph Lister was raised in quiet Quaker family surroundings. Undoubtedly, his father's scientific interests contributed to the boy's early decision that surgery should be his life's work. Joseph Lister received the degree of Bachelor of Arts from London's University College in 1847, and continued his studies in medicine at the same institution. There, Lister had opportunity to observe, on December 21, 1846, the first operation performed in Great Britain with the aid of ether anesthesia by the famous surgeon, Robert Liston.

In 1852, Lister obtained the Bachelor of Medicine degree from University College, and Fellowship in the Royal College of Surgeons of England. In this year, too, his first original work, "On the Contractile

270

Tissue of the Iris," appeared in the *Quarterly Journal of Microscopical Science*, followed a few months later by another, "The Muscular Tissue of the Skin." His familiarity with microscopes served him well.

In September, 1853, with a letter of introduction from a former teacher, Lister called upon James Syme, who was Professor of Clinical Surgery in the Medical School of the University of Edinburgh, Scotland. The visit to Edinburgh was to have been one of a series to medical centers, but Syme was immediately attracted to the enthusiastic young surgeon and persuaded Lister to stay on as clerk, and, shortly thereafter, as resident house surgeon in Syme's wards in the Old Royal Infirmary of Edinburgh. Within a short time, Lister became affectionately known as "The Chief" among students; and Syme was known as "The Master."

Within a year after Lister's arrival in Edinburgh, a series of circumstances created vacancies, not only at the Infirmary, but on the teaching staff of the Royal College of Surgeons of Edinburgh. Persuaded to take these appointments, Lister began his teaching career, and opened an office for consultation practice.

By 1856, Lister had been appointed Assistant Surgeon at the Royal Infirmary. In that year, too, he married Agnes Syme, the Professor's daughter. She proved to be an ideal wife, helpmate, and companion for the busy teacher, researcher, and surgeon. Though the Listers had no children, theirs was a long, happy life of sharing work and leisure.

In his prime, Lister was described as nearly six feet in height, upright, well knit, compactly built, deep chested. He wore the so-called "mutton-chops" sideburns, shaving his face and chin. His bearing was dignified and his manner always restrained; he was ever kindly and considerate; his voice was soft and musical. He wore a black frock coat with a waistcoat of the Victorian type, and a chimney-pot silk hat of the period. He was invariably courteous and polite; but not a "good mixer." Generally he was serious and somewhat formal. He never scolded assistants, but gently made any correction that was required. Usually in operating he was slow and deliberate, but when occasion demanded, he showed that his dexterity was equal to that of other surgeons.

At about this time, Lister is credited with having invented several ingenious surgical instruments, including: a needle for silver wire used as suture material; a hook for removing foreign bodies from the ear;

forceps for use in sinuses; blunt-pointed bandage scissors; and a screw tourniquet for compressing the abdominal aorta. Some instruments associated with his name are used by surgeons even today.

Opportunity again knocked at Lister's door when the Professorship in Surgery at Glasgow University was vacated. He was the successful one among seven applicants for the appointment. He took over his new post March 9, 1860. The teaching position did not include a hospital appointment, and another year elapsed before Lister was placed in charge of wards at the Glasgow Royal Infirmary.

It was at the Glasgow Royal Infirmary that Lister was to make his most important studies. Along with teaching and clinical duties, Lister, appalled by conditions and sufferings of patients in surgical wards, began studies on the cause of inflammation. The first changes he made —introduction of ordinary cleanliness and of liberal use of soap and water—met with resistance; but the quiet, mild Quaker got his way. Then, seeking to reduce suppuration, he began study of various methods of wound treatment—open, closed, water dressings, poultices, irrigations, collodion—all to little avail. Suppuration defeated each method. In an early paper, he attributed hospital gangrene to the "impure state of the atmosphere produced by overcrowding of patients with decomposing sores," and later he wrote that the essential cause of suppuration is decomposition. Certain questions kept recurring to him: Why does a simple fracture heal and a compound fracture prove almost always fatal? Why is mortality greater among patients in hospitals than among those in private homes? Why must there be suppuration?

Publication of Pasteur's work on fermentation and on decomposition, demonstrating that these processes are due to living organisms, provided Lister with his essential clue. He repeated some of Pasteur's experiments. He experimented further with prevention of putrefaction of blood. He satisfied himself that Pasteur was indeed right: it was not air, but something in the air, which produced fermentation. Was it not likely that these minute organisms, these germs, were the cause of putrefaction in wounds? If living organisms cause suppuration, then a way must be found to kill them in the wound, or better still, to keep them out of it. Lister knew that heat would kill germs—and kill living cells, too; filtering could remove germs—but how could it be done practically? He knew, too, that some chemicals destroy germs. This approach seemed most logical. "It appears," Lister wrote in the *Lancet*, "that all that is requisite is to dress the wound with some material capable of killing these septic germs, provided that any substance can be found reliable for the purpose, yet not too potent as a caustic."

Lister had been intrigued by an account of effects produced by carbolic acid upon sewage from the town of Carlisle, and it occurred to him that this antiseptic might be used in treatment for compound fractures. First samples, in the form of crude creosotes, were unsatisfactory; but Lister was happy to find that purified crystalline phenol was miscible with water, and that addition of a small amount of water caused the substance to remain in liquid state. It proved to have local sedative qualities, and, reacting with blood, formed a hard, tenacious, protective crust. Lister's first trial was a failure, but he attributed that to improper management.

On August 12, 1865, James Greenlees, a boy aged eleven years, was admitted to one of Lister's wards in Glasgow Royal Infirmary, with a compound fracture of his left lower leg. The wound was about one and one-half inches long, and three quarters of an inch wide. Little bleeding had occurred.

Lister treated the wound first by thorough application of carbolic acid, then dressed it with lint and cloth soaked in the solution. The dressing was covered with tin foil to prevent evaporation, and the leg splinted. Dressings saturated with carbolic acid in water, or in oil, were continued. In six weeks, the bones had united, and two days thereafter the wound was found to be entirely healed. Lister reported modestly: "The remarkable retardation of suppuration, and the immediate conversion of the compound fracture into a simple fracture with a superficial sore, were most encouraging facts."

Ironically, Ignaz Semmelweis, who had blindly sought to apply antiseptic principles to obstetric and to surgical procedures in hospitals in Vienna and in Budapest, died of septicemia, August 13, 1865—the day after Lister began his first successful antiseptic treatment for a wound. At the time, Lister had not heard of Semmelweis. In later years,

Lister's writings generously accorded the Hungarian physician credit for his earlier work.

By 1867, Lister was able to report on a series of eleven patients treated for compound fractures, all but two of whom regained use of their limbs. One man, during Lister's absence, had to have an amputation, after which he recovered. Another, though he progressed satisfactorily at first, died of hemorrhage caused by perforation of an artery by a fragment of bone.

Lister began to apply his antiseptic principle to treatment for ordinary wounds, and for carbuncles, for boils, for whitlows, and for acute abscesses. Results were equally remarkable. In 1867, Lister published a series of reports in the *Lancet* entitled, "Papers on a New Method of Treating Compound Fracture, Abscess, etc., With Observations on the Condition of Suppuration." To the Surgical Section of the British Medical Association, meeting in Dublin the same year, Lister reported more fully "On the Antiseptic Principle of the Practice of Surgery." In this he made the remarkable observation:

"Previous to its (the antiseptic method) introduction the two large wards in which most of my cases of accident and of operation are treated were among the unhealthiest in the whole surgical division of the Royal Glasgow Infirmary . . . But since the antiseptic treatment has been brought into full operation, and wounds and abscesses no longer poison the atmosphere with putrid exhalations, my wards, though in other respects under precisely the same circumstances as before, have completely changed their character; so that during the last nine months not a single instance of pyemia, hospital gangrene, or erysipelas has occurred in them."

Soon convinced that pure carbolic acid was too strong, Lister experimented with dilutions. He found 1:20 to 1:40 solutions in water, and 1:4 solutions in oil, satisfactory. He experimented also with various other formulations, such as paste, putty, and solid dressings; and with other antiseptics, ranging from bichloride of mercury (corrosive sublimate) to boric acid.

Lister, observing that suppuration took place around sutures in wounds despite antiseptic procedure, next turned his attention to suture material. Customarily, surgeons had carried silk suture threads in coat lapel buttonholes for convenience. Lister experimented on animals, and found that silk sutures soaked in antiseptic could be left in wounds without suppuration. Further, he experimented with suture material from animal sources, developing sterile "catgut" sutures (made from sheep's intestine). He proved that they are superior, in some respects, to silk, and that they are absorbed, *in situ.*

New events were to change the course of Lister's life. His father-in-law, Professor Syme, became ill and the Chair of Clinical Surgery at the University of Edinburgh became vacant. Lister was elected to the post, and returned to Edinburgh in October, 1869. Professor Syme died the following June.

In Edinburgh, Lister had more free time, so his experiments continued. His microscope was an invaluable aid; and with it he learned many new things about germs. Although he never wrote a book, Lister continued to teach and to write about his findings for medical journals. Typically, his views were accepted more readily by Continental surgeons than by British. Though his students loved him and put his methods into practice, most British surgeons of Lister's generation were apathetic, indifferent, or antagonistic toward his concept of antisepsis.

Undiscouraged, Lister calmly forged ahead. He began to apply the antiseptic technique to surgical wounds. Operators and assistants were directed to scrub their hands with soap and water, then dip them frequently in carbolic acid solution. Instruments were immersed in carbolic acid solution for twenty minutes before use. The skin of the field of operation was scrubbed with soap and water and with carbolic acid solution, and towels wrung out in the solution were used to surround the operative site. In addition to these precautions, Lister was concerned about germs floating in the air. Seeking a remedy, he developed the spray technique: carbolic acid 1:100 was placed in a sprayer and disseminated as vapor in the operating room. Early hand-operated sprays soon gave way to steam sprays. Needless to say, a cloud of carbolic vapor created difficulties for patients, for surgeons, and for assistants; but operations could now be undertaken that previously had not been thought possible. Lister reported on use of this spray method to the British Medical Association in 1871, and continued the spray technique in his operating rooms until 1887, after which time he concluded that, with proper aseptic procedures, surgeons could dispense with the irritating cloud of phenolic vapor.

Lister's star continued to rise. He was called to treat Queen Victoria for an abscess. He became a friend of Pasteur, and was instrumental in smoothing out differences that threatened to become acrimonious between Pasteur and the rapidly rising young German scientist, Robert Koch, who had proved that each infectious disease is the product of a particular microorganism; and whose work had given medicine the new science of bacteriology.

In 1877, Lister was invited to take the Chair of Surgery at King's College Hospital, in London. While Lister was happy in Edinburgh, where his classes were large and well attended, he decided to accept the London position. London physicians had been particularly cold to his concept of antisepsis and he hoped to convince them by working among them. His was a hard task. He acquired only a small personal practice in London, though patients were sent to him from all over the world. His classes were small and poorly attended. Hospital staff members resented his procedures. He accepted patients given up by other surgeons, operated aseptically with success, and saw them restored to health. At the International Congress of Medical Science in Amsterdam in 1879, Lister was acclaimed with enthusiasm by surgeons from all over the world; but it took ten years of patient, brilliant work for Lister to win over his colleagues in London. Meanwhile, his antiseptic technique was developed into aseptic technique by surgeons in Germany and in France, during the 1880's.

In his later years, Lister was showered with honors. His visits to Continental Europe were like triumphal marches. He received numerous degrees from universities and honors from nations. He was made surgeon-in-ordinary to Queen Victoria in 1878; made a baronet in 1883; elected Foreign Secretary to the Royal Society in 1893; and created a peer by Queen Victoria in 1897—the first medical man to have been thus honored in Britain. He participated actively in the celebration of Pasteur's seventieth birthday at the Sorbonne in Paris in 1892. He visited the United States of America in 1876. As an indirect result of Americans' acceptance of his doctrine, rubber gloves were first used as a requisite to asepsis in surgery by Professor William Stewart Halsted of Johns Hopkins University School of Medicine and Johns Hopkins Hospital in Baltimore, about 1890.

Lord Lister's triumphs in his later years were clouded by the loss of Lady Lister, who died suddenly in 1893. Lister had held his teaching position at King's College for fifteen years. The next twelve years were spent largely in traveling, in lecturing, and in writing. Then, in 1903, he saw the Lister Institute of Preventive Medicine open its doors. The same year, however, brought illness that curtailed his activities. His eightieth birthday, April 5, 1907, was occasion for widespread acknowledgment. Lister was deeply moved, commenting: "What a change of opinion has taken place during the years in which I have been doing nothing."

Though physically frail, Lister's mind continued active. His last publication, on improved catgut ligatures, was published in *Lancet* and in the *British Medical Journal* in 1909. Cared for by his wife's sister, Lucy Syme, he lived out his last years at the seaside town of Walmer, in Kent. There he passed away quietly, February 10, 1912.

How Lister's work has served medicine and has benefited the public has been told many times. Dr. Irving I. Edgar summed it up well in a recent article: "Preventive medicine," wrote Edgar, "really began when Lister introduced his great principles . . . The treatment of our water supply, the preservation of foods, and numerous other important procedures all draw upon the principles of antisepsis . . . Lister raised surgery from a lottery, a game of chance and a craft, to a safe scientific art and science . . . He removed the obstacle limiting surgery to a small sphere of application and made only the skill and dexterity of the surgeon its real limits . . . The present hospital system exists because of Lister, for without antisepsis hospitals were houses of torture and death . . . Lord Lister's discoveries . . . gave hospitals all over the world a new lease on life, making them houses of healing and cure."

CHARCOT
MASTER OF NEUROLOGY

ON THE LEFT BANK of the Seine, in Paris, not far from the Gare d'Orléans, there stands a large and venerable group of buildings on spacious grounds: the Salpêtrière. Some of its structures are centuries old; they have witnessed many stresses during French history, and have served Paris in many ways. They have experienced periods of intense activity, and of neglect. Their uses have been sometimes glorious, sometimes ignominious. Once far out on the outskirts of the city, the Salpêtrière today is within the heart of France's capital city and is one of the city's largest and most respected hospitals.

The Salpêtrière had its beginning when the French ruler, Louis XIII (1610-1643) ordered construction of a little Arsenal on the remote site, so that citizens of Paris might be spared the danger of storage of explosives near their homes. Some time later, the Little Arsenal was abandoned, and the buildings fell into disrepair.

Toward the middle of the seventeenth century, Paris was plagued with an influx of thousands of persons rendered destitute by a series of intermittent civil wars, and with an alarming rise in acts of crime and violence. The President of the Parliament placed the buildings of the Salpêtrière at the disposal of Vincent de Paul, a priest noted for organization of charitable movements. It became, along with the Bicêtre, a part of the Hospice Général, for housing of indigents. In 1656, by royal decree, the Salpêtrière became a place for confinement of insane women and beggers. Soon, arrests built its population to overflowing, and new buildings had to be constructed. During the seventeenth and eighteenth centuries, the Salpêtrière was the largest asylum in Europe, having from 5,000 to 8,000 inhabitants. Primitive, unsanitary cells in a section called "les Loges des Folles" were reserved

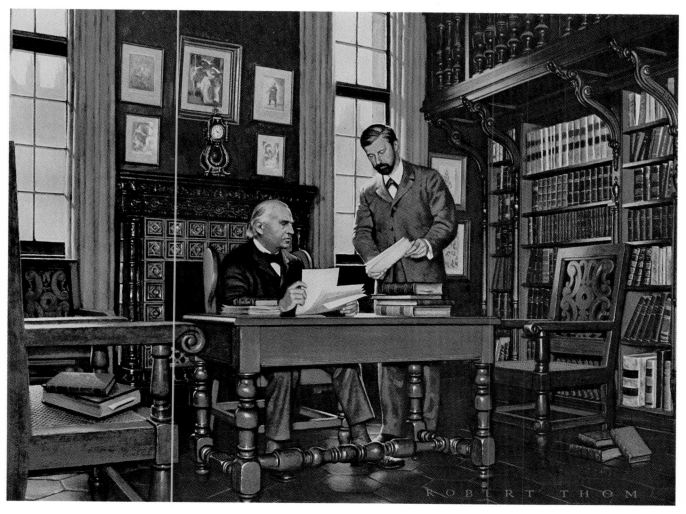

CHARCOT: MASTER OF NEUROLOGY

Greatest neurologist of the 19th century, Parisian physician Jean-Martin Charcot

(1825-1893) developed La Salpêtrière from an asylum for indigent women to one of

France's leading hospitals. Charcot's study and care of its vast patient population led to

teaching, research, and the creation of the world's leading neurological clinic; attracted

students from many nations; raised neurology to a respected medical science. Some of

Charcot's teachings inspired Sigmund Freud of Vienna (Charcot's student, 1885-1886)

to develop the world-famous Freudian hypothesis on psychoanalysis and psychotherapy.

279

for demented women; and it was there that, beginning in 1795, Philippe Pinel pursued his efforts at rehabilitation of the insane.

During the early part of the nineteenth century, medical and surgical men were regularly appointed to the staff of the Salpêtrière. It was still a muddled, disordered home for infirm old women when Jean-Martin Charcot became chief of medical services, in 1862. When death ended his career, in 1893, he left at the Salpêtrière the largest, best organized and appointed neurological clinic in the world. During the same peroid, too, Dr. Charcot had brought the practice of neurology from a rudimentary, undeveloped state to that of a disciplined medical specialty; and, through well-trained pupils, had laid foundations for world-wide modern psychiatric and neurological services.

Jean-Martin Charcot was born November 29, 1825, in Paris. His father was a carriage maker of modest means. He received his early education at the Lycée Bonaparte. Early in life, he showed a better than average talent for art—an ability that was to be of great advantage to him during his teaching career. Young Jean-Martin was not the sociable type, and from an early age possessed the cold, taciturn personality that was to become so identified with him in later years. During his entire life he was a penetrating observer, and he loved to sketch. When he traveled, he made drawings of people and places. In the hospital, he sketched patients who exhibited unusual anatomic features. With a few pen strokes he could unmercifully caricature his contemporaries.

At age nineteen, Charcot began the study of medicine at the Faculté de Médecine associated with the University of Paris (the Sorbonne). He rose rapidly through the stages of extern and of intern. During his internship, he was particularly influenced by Professor Rayer, a friend of Claude Bernard, of Brown-Séquard, and of Berthelot. Charcot became an intern at the Salpêtrière in 1848, and there prepared his doctoral thesis, which he defended successfully in 1853. It was on the subjects of rheumatism and of gout. From 1853 to 1855, he was chief of clinics under Rayer at the Faculté de Médecine; and, in 1856, Charcot was appointed to the rank of hospital physician. In 1857, he became a candidate for the competitive examinations for a faculty position; but it was not until 1860 that he was successful and earned the right to teach at university level.

In 1862, Charcot became chief of the medical services at the Salpêtrière. At that time, he was 37 years old, and, while well trained, would not have been recognized by his contemporaries as having the experience from which greatness might be born. Within the next decade he was to win an international reputation as a researcher and teacher through his work at the great hospital. To many young physicians, assignment to this superannuated "old ladies' home" would have seemed deadly to ambitions. To Charcot, it was the opportunity of his lifetime. Here, virtually, was a small town within the big city: it had about 5,000 inhabitants, of whom 3,000 were neurotic paupers and epileptic patients; 800 were insane; and 250 incurable. This "pandemonium of infirmities" offered a veritable mine of neurological material, extraordinary in its variety and its extent. Almost every type of abnormal neurological manifestation could be found here—not in one, but in many patients. Furthermore, due to the advanced age or incurable status of many, there were multiple opportunities for verification of clinical hypotheses.

Charcot's first step was to establish a pathological laboratory. He felt that a good physician first of all had to be a good pathologist; and he proceeded to earn a reputation in this field before he began to concentrate on nervous disorders. His first book, based on his lectures, was on diseases of old age. By 1866, he had established his free public lectures on clinical subjects, using a hall in the old pharmacy as a forum. His teaching took two forms: these public lessons, given once a week; and daily lessons to his private pupils. Not a fluent speaker, Charcot was a man of few words; but those he uttered were carefully chosen and direct. He supplemented his lectures by a rare power of mimicry, by which he emphasized the various movements, gaits, and symptomatic clues to be observed in patients. His aim was, first of all, to make his pupils see for themselves. Patients were brought into the lecture room, one by one. The patient's history was briefly summed up by an assistant. If pertinent, Charcot asked the patient to disrobe. He would observe keenly, directing the patient to move or to respond so as to reveal some unexpected sign. At the end, he would quickly state his diagnosis; support it, if necessary, with comments and citations to literature; and follow with his therapeutic suggestions. He was quick to discern the difference between true epilepsy and hysteria; and he could spot malingering at a glance. It came to be a legend among patients at the Salpêtrière that "you can't fool Dr. Charcot."

Charcot insisted upon the "anatomicoclinical method" in his classes. Every description of a pathological condition was preceded by a discussion of normal histology of the part. Then the patient was examined.

Charcot is credited with introduction of use of the clinical thermometer in France; and in time he introduced to his clinic the services of ophthalmologists, laryngologists, otologists, psychologists, and other specialists. He established special laboratories for microscopic work and for photography; a museum of pathology; and a section on artistic anatomy. In 1872, he succeeded Vulpian as professor of pathology at the Faculté de Médecine, but his principal teaching and research were carried on at the Salpêtrière.

It was said by Charcot's students that each year was marked by discovery of some new neurological entity. In 1864, Charcot studied muscular atrophy caused by poliomyelitis. In 1868, he went into miliary aneurysm and its role in cerebral hemorrhage. Amyotrophic lateral sclerosis (which became known as Charcot's disease) held his interest in 1869. He did particularly brilliant work on multiple sclerosis (1863-1866) and on differentiation of this disease from parkinsonism. For years, he retained the services of a maid afflicted with multiple sclerosis so that he might better observe the condition. In 1880 came his important book on localization of disease-producing lesions in the brain.

Basically, Charcot's contributions to neurology fall into five groups: original descriptions of various nervous diseases having definite pathological basis; discovery of localization of functions of the brain and of the spinal cord from clinical and pathological examinations, mapping for future neurosurgeons the areas where they should look for these correlations; establishment that there are types of nervous diseases caused by psychic trauma, without physical lesions; investigation of hysteria, of hypnotism as the psychic equivalent of hysteria, and development of psychotherapeutic measures for treatment; and an exhaustive survey of paintings, photographs, engravings, and sculptures illustrating manifestations of nervous diseases, constituting an important contribution to the history of neurology. In addition to publication of many papers and books, he also found time to edit journals having relationship to his fields of interest.

It was through an administrative accident that Charcot began to study hysteria intensively. The Pavillon Sainte Laure in the Salpêtrière, which housed both hysterical insane and epileptic patients, was deteriorating, necessitating evacuation of patients. It became Charcot's duty to "sort them out." He found that hysterical young girls, housed with epileptic patients, soon began to mimic the convulsions and attitudes of epilepsy. In separating these patients from true epileptics, Charcot became interested in the causes and possible treatment of these patients. Many of his ideas have since been outmoded by newer concepts, but at their time they constituted a beginning of concern for these psychiatric patients. Employing isolation, understanding, and psychologic suggestion, he was able to improve the condition of an appreciable number of them.

Charcot's investigations into hypnotism (then regarded only as in the domain of charlatans) were impelled by his desire to study comparisons with hysterical states, and by the hope that patients suffering from hysteria might be treated by hypnotism. He finally discarded hypnotism as a suitable therapeutic tool in care for such patients.

Charcot attracted students from many foreign nations to his lectures at the Salpêtrière (where, in 1882, a special professorial chair in clinical neurology was established for him). Among them were gifted, original men like Joseph Déjerine, Pierre Marie, Joseph Babinski, Gilles de la Tourette, F. Raymond, H. Meige, and P. Richer. These men did much to carry forward the science of neurology from foundations laid by Charcot. Another famous student was Sigmund Freud, who studied under Charcot in 1885 and 1886. Freud himself admitted that his ideas concerning psychoanalysis grew out of one of Charcot's remarks about the importance of sexual incompatibility in marital unhappiness. Charcot's ideas of stimulating the patient to talk about his problems was the germ from which grew the Freudian concept of "mental catharsis" by psychoanalytic methods as a means of relieving disturbed minds. Freud also translated some works of his teacher into German. Charcot thus could be called the "grandfather" of modern psychotherapy.

Shortly after Charcot assumed responsibility for services at the Salpêtrière, in 1862, he married Madame Durvis. She was a woman of beauty, wealth, and social charm; their home life was a happy one. Madame Charcot's daughter by her first marriage eventually married one of Charcot's interns, Henri Liouville. The Charcots had one daughter, Jeanne, born in 1865, and a son, Jean, born in 1867. Though Jean Charcot studied medicine and became a physician, after his father's death he turned to his first love, the sea, commanded several ships, and earned fame for himself as an arctic and antarctic explorer.

Despite his cold exterior and autocratic mien, Charcot, a handsome man, was kind to his interns, and treated them almost as sons. Like all persons who attain fame, he had his enemies and his detractors; but he also had influential friends, and he was recognized internationally for his work. In perspective, he looms as the greatest neurologist of the nineteenth century, and one of the most eminent clinicians in the latter half of that century.

Only in his last years did Charcot lose the speed and physical vigor for which he was noted. His heart began to trouble him, but his mind remained clear, and he maintained his autocratic dominance over clinics at the Salpêtrière. In August, 1893, with two friends who had been former students, Charcot went on a vacation trip into the Morvan, a district southeast of Paris. There, he died suddenly, on August 16, 1893, following an attack of angina pectoris and congestion of the lungs. His funeral was held at the chapel of the Salpêtrière, and he was buried in the Cimetière Montmartre. A bronze statue, erected by commission of his former students, stood before the entrance of the venerable hospital until it was pulled down and melted as scrap metal by Nazi occupation troops during World War II.

WORLD EVENTS AND MEDICAL HISTORY

Dates, persons, and events of significance to the evolution of Medicine include:

1926   Minot and Murphy introduced raw liver diet in pernicious anemia.

1926   Harvey Cushing received the Pulitzer prize for his *Life of Sir William Osler*.

1926   Vitamin B$_1$ isolated.

1926   C. R. Harington effected synthesis of thyroxin.

1926   E. L. Kennaway extracted first known cancer-causing chemical, 3, 4-benzpyrene.

1926   Collip isolated parathyroid hormone.

1926   Vitamins B$_1$ and B$_2$ described.

1926   Förster developed the brain-function chart.

1926   Busch developed electron optics.

1926   Nobel prize awarded to Fibiger for his discovery of the spiroptera carcinoma.

1927   Windaus identified ergosterol.

1927   Lindberg crossed Atlantic in aëroplane.

1927   Ramon (France) developed active immunization against tetanus; and later, diphtheria.

1927   Nobel prize awarded to Wagner-Jauregg for his use of malaria inoculation in treatment for dementia paralytica.

1928   Noguchi discovered pathogen of trachoma.

1928   Vitamin C (ascorbic acid) isolated.

1928   Penicillin discovered by Alexander Fleming (England).

1928   Forssmann performed the first heart catheterization.

1928   Nobel prize awarded to Windaus for vitamin research and Nicolle for his work on typhus fever.

1928   Raman reported on light dispersion of molecules.

1929   W. H. Welch appointed Professor of Medical History at The Johns Hopkins University.

1929   Joseph Goldberger died.

1929   Alexander Fleming announced discovery of penicillin.

1929   Hans Berger constructed the electroencephalograph.

1929   World-wide stock market crash—Black Friday.

1929   Nobel prize awarded to Eijkman and Hopkins for discoveries of antineuritic and growth-stimulating vitamins.

1930   Beginning of plastic chemistry.

1930   Nobel prize awarded to Landsteiner for discovery of human blood groups.

1930   Theiler developed immunization against yellow fever in animals.

1931   Vitamin K studied.

1931   Biotin described by György.

1931   Nobel prize awarded to Warburg for discovery of respiratory enzymes.

1931   Development of electron microscope.

1932   Gerhard Domagk (Germany) discovered prontosil (first of sulfa drugs).

1932   Riboflavin discovered.

1932   Chadwick discovered the neutron.

1932   Joliot-Curie discovered the positron.

1932   Urey discovered "heavy hydrogen."

1932   Lawrence developed the cyclotron.

1932   Zernike developed the phase-contrast microscope.

1932   Nobel prize awarded to Sherrington and Adrian for discovering the function of the neuron.

1932   High point of the depression. 30 million jobless. Beginning of Roosevelt era.

1933   Hitler rises to power in Germany. Beginning of the Third Reich.

1933   Nobel prize awarded to T. H. Morgan for his studies on chromosomes.

1934   Santiago Ramón y Cajal died.

1934   György reported vitamin B$_6$ (pyridoxine).

1934   Joliot-Curie reported on artificial radiation and radioactive isotopes.

1934   Nobel prize awarded to Urey for discovering heavy hydrogen. Whipple, Minot, and Murphy awarded Nobel prize for discovery of liver treatment of anemia.

1935   Trefouël, Nitti, and Bovet (France) discovered prontosil's action to be due to sulfanilamide.

1935   Filatov improved corneal transplantation.

1935   Kendall and Reichstein isolated cortisone.

1935   Stanley discovered the virus agent of tobacco mosaic, a "living" molecule.

1935   Nucleic acids found to be principal components of viruses and genes.

THE HOPKINS: A REVOLUTION IN MEDICAL EDUCATION

ON CHRISTMAS EVE, 1873, the city of Baltimore, Maryland, lost its richest man: Johns Hopkins. The bachelor merchant and financier, aged 78, had willed his substantial fortune to found a hospital and a university within which a medical school was to be organized. Each of these institutions, he decreed, was to bear his name. The shrewd and far-sighted Quaker regarded his fortune as a trust, and had spent considerable time planning its use for the good of humanity. As early as 1867, bills had been passed in the Maryland General Assembly authorizing formation of two corporations, The Johns Hopkins Hospital, and The Johns Hopkins University; carefully selected boards of trustees had been established to carry out the donor's wishes; and various plots of real estate, trust funds, and stocks had been earmarked to endow the institutions.

Altruistic as had been Johns Hopkins' motives and plans, neither he nor his trustees could have envisioned the tremendous impact that the forces thus set in motion would have on the social and cultural life of the nation; or the revolution that would be brought about in methods of medical education and in standards prerequisite to qualification for medical practice. Abraham Flexner, writing in 1940, said of The Johns Hopkins University Medical School: "It possessed ideals and men who embodied them, and from it have emanated the influences that in a half century have lifted American medical education from the lowest status to the highest in the civilized world."

In the North American colonies, medical education in the seventeenth and eighteenth centuries had largely followed the apprenticeship system. First attempt to establish a medical school came at the College of Philadelphia in 1765. Medical students who could afford it finished their training in Germany, France, Holland, Great Britain, or Denmark. In the early years of the 1800's, less than ten per cent of physicians in the United States were graduates of medical schools, and

286

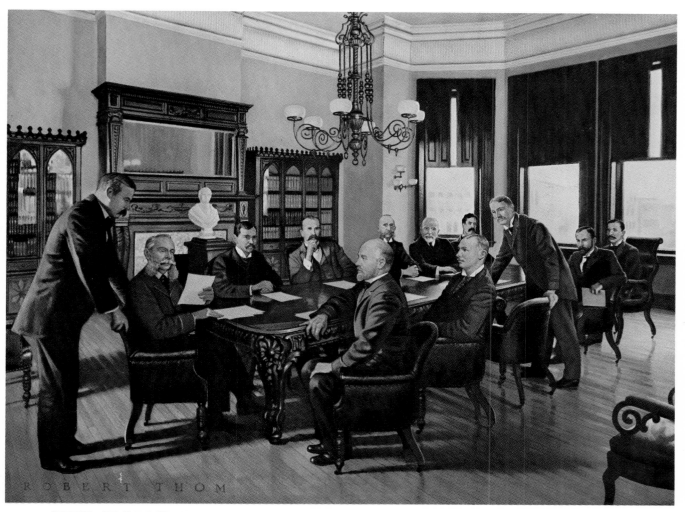

ROBERT THOM

THE HOPKINS: A REVOLUTION IN MEDICAL EDUCATION

Success of The Johns Hopkins University School of Medicine, opened in Baltimore, Maryland, in 1893, stemmed from policies developed at meetings of the Faculty of Medicine and its advisors during formative years. The School, with cooperation of The Johns Hopkins Hospital, was to become world renowned for emphasis on research, for high admission standards, and for innovations in medical training. These advanced teaching methods influenced a revolution in medical education, led to higher requirements for medical licensure, brought about closure of many substandard schools of medicine, and helped raise the status of medicine in the United States to a position of world leadership.

287

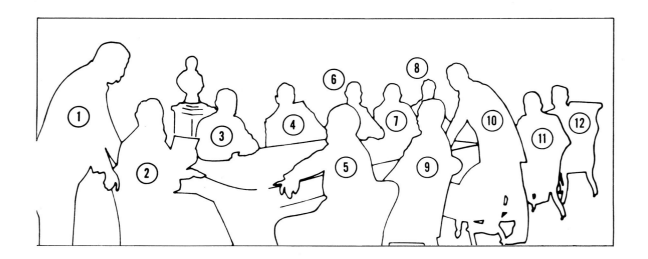

Identity of Persons in the Picture
THE HOPKINS: A REVOLUTION IN MEDICAL EDUCATION

1. John Shaw Billings, member, U. S. Army Surgeon General's staff, who served as advisor concerning construction of the Hospital and establishment of the Medical School.

2. Daniel Coit Gilman, President of the University.

3. Howard A. Kelly, Professor of Gynecology and Obstetrics.

4. William Osler, Professor of the Principles and Practice of Medicine.

5. William H. Welch, Dean, and Professor of Pathology.

6. Henry M. Hurd, Professor of Psychiatry, and Superintendent of the Hospital.

7. Ira Remsen, Professor of Chemistry.

8. J. Whitridge Williams, Associate in Obstetrics.

9. William S. Halsted, Professor of Surgery.

10. Franklin P. Mall, Professor of Anatomy.

11. John J. Abel, Professor of Pharmacology.

12. William H. Howell, Professor of Physiology.

The bust of Johns Hopkins, founder of the institutions,
holds a place of honor in the Hospital Board Room.

more than eighty per cent had never attended a lecture in a school of medicine.

Early in the nineteenth century, some 460 proprietary schools came into being. The primary aim of many of them was to collect tuition fees from students for the privilege of attending lecture courses running ten to twenty weeks. There were virtually no entrance requirements beyond ability to sign a promissory note or to pay for the course; and, in absence of any state regulation, a diploma from such a school was accepted as a license to practice medicine.

The aim to improve this deplorable state of medical education was one of the pillars upon which The American Medical Association was founded in 1847; but without vested authority, the Association could do little but point the way toward reform. Though Nathan Smith Davis, "father" of the AMA, introduced a graded curriculum in the Northwestern University School of Medicine in 1859, the Association itself has published the statement: "True university orientation of medical education really began with the Johns Hopkins University Medical School in 1893."

The philosophical (arts and sciences) faculty and the graduate school of The Johns Hopkins University opened their doors three years after the death of the man who made them possible. Significantly, this year, 1876, marked the centennial of the declaration of political independence by the United States of America. Shryock has observed that opening of The Hopkins "in effect announced American independence in scholarship and science."

The trustees selected by Johns Hopkins took their responsibilities seriously and did their work well. They persuaded Daniel Coit Gilman to leave the presidency of the University of California to organize the new university in Baltimore and to become its president. Gilman believed in the value of advanced training and of encouragement of research; as Shryock stated, "The Hopkins had neither antiquated notions nor obsolescent staff to handicap it at the start . . . The results: Hopkins products were soon in demand all over the country. Within twenty years (1896) over sixty American colleges or universities had three or more professors holding Hopkins degrees on their staffs."

While the University was getting under way, the trustees of The Johns Hopkins Hospital sought to carry out their first assignment: to build the Hospital. Members of this board depended greatly on John Shaw Billings, whom they had chosen as their official advisor. Dr. Billings was a military physician and librarian attached to the Army Surgeon General's office, who had acquired wide hospital experience during the Civil War. Dr. Billings designed The Johns Hopkins Hospital buildings, and assisted President Gilman in preparing plans both for hospital management and for integration of the Hospital with the proposed Medical School. Billings included plans for a school of nursing, and for various supporting services, among them pharmacies. It was he who recommended small classes, actual clinical teaching, laboratory facilities, and that professors heading departments in the school should also head the appropriate services in the Hospital. He also envisaged creation of departments of public hygiene, psychiatry, pediatrics, and medical history.

Funds for construction of the Hospital came largely from income from real estate, bank stock, and the Johns Hopkins town house. The aggregate from these income sources did not permit rapid fulfillment of the donor's plans. Building only as they had accrued income to do so, the Hospital trustees resisted pressures of persons who wished them to operate an incomplete hospital; it was not until May 7, 1889, that the doors of The Johns Hopkins Hospital were formally opened. In absence of a suitable professional administrator, the Hospital trustees asked President Gilman of the University to direct the Hospital. This he did during the first four months following its opening. Then the trustees secured the services of Henry M. Hurd, M.D., to superintend the Hospital, and Dr. Gilman returned to his University duties.

The University trustees had hoped to open the Medical School at the same time as the Hospital was opened. Several years previously, President Gilman had surveyed British medical opinion regarding educational standards that should be required of applicants prior to admitting them to study of medicine. He actually established, as early as 1878, a so-called "Preliminary Medical Course" in the University.

In 1883, the trustees of the University created a Faculty of Medicine, which in addition to President Gilman, consisted of Ira Remsen, Professor of Chemistry; H. N. Martin, Professor of Physiology; and J. S. Billings, Professor of Hygiene. Though none of these men actively taught in the Medical School after it was officially opened, they were influential in establishment of certain general policies of the school, notably in recommendation of high admission requirements.

It is significant that all members chosen for the faculty of The Johns Hopkins University Medical School were comparatively young. First to be chosen was William H. Welch, M.D. (1850-1934), as pathologist, in 1884. Then 34 years of age, Dr. Welch was to serve the University in various capacities for fifty years, and was the most influential of the faculty members. Dr. Welch was a graduate of Yale and of the College of Physicians and Surgeons of New York, and had studied for some time in Germany. Dr. Welch at once began to organize postgraduate courses in bacteriology and pathology for practicing physicians, using hospital facilities for teaching, since there was as yet no medical school. The greater part of responsibility for selection of his associates on the Medical School faculty fell upon Dr. Welch's shoulders.

Next to come, in 1888, was Canadian-born William Osler (1849-1919), called from a post at the University of Pennsylvania to become Physician-in-Chief at the Hospital and Professor of the Theory and Practice of Medicine at the University. Dr. Osler's services continued until 1905, when he was called to England to become Regius Professor of Medicine at Oxford University. Prior to opening of the Hospital in 1889, a New York surgeon, William S. Halsted (1852-1922), temporarily working in Dr. Welch's laboratory, was made Acting Surgeon to the Hospital; and Howard A. Kelly (1858-1943) was called from the University of Pennsylvania to become Gynecologist and Obstetrician to the Hospital.

The best of plans go awry, however. A substantial proportion of The Johns Hopkins University's endowment consisted of shares in the Baltimore and Ohio Railroad. These shares, which paid as high as ten per cent dividends when first received by the University trustees, dwindled in value within a decade to provide virtually no income at all. In 1889, President Gilman faced a seemingly insurmountable problem: there were not sufficient funds available to permit opening of the Medical School. The trustees had agreed that a minimum endowment of $500,000 should be accumulated to guarantee successful operation of the school—and when the Hospital opened, in 1889, the Medical School goal seemed far away, due to shrinkage in revenues from the original University endowment.

Fortunately, a group of young women in Baltimore, interested in a country-wide movement to provide higher education for women, and particularly desirous of assuring opportunities for women in medical education, formed a committee to raise funds. Among the leaders in this movement were the Misses M. Cary Thomas, Mary E. Garrett, Mary Gwinn, and Elizabeth T. King—all daughters of trustees or former trustees of the University. This women's committee succeeded in raising more than $100,000 in 1890, which was made available to the trustees of the University for the Medical School, on stipulation that women be admitted to the study of medicine on the same terms as men. Efforts to raise further funds languished during the next two years; but in December, 1892, Miss Garrett offered the trustees the balance required to make up the $500,000 needed to open the Medical School, subject to two conditions: admission of women on the same terms as men, and maintenance of admission qualifications for all students of a Bachelor's degree or equivalent work in chemistry, in physics, in biology, and in modern languages. Though some faculty members had misgivings about this admission standard, the trustees accepted Miss Garrett's gift and terms.

When The Johns Hopkins University School of Medicine opened, October 2, 1893, its catalogue listed the faculty as follows: Daniel C. Gilman, LL.D., President; William H. Welch, M.D., Professor of Pathology and Dean; Ira Remsen, M.D., Ph.D., Professor of Chemistry; William Osler, M.D., F.R.C.P., Professor of the Principles and Practice of Medicine; Henry M. Hurd, M.D., Professor of Psychiatry; William S. Halsted, M.D., Professor of Surgery; Howard A. Kelly, M.D., Professor of Gynecology and Obstetrics; Franklin P. Mall, M.D.,

292

Professor of Anatomy; John J. Abel, M.D., Professor of Pharmacology; William H. Howell, Ph.D., M.D., Professor of Physiology; George H. F. Nuttall, M.D., Ph.D., Associate in Bacteriology and Hygiene; Simon Flexner, M.D., Associate in Pathology; John M. T. Finney, M.D., Associate in Surgery; Hunter Robb, M.D., Associate in Gynecology; J. Whitridge Williams, M.D., Associate in Obstetrics; and B. Meade Bolton, M.D., Acting Associate in Bacteriology and Hygiene.

This fifteen-member opening faculty was in charge of seven active departments (Dr. Abel also directed physiological chemistry; Dr. Welch taught bacteriology; and as yet there was no department of psychiatry). Students beginning first-year medicine included fifteen men and three women. The Medical School had no buildings exclusively its own. The 225-bed Hospital afforded clinical facilities. Of this first class, fourteen men and one woman graduated and received degrees of Doctor of Medicine in June, 1897. Four members of this first graduating class eventually became heads of departments in four of the nation's leading medical schools.

In 1962, sixty-nine years after its opening, The Johns Hopkins University School of Medicine had 282 full-time salaried members on its faculty; a student body of 344; and The Johns Hopkins Hospital had a capacity of 1,100 beds. The School of Medicine graduated 4,673 students with the degree of Doctor of Medicine during the period from 1897 through 1961.

When it opened in 1893, The Hopkins was a school of medicine unlike any that had previously existed in the United States. It was the first medical school in the country which was constituted as a graduate school.

Conservatives had doubted that the new Hopkins program would succeed; but its success was phenomenal. It immediately attracted patients in great numbers, as well as the best of students, of residents, and of teachers. Its example stimulated other schools and acted as a catalyzer in the great reaction of reform in medical education that was beginning to shape up in the United States as the twentieth century began.

The Johns Hopkins University School of Medicine was to make six significant contributions to the field of medical education, each of which was to have a profound influence on practices in other medical schools, and, eventually, on elevation of the quality of medical practice in the United States. Three of these were evident when the School opened in 1893:

1. Elevation of standards of admission, requiring college graduation or its equivalent, with predominance of credits in premedical subjects.
2. Acceptance of both men and women students.
3. Provision for full-time instructors, selected from among the best men available, nationally and internationally (rather than, as was the custom, local practitioners employed on a part-time basis), for the preclinical disciplines, such as anatomy, physiology, physiological chemistry, pharmacology, pathology, and bacteriology.

(Credit for establishment of these high beginning standards is due primarily to the foresight of President Gilman and Dr. Billings, with the cooperation of the medical faculty as it was assembled.)

The next innovation of nationwide importance, initiated primarily by Dr. Osler as the first classes got under way, was:

4. Introduction of medical students to an active part in the clinical care of patients in the hospital wards as a regular feature of ward operation.

(Thus students gained actual experience in patient care, rather than merely "walking the wards" at the heels of instructors.)

Two further contributions were to follow. These were:

5. Introduction (by Osler, in 1889) of the residency system in postgraduate clinical teaching.

(This was the foundation upon which competent specialization was built.)

6. Introduction (in 1913) of full-time faculty members responsible for teaching in, and conduct of, three main clinical departments —medicine, surgery, and pediatrics.

(Until then, clinical instruction traditionally had been carried on by physicians who also maintained active private practices.)

The influence exerted upon medical educational practices by The Johns Hopkins School of Medicine and by the Hospital, as Shryock

294

has pointed out, "resulted, first, from the setting of an example." Welch and his associates "insisted that the School become . . . a center of basic as well as of applied science . . . Not only did able men accept the chairs, but their work promptly set such standards that no good school was content thereafter with part-time lecturers . . . Whatever their effect on average students, Hopkins methods certainly stimulated the more original men."

Despite the beneficial influences of The Hopkins and of its graduates on better schools of medicine, proprietary medical schools continued to flourish and through release of inadequately trained physicians to endanger the health of patients. By 1900, only twenty-six states required state examinations for licensure of medical school graduates. The American Medical Association, reorganized in 1901, solidified state and county medical societies into a unified organization; and in 1904, it established a Council on Medical Education. This body, in 1906, undertook the first classification of medical schools as A (acceptable), B (doubtful), and C (unacceptable).

To avoid charges of prejudicial reporting, the AMA in 1908 set in motion what proved to be the most stimulating, as well as most shocking, action in the educational reform program: the AMA Council invited the Carnegie Foundation for the Advancement of Teaching—a privately endowed foundation—to make a survey of the status of medical education. Abraham Flexner, a young educator and a brother of Simon Flexner, was commissioned by the Foundation to make a study of medical schools in the United States and in Canada.

Flexner personally visited 155 medical schools in eighteen months. He talked at length at The Hopkins with Drs. Welch, Halsted, Mall, Abel, and Howell, and "with a few others who knew what a medical school ought to be, for they had created one." Flexner's survey was published in 1910. It was scathingly critical of many schools, suggested major improvements in others, and commended only a few. The shock of his forthright and honest report mobilized both the medical profession and the public in an assault on inferior medical schools. The Flexner report was directly responsible for closing down twenty-nine medical schools within the next four years. Still more schools were to close when state licensing boards agreed to accept for examination only students from the list of 66 medical schools then approved by the AMA Council on Medical Education. As a means of meeting the demand for higher standards, most medical schools have become a part of, or associated with, universities. In 1962, all of the eighty-one schools of medicine in the United States were fully accredited, and four more were schools limited to premedical basic sciences. In the course of fifty years, progress in medical education has moved westward, and medical teaching centers in the United States now are attracting many students from abroad.

The Hopkins School of Medicine and the Hospital continued to inspire, to experiment, to innovate. Osler, Kelly, and Howell wrote famous medical textbooks, founded new journals, formed new medical associations, and rejuvenated old ones. Osler and Welch inspired founding of the Rockefeller Institute for Medical Research, in 1901, of which Welch later became President of the Board of Scientific Directors, and of which his one-time pupil and faculty member, Simon Flexner, became Director in 1903. Dr. Welch took over direction of The Johns Hopkins School of Hygiene and Public Health when it opened, in 1916; and he became The Hopkins' first Professor of Medical History in 1929, at the age of 79. Dr. Halsted became a surgeon of international fame, and is credited with introduction of rubber gloves in surgical operating rooms. New faculty members were added, and new chairs and institutes were created: J. W. Williams, in obstetrics, 1899; Walter Jones, in physiological chemistry, 1908; Adolph Meyer, in psychiatry, 1908; John Howland, in pediatrics, 1912; Hugh H. Young, in urology, 1915; and William H. Wilmer, in ophthalmology, 1927. In 1904, Harvey Cushing created the Hunterian Laboratory of Experimental Surgery. Clinical social services were introduced in 1907. Another "first" for Hopkins was the Department of Art as Applied to Medicine, inaugurated by Max Broedel.

Perhaps the truest measure of the influence of The Johns Hopkins University School of Medicine and of the strong faculty men who created it is to be found in the fact that its methods of medical and clinical teaching are no longer regarded as unique, but have become standard for medical schools throughout the United States. To Welch, Osler, Halsted, Kelly, Mall, Abel, Howell, and Williams, and others who were associated with them, and to those who have followed them, must go credit for having envisioned new goals for medical education: they trained men who achieved world-wide recognition for research, for teaching, and for practice of medicine in the United States; and they created an atmosphere of competence and of cooperation in which such training could take place.

WORLD EVENTS AND MEDICAL HISTORY

Dates, persons, and events of significance to the evolution of Medicine include:

1935	Witzleben developed the ultra-short-wave transmitter.
1935	Nobel prize awarded to Spemann for his studies in experimental embryology.
1935	H.W. Dudley isolated ergometrine.
1936	Bittner discovered agent of mammary tumor.
1936	Vitamin P announced.
1936	Nobel prize awarded to Dale and Loewi for their work on neuro-chemistry.
1936	Yeast hormone biotin (vitamin H) discovered by Kögl.
1937	Max Theiler developed yellow fever vaccine.
1937	Nicotinic acid announced.
1937	Sourdille improved fenestration operation.
1937	Sulfonamide therapy for gonorrhea.
1937	Nobel prizes awarded to Haworth and Karrer for their work in vitamin research, and to Szent-Györgyi for his discoveries in biological combustion.
1938	Harvey Cushing published *Meningiomas*.
1938	Vitamin E reported.
1938	Florey, Chain, and associates began work on penicillin.
1938	Dustin discovered the growth-stimulating effect of colchicine.
1938	Hess discovered the regulatory function of the midbrain.
1938	Hahn developed a device for nuclear fission.
1938	Carothers developed nylon.
1938	Heinkel adapted the turbine engine for use in aviation.
1938	Nobel prizes awarded to Kuhn for vitamin research and to Heymans for his discovery of the vascular regulation of respiration.
1939	Harvey Williams Cushing died.

1939	R. J. Dubos described tyrothricin.
1939	R. E. Gross operated on open ductus arteriosus.
1939	World War II began, Sept. 1. (Many advances in the treatment of wounds and traumatic infections, sanitation methods, and improvements in prosthetic limbs.)
1939	P. Muller (Switzerland) introduced DDT insecticide.
1939	Florey and Chain (England) developed penicillin to stage of therapeutic use.
1939	More than 150 different kinds of synthetic materials known.
1939	Gibbons developed blood circulation apparatus, "artificial heart."
1939	Nobel prizes awarded to Domagk for his discovery of the anti-bacterial action of prontosil, and to Butenandt for his work on sex hormones.
1940	Florey, Chain, and associates published work on penicillin as chemotherapeutic agent.
1940	Pantothenic acid synthesized.
1940	Inositol proved essential vitamin by Woolley.
1940	Karl Link (U.S.) discovered dicumarol.
1940	Landsteiner and Wiener discovered the Rhesus factor in blood.
1940	Development of plastic facial surgery.
1940	Euthanasia practiced in Germany.
1941	Frederick G. Banting died.
1941	Charles Huggins (U.S.) arrested prostatic cancer with female hormone.
1941	U.S.A. entered World War II after Japanese attack on Pearl Harbor.
1941	Sinizin transplanted a second heart.

RÖNTGEN: INVISIBLE RAYS
THAT SAVE LIVES

THE NEW YEAR of 1896 had dawned, and the postholiday party at the home of Franz Exner was a gay one. The Professor of Physics at the University of Vienna looked about to see that his guests were well cared for, then turned to a young colleague, physicist Ernst Lecher, and said: "You'll be interested to know that I have just received a most remarkable pamphlet from my good friend, Professor Röntgen, in Würzburg. You remember, we used to work together in Professor Kundt's laboratory. It seems that Professor Röntgen has discovered a remarkable new ray. You can't see it—but it passes right through wood, paper, and almost anything. You can photograph weights in a box without opening the lid. You even can see the bones in your own hand. Here, let me show you the photographs he sent along—"

Ernst Lecher looked at the photos; read a few lines from the little pamphlet which bore the title: *On A New Kind of Rays*. Excitedly, he called to his father, who was standing near by. Z. K. Lecher, the father, was editor of the Vienna *Presse*. At first astounded, he soon recovered his aplomb and recognized the ingredients for a great news story.

The story appeared on the front page of the *Presse*, Sunday, January 5, 1896. To the facts set forth in Professor Röntgen's pamphlet, the editor added a few enthusiastic conjectures of his own. He predicted many possible uses for these mysterious, newly discovered "x-rays," as they were called. He even contended that they might find a place in medicine, perhaps in diagnosis of diseases and in treatment of injuries of bones.

The Vienna representative of the London *Daily Chronicle* cabled the story to his paper, wherein it appeared the following day. The *Frankfurter Zeitung*, the Paris *Matin*, and many others soon had the story, as did New York newspapers. By the second week in January, leading medical journals world-wide were commenting on the possibilities of

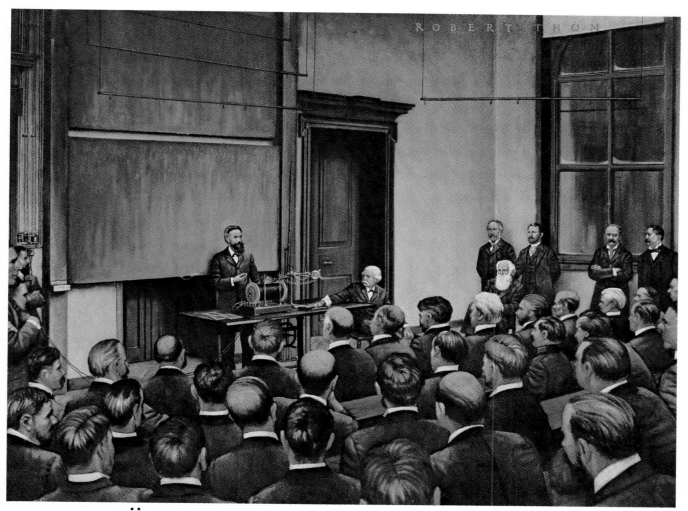

RÖNTGEN: INVISIBLE RAYS THAT SAVE LIVES

At his first public demonstration of newly discovered x-rays, the evening of January 23, 1896, Wilhelm Conrad Röntgen (1845-1923) astounded scientists who filled the room. Professor of Physics and Rector of the University of Würzburg, Germany, Röntgen completed his demonstration by taking an x-ray photograph of the hand of the famed Professor of Anatomy, Albert von Kölliker. This led to discussion of possible medical applications. The news traveled fast, and within a year, x-ray equipment was being employed by medical men around the world as a diagnostic tool. Later research revealed many therapeutic and industrial applications, as well as the hidden dangers, of x-rays.

x-rays. Physicians, physicists, and photographers were repeating Röntgen's experiments, and devising new ones. Within four days after arrival of the news in the United States, x-rays had been employed by a physician to locate a bullet lodged in a patient's hand.

Thus in a few weeks was Wilhelm Conrad Röntgen, Professor of Physics, Director of the Physical Institute, and Rector of the University of Würzburg, Germany, catapulted from the semiobscure, quiet life of a researcher and teacher to that of an international celebrity. It came about because his research-trained mind demanded that he look into the cause of what at first seemed a minor laboratory curiosity.

Professor Röntgen had first observed the phenomenon he named x-rays, on Friday, November 8, 1895. Over the week end, he took advantage of absence of students to reconfirm his findings. Then came weeks of feverish experimentation, and writing of notes on findings. Röntgen did not tell students or fellow teachers of his experiments for fear they would think him out of his mind: rays that could penetrate flesh, paper, wood, most metals; that could cause a screen coated with barium platinocyanide to fluoresce, even in the next room, with the door closed! Röntgen himself could hardly believe his eyes. Cathode rays, created in the Hittorf-Crookes tube he was using, would cause fluorescence if the screen were held only a few centimeters from the tube. When the tube was covered with a black cardboard mask, such as he was now using, cathode rays were shut in, just as were visible light rays. But the x-rays—they penetrated the cardboard; they penetrated a 1,000-page book; they penetrated wood; they penetrated flesh, showing bones clearly as darker shadows; they exposed photographic plates that were securely protected from visible light. Here, indeed, was a phenomenon unheard of before.

Convinced at last that his observations were sound, proved by repeated experimentation, Röntgen realized the need for immediate publication. Just after Christmas, he presented his manuscript to the secretary of the Würzburg Physical Medical Society. It was published in the last pages of the year's final issue of the *Sitzungsberichte der Physikalisch-Medizinischen Gesellschaft zu Würzburg*. On New Year's Day, 1896, Professor Röntgen mailed reprints, together with prints of his photographs, to a number of his physicist friends. Among them was Professor Exner of Vienna.

The fame that was about to come to Professor Röntgen in his fiftieth year of life was not achieved easily. Born March 27, 1845, in the German town of Lennep in the Ruhr valley, the son of a textile merchant, Wilhelm Conrad Röntgen grew up in Apeldoorn, Holland, to which city his parents had moved when he was three years old. An only child, his schooling was somewhat erratic. He demonstrated an ability for making mechanical gadgets, and had no difficulty with schoolwork until the prank of a schoolmate got him into trouble. Refusal to reveal the name of the offender resulted in Röntgen's expulsion without being admitted to examinations so necessary to accreditation for higher education. Röntgen was allowed to study, without credit, at the University of Utrecht, and was accepted at the Polytechnical School at Zurich, Switzerland, from which he received a degree in mechanical engineering, August 6, 1868. Strangely enough, Röntgen, the great experimental physicist, never had a basic college course in physics.

Staying on at the Polytechnical School in Zurich after graduation, Röntgen took some additional courses, and attracted the attention of August Kundt, professor of physics. After a year in Kundt's laboratories, Röntgen submitted a thesis on *Studies on Gases* to the University of Zurich, and on June 22, 1869, received a doctor of philosophy degree from that institution. In Zurich, too, he met Bertha Ludwig, whom he married in 1872.

Röntgen's relations with Kundt were such that when, in 1870, the professor was called to the chair of physics at the University of Würzburg, he took Röntgen along as his assistant. At Würzburg, Röntgen met with double disappointment: first, the surroundings of the physics laboratories were poor, and the equipment meager; second, Röntgen was denied appointment as *Privatdozent*, or unpaid instructor (first step in the academic ladder) because of lack of the diploma denied him when he was expelled from preparatory school.

However, in 1872, a few months after Röntgen's marriage, Kundt took his assistant with him to the newly reorganized Kaiser-Wilhelm's University at Strassburg. In this new and broader minded university,

Röntgen, after two years of hard work, was appointed a *Privatdozent* in 1874. By that time, his interest in conducting physical experiments equaled that of teaching. Consequent to investigations he had conducted with Kundt, Röntgen was offered a full professorship in physics and mathematics at the Agricultural Academy in Hohenheim. Due to inadequate equipment and facilities there, Röntgen was happy to return to Strassburg a year and a half later to accept appointment as an associate professor.

Meantime, Röntgen was developing a remarkable ability for conducting research, and for measurement of minute quantities of substances and of changes in their temperature due to altered physical conditions. His publications began to appear regularly in leading journals on physics.

In 1879, friends, including von Helmholtz, recommended Röntgen for the chair of physics at the University of Giessen. In 1880, a new physics building was built there, and Röntgen headed the institute.

Röntgen's interests were rapidly turning to problems of electricity. In 1888, his reputation was enhanced by experiments that proved and measured magnetic effects produced when a glass plate, or other suitable medium, was moved between two electrically charged condenser plates.

Röntgen received several flattering invitations to take professorships in physics at other universities, including Jena, and Utrecht (where he had once been denied enrollment as a regular student). These offers he declined; but when, in 1888, the University of Würzburg (which had denied him *Privatdozent*) offered him the post of professor of physics and director of the newly built physical institute, Röntgen could not resist. The Röntgens returned to Würzburg. Six years later, Röntgen was elected Rector of the University—its highest office.

As he reached his fiftieth year, Röntgen was a typical successful professor in a large university. His publications had made him well known among his colleagues. His abilities as researcher and teacher were recognized by his university, and flattering offers came from others; but the Röntgens preferred Würzburg. It was in this setting that Röntgen, in 1895, became interested in cathode rays, and in the work that had been done on them by Hertz, Lenard, Hittorf, and

Crookes. Röntgen secured several types of cathode ray tubes, a Ruhmkorff induction coil, a Depres interrupter, and other apparatus, including a Raps vacuum pump. Repeating experiments of his colleagues with cathode rays, Röntgen confirmed them, and made some additional observations: the rays from the tubes darkened photographic plates, and they produced fluorescence in certain salts, notably, barium platinocyanide.

Working alone, as was his habit, on the afternoon of November 8, 1895, he had covered a tube completely with black cardboard. Wishing to test the opacity of the cover, he darkened the room. It was then that he discovered the screen, across the room, fluorescing. Unbelieving, Röntgen searched for an overlooked light source. Cathode rays could not be the cause of fluorescence. He checked and rechecked his experiments; he hardly took time to eat and sleep. This must be a new kind of ray—no known rays would penetrate opaque substances so readily; nor would they travel in a straight line, as did those produced in his experiments. The new rays also differed from cathode rays in that they were not deflected by a magnetic field. To them, Röntgen attached the mathematician's symbol for the unknown: he thought of them as x-rays; and as such, he reported them in his first paper, *On a New Kind of Rays*.

Reactions were not long in coming. In addition to newspapers and medical journal reports, electrical, photographic, and general interest publications carried articles of varying reliability. From physicists and other scientists came congratulations, in the main; and a few disagreements, as well as insubstantial claims to priority. On January 13, 1896, Röntgen was called to Berlin to demonstrate his apparatus before the Emperor, Wilhelm II, and his guests. The Emperor decorated Röntgen with the Prussian Order of the Crown, II Class.

Meantime, Röntgen's colleagues at Würzburg were urging him to reveal his discovery to them. This event took place in the auditorium of Röntgen's own institute, the night of January 23, 1896. Every seat in the auditorium was filled. After explaining his experiments and demonstrating various properties of x-rays, Röntgen invited Albert von Kölliker, famous anatomist at the University, to have his hand photographed. Von Kölliker agreed, and within a short time an excellent photograph, revealing bones, flesh, and a ring in graduated shadows, was shown to the audience. Von Kölliker praised Röntgen's work as of the greatest significance, and suggested that the new force be designated "Röntgen rays." He also conjectured as to the possibility of photographing other structures of the body. Röntgen, who himself was never to use the term, Röntgen rays, expressed his willingness to give the benefit of his experience to anyone wishing to carry on further research in medical institutions. He refused to apply for patents, or to realize any commercial gain either from the rays or apparatus for their production.

Though Röntgen thus contributed to medicine a great diagnostic aid, and one that later became adapted to therapeutic procedure, he did no further work on the medical aspects of x-rays. His closest tie with the profession was an honorary degree of Doctor of Medicine conferred upon him, March 3, 1896, by Würzburg University.

Within the first year, experimenters learned to respect x-rays, and that they are agents of destruction and of death as well as being useful in diagnosis and in therapy. Physicians learned to shield themselves, as well as their patients, from unwanted effects—but not before several dedicated experimenters had become martyrs to x-ray research.

Two further papers were published by Röntgen on the physical aspects of the new kind of rays: the second, March 9, 1896, in the same journal as was his first; and the third, March 10, 1897, in the bulletin of the Prussian Academy of Sciences, in Berlin. Meanwhile, dozens of honors were bestowed upon him. Röntgen was made an honorary citizen of Lennep, the town of his birth; he received the Royal Order of Merit of the Bavarian Crown, but turned down a proffered grant of nobility, which would have added the prefix *von* to his name. He continued his work in Würzburg until April 1, 1900, when he accepted an appointment as Professor of Physics and Director of the Physical Institute at Ludwig-Maximilian's University in Munich. In December, 1901, he traveled to Stockholm, and, in the year of its inception, he received the Nobel prize for his contribution to physics.

Röntgen continued his work at the University in Munich until retirement in 1920. Even then, two small laboratories were made available to him for continued work. At seventy-five years of age, however, he was a tired and lonely man. Once comparatively secure financially, World War I and the collapse of the German economy virtually impoverished him; and Mrs. Röntgen had died, October 31, 1919. Many of his friends were gone, too. Honors still came to him, but now they meant little. He experienced a feeling of great satisfaction from the progress that had been made in use of x-rays in medicine, and in industry. The demands of World War I had proved their value.

A victim of carcinoma, Röntgen died February 10, 1923.

What of Röntgen rays—or x-rays—over the ensuing years? Their diagnostic applications offered almost endless possibilities for development—but virtually all basic physical facts about the rays were established within two years after their discovery. As a medical student, Walter B. Cannon (later to become a famous physiologist at Harvard) demonstrated experimentally that a contrast meal could be followed through the stomach and the intestinal tract by use of x-ray equipment. Along with radium, discovered by Mme. Curie some three years later, x-rays were found to be valuable as a therapeutic agent.

The first twenty years of employment of x-rays were years of trials and errors, due to crudeness of equipment and to lack of understanding of their behavior. The next decade, which began with World War I, brought many advances. The 1930's placed a firm foundation under radiotherapy; and by 1940, reliable systems for calculation and control of x-ray dosage had been devised. The next twenty years, encompassing World War II, brought still greater advances in application of x-rays. Powerful machines that would have astounded Röntgen were developed, the rays of which may be focused effectively to alter malignant growths deep in the body.

From the pioneer research begun by Röntgen came the science of roentgenology. Following in rapid succession came related discoveries by other scientists: radium, the electron, radioactivity, nuclear fission, nuclear fusion, and preparation of radioisotopes. Each has been demonstrated to have power to improve and to save lives—as well as to destroy them. Only history, with benefit of perspective of centuries to come, will be able to evaluate truly the use which man will have made of the forces unleashed when Wilhelm Conrad Röntgen saw a ghostly green glow in his darkened laboratory.

THE CONQUEST
OF YELLOW FEVER

"I THANK GOD that I did not accept anybody's opinion on this subject, but determined to put it to a thorough test with human beings in order to see what would happen . . . actual trial has proven that I was right . . . "

Thus wrote Dr. Walter Reed, 49-year-old surgeon with rank of Major, United States Army, stationed at Columbia Barracks, Quemados, Cuba, on December 9, 1900, in a letter to his wife. Dr. Reed had been sent to Cuba by the Army's Surgeon General to head a commission to study yellow fever, and he was on the threshold of discoveries that would unlock secrets of propagation of that dread disease.

Not far away, in Havana, undoubtedly another prayer of thanksgiving was in the mind of 67-year-old Dr. Carlos Juan Finlay, who at long last was witnessing men of science accepting and proving, beyond doubt, that his theories regarding transmission of yellow fever were correct.

The story of yellow fever is one of many men, as Dr. Joseph E. Smadel has pointed out. Dr. Reed and his associates gave the facts to the world. Surgeon Major William Gorgas transformed facts to action, freeing Havana of a scourge it had known for almost 400 years. It would be another forty years before Max Theiler would develop vaccines against yellow fever. But Carlos Finlay was first to have given the Reed commission the idea that mosquitoes transmitted the disease.

Where yellow fever originated is still a controversial question. Some authorities trace it back in Mexico to the fifteenth century; others believe it to have been reported in Africa as early as 1585. It has been said that no European writer mentioned the disease before Columbus' day; but older records are not easily interpreted—and yellow fever has borne at least 152 names during the course of history. A most dramatic record of its devastation is to be found in the writings of Dr. Benjamin Rush and others concerning the epidemic of yellow fever

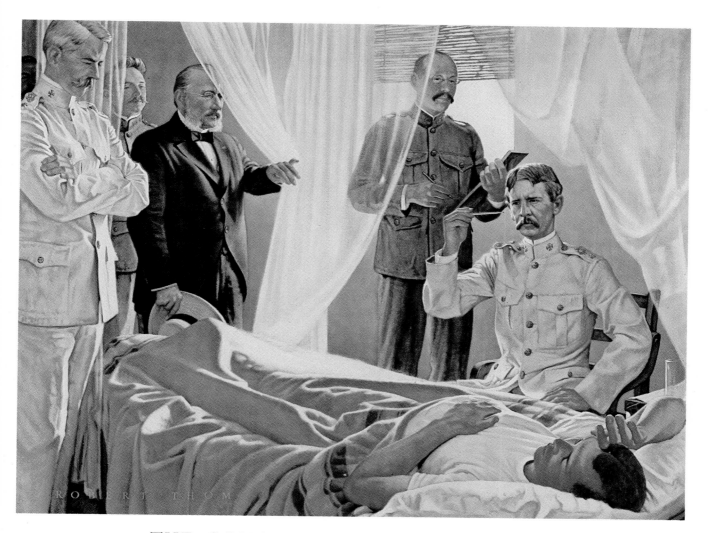

THE CONQUEST OF YELLOW FEVER

Methods of controlling and preventing yellow fever resulted from investigations conducted in 1900 at Camp Lazear, Cuba, by a United States Army commission led by Major Walter Reed (1851-1902). This research proved conclusively that mosquitoes carry the yellow fever virus from person to person. First volunteer patient to be infected by mosquito bites was Private John Kissinger. Examining physicians were Major W. C. Gorgas, Havana sanitation officer; Dr. A. Agramonte, pathologist; Dr. Carlos J. Finlay, chairman of the cooperating Cuban Yellow Fever Commission and first man to point to the possible inefective role of mosquitoes; Dr. James Carroll, bacteriologist; and Dr. Reed, commission chairman.

in Philadelphia in 1793; this was but one of the fever's visits to United States ports. In the eighteenth century, yellow fever is reported to have caused 41,000 deaths in New Orleans, 10,000 in Philadelphia, and 3,400 in New York; and the United States losses in the nineteenth century approached 100,000. Epidemics periodically devastated cities in the Caribbean islands, Central and South America, and frequently visited the shores of Spain, Portugal, and France. It helped shape the future of the new republic of the United States: Napoleon was forced to sell Louisiana after yellow fever had destroyed nine-tenths of his expeditionary force in San Domingo in 1802. Yellow fever, or "black vomit," as it was known, defeated more Spanish, French, and English expeditions in the New World than did military action.

Dr. Rush believed the Philadelphia epidemic of 1793 to have arisen from the fumes of a shipment of coffee spoiling on the docks. He noted that mosquitoes were numerous that summer, but failed to realize the significance. In 1797, he recorded the observation that one patient developed the fever after smoking a cigar; and that wind direction seemed to have some influence on the number of persons becoming ill of the disease.

The idea that insects might have a part in spreading disease came to acceptance only with great difficulty. Bishop Knud of Denmark alluded to it in 1498 in *De Regimine Pestilentico*. Ambroise Paré, at St. Quentin in 1557, said of battlefield flies: "Where they settled, they infected the air, and brought the plague with them." First scientific establishment of insects as carriers of disease was published by Dr. Patrick Manson, in 1880, concerning the mosquito as intermediary host in filariasis. In 1894, Manson communicated his theories concerning mosquitoes to Major Ronald Ross of the British Army. Two and a half years later, in India, Dr. Ross was able to pinpoint responsibility upon female mosquitoes of the genus *Anopheles* for a part in the life cycle of the parasites causing malaria.

First persons to suggest that insects play a part as carriers of yellow fever were Dr. J. Crawford of Baltimore, in 1807; Dr. J. C. Nott of Mobile, Alabama, in 1848; and Dr. L. Beauperthuy, in 1854. The mosquito was not specifically accused until Dr. Finlay's paper, "The Mosquito Hypothetically Considered as the Agent of Transmission of

Yellow Fever," was read before the Royal Academy in Havana, Cuba, August 11, 1881. But for two decades no one paid attention to Dr. Finlay's claims.

Havana, Cuba, historically had been a focus of yellow fever. After its occupation in 1898 in the course of the Spanish-American War, losses among United States troops became so great that Surgeon General Sternberg named a commission to go to Cuba to study the mystery concerning the cause and transmission of yellow fever. Thus, in the year 1900, were persons most responsible for conquest of yellow fever brought together upon that tropical Caribbean isle.

Chairman of the commission was one of Sternberg's most trusted officers, Major Walter Reed. Born the son of a minister, in Virginia, September 13, 1851, Reed had graduated in New York from Bellevue Hospital Medical College in 1870; he interned and practiced in New York for a time, then entered the Army with a commission as Assistant Surgeon and rank of First Lieutenant, in 1875. In 1876, he was assigned to his first post at Fort Lowell, Arizona. There his new bride joined him at the first of fifteen posts he was to hold in the "Old West." Returning East in 1889, he was assigned to be Attending Surgeon and Examiner of Recruits in Baltimore, with permission to pursue professional work at The Johns Hopkins Hospital. This brought him under the influence of Professor William H. Welch, and he received special training in pathology and bacteriology.

Dr. Reed was ordered to another two-year field assignment in the Dakotas; then, in 1893, he returned to Washington, D.C., to become curator of the Army Medical Museum and professor of bacteriology and clinical microscopy at the United States Army Medical School, with the rank of major. He published a significant work on the contagiousness of erysipelas in 1892; and, in 1898, headed a commission to study typhoid fever in army camps, reporting the importance of flies as probable carriers. With Dr. James Carroll, another of the Surgeon General's staff, he studied *Bacillus icteroides*, claimed by its Italian discoverer, Guiseppe Sanarelli, to be the cause of yellow fever. Reed and Carroll's findings were negative.

The yellow fever commission which Dr. Reed was appointed to head included Dr. Carroll, in charge of bacteriologic work; Dr. Jesse

W. Lazear, specialist in insect work; and as pathologist, Dr. Aristides Agramonte, a native of Cuba serving in the U.S. Army. Drs. Agramonte and Lazear already were in Cuba; Drs. Reed and Carroll joined them in Havana in June, 1900. First work of the commission was directed toward determining whether *Bacillus icteroides* had a part in yellow fever. It soon was decisively ruled out.

At this time, Dr. Reed and his commission members met Dr. Finlay, who was to point them toward another important aspect of the yellow fever puzzle—the mosquito.

Dr. Finlay had been born in Camagüey, Cuba, in 1833, the son of a Scotch physician and a French mother. Following early education in Cuba, he enrolled in Jefferson Medical College in Philadelphia, receiving his doctorate in 1855, entering medical practice in Havana in 1864. He became expert in epidemiology, and made contributions in the fields of leprosy, beriberi, filariasis, trichinosis, relapsing fever, cholera, and tuberculosis; but yellow fever held his greatest interest. Dr. Finlay began his long series of papers on yellow fever in 1872. In 1881, he first pointed out necessity for consideration of an intermediate agent to explain transmission of yellow fever; and later that year, declared the vector to be a mosquito, then known as *Culex fasciatus.* He supported his claims with reports of experiments in humans. Though firm in his convictions, Dr. Finlay failed to gain support of medical men. When the Spanish-American War broke out, Dr. Finlay, then 65 years old, went to Washington, offered his services to the United States Army, and served in the Santiago campaign. In 1899, the provisional government of Cuba appointed him chairman of its Yellow Fever Board. It was in this capacity that he received Dr. Reed courteously, and patiently reiterated his theories regarding transmission of yellow fever by mosquitoes. Dr. Finlay's proofs failed to convince Dr. Reed; but nevertheless Dr. Finlay and his Cuban commission offered full cooperation with the United States commission.

Unable to find a bacterial cause for the fever, Reed and his associates determined to try to clear up two remaining questions: Dr. Finlay's controversial mosquito theory, and the ideas generally embraced by the medical profession that the disease was spread by personal contact and by fomites—a term applied to clothing, bedding, and personal effects of the sick.

Dr. Reed frequently was called away from work in Cuba for special assignments from the Surgeon General. However, three events soon emphasized the importance of checking the mosquito theory more fully: Dr. Carroll deliberately allowed an infected mosquito to bite him, developed yellow fever, and nearly lost his life; Dr. Lazear accidentally was bitten and died September 25, 1900, of fever; and, Dr. Reed observed, nonimmune nurses in attendance of very sick yellow fever patients seldom contracted the disease.

With the permission of Major General Leonard Wood, Military Governor of Cuba, Dr. Reed established a heavily quarantined experimental headquarters, named Camp Lazear, a mile outside Quemados. Dr. Reed and his associates determined to seek answers to the puzzling questions by daring use of human volunteers. Two wooden structures were built and heavily screened. In one, deliberately poorly ventilated, enlisted volunteers spent twenty nights in beds, bedclothes, and personal wear that were heavily saturated and stained with excrement and with "black vomit" of patients who had died of yellow fever. Revolting and uncomfortable as were their experiences, two groups of volunteers came through the tests healthy and unharmed.

The other experimental building at Camp Lazear was light and well ventilated. It was divided by a screen wall into two compartments. Equipped alike, one side was used by volunteers who allowed themselves to be bitten by mosquitoes; the other by control volunteers carefully protected from mosquitoes, but living under identical conditions and breathing the same atmosphere.

First man to be exposed to contaminated mosquitoes was Private John Kissinger. On December 8, 1900, Kissinger had the beginning of a well-defined attack of yellow fever. But Dr. Reed did not depend on diagnoses by his staff alone: the Havana commission, led by Dr. Finlay and including Drs. Juan Guiteras, W. C. Gorgas, and A. Diaz Albertini, was invited to examine Kissinger. All agreed beyond doubt that he had yellow fever.

Reporting the experiments to the Medical and Chirurgical Faculty of the State of Maryland, in Baltimore, April 24, 1901, Dr. Reed said of Kissinger: "In my opinion this exhibition of moral courage has never been surpassed in the annals of the Army of the United States."

In addition to Kissinger, three other volunteers were bitten by mosquitoes which previously had fed on yellow fever victims. Each developed typical yellow fever, and diagnoses were verified by physicians of the combined commissions. Meanwhile, nonimmune controls, sleeping in the other half of the building and sharing a common atmosphere, suffered no ill effects. Results of the experiments at Camp Lazear were so clear cut that Dr. Reed, at the conclusion of his report, "The Etiology of Yellow Fever, an Additional Note," read before the Pan-American Medical Congress at Havana, in February, 1901, was able to make eleven statements, of which the most important were:

"1. The mosquito—*C. fasciatus*—serves as the intermediate host for the parasite of yellow fever.

"2. Yellow fever is transmitted to the nonimmune individual by means of the bite of the mosquito that has previously fed on the blood of those sick with this disease.

"5. Yellow fever can also be experimentally produced by the subcutaneous injection of blood taken from the general circulation during the first and second days of this disease.

"Yellow fever is not conveyed by fomites, and hence disinfection of articles of clothing, bedding, or merchandise, supposedly contaminated by contact with those sick with this disease is unnecessary.

"10. The spread of yellow fever can be most effectually controlled by measures directed to the destruction of mosquitoes and the protection of the sick against the bites of these insects."

Two months later, in Baltimore, Dr. Reed also made this statement:

"To Dr. Carlos J. Finlay, of Havana, must be given . . . full credit for the theory of the propagation of yellow fever by means of the mosquito . . ."

Further experimental work of the United States commission, carried out largely by Dr. Carroll in 1901, proved that the causative agent of yellow fever was not a bacterium, but a filterable virus which could be transmitted either by mosquito bite or by injection of blood from a sick patient into a nonimmune subject. The conclusive, courageous, rapid, and brilliant work of the commission added greatly to the prestige of medical science in the United States.

Practical consequences of the work of the Reed commission were tremendous. Dr. William Crawford Gorgas, Havana's chief sanitary officer, applying rigid, vigorous antimosquito measures, was able to rid the city of yellow fever within ninety days, in 1901, freeing its people of a centuries-old rule of terror. In 1903, Dr. Guiteras freed Laredo, Texas, of the scourge; New Orleans combated an epidemic in 1905; and other cities in North, Central and South America soon adopted measures that wiped out epidemics and controlled new cases as they arose. Drs. Licéaja, in Mexico, and Oswaldo Cruz, in Brazil, did outstanding work in ridding their countries of the fever. In 1904, Dr. Gorgas, now a General, applied his antimosquito measures to the Panama Canal Zone, making possible completion of that monumental engineering project.

It was not Dr. Reed's fate to live long in the light of his triumph, or to add further to scientific knowledge of medicine. He died suddenly in Washington of appendicitis, November 22, 1902.

Of him, General Wood said, at a memorial service: "I know of no man who has done so much for humanity as Major Reed. His discovery results in the saving of more lives annually than were lost in the Cuban war and saves the commercial interests of the world a greater financial loss in each year than the cost of the entire Cuban war." Today, near Washington, D.C., a great research hospital bears Walter Reed's name.

Fate dealt more kindly with Dr. Finlay. In 1902, he became Chief Sanitary Officer of Cuba, a position from which he retired in 1909. Before his death in 1915, at 82 years of age, he had become an international hero, and several institutions have been named for him.

Romantically, the yellow fever story might end here. But the tiny virus that causes the death-dealing disease is not romantic; nor is it choosy about whom it attacks. The most common insect host in its man-mosquito-man cycle has been renamed—Dr. Finlay called it *Culex fasciatus;* later, it became known as *Stegomyia fasciata;* today, it is known world-wide as *Aedes aegypti.* This mosquito is definitely of domestic inclination, living near man and depositing its eggs in small bodies of water—in rain barrels, in tin cans, in hollows of roofs, in puddles, and in swamps. Sanitation experts succeeded in combating yellow fever by rigid inspections and measures to eliminate breeding places for mosquitoes, by adequate closure and screening of living quarters, and by preventing mosquitoes from biting yellow fever patients. Like measures applied to ships, plus health inspections of passengers at ports of arrival, minimized transportation of the disease to far-distant communities.

The Rockefeller Foundation, in New York, taking a cue from the work of Drs. Reed and Gorgas, appointed General Gorgas to head its Yellow Fever Commission, when his work in Panama was completed upon opening of the Canal in 1914. Between 1916 and 1949, the Foundation spent over $14,000,000 on research and on grants to help various countries stamp out yellow fever. For a while, it seemed that the fever fighters were to be crowned with success. *Aedes aegypti* could be wiped out, or controlled. But from time to time, unaccountable new outbreaks occurred. Thus, yellow fever presented scientists with a new mystery. As in the first instance, the fever was not quick to give up its secrets. Hideyo Noguchi, a Rockefeller investigator, searching vainly for a spirochete as cause of yellow fever, was a victim of the fever in 1928. Researchers both in Africa and in South America discovered that yellow fever existed in the jungle, that monkeys and marsupials are susceptible to the disease, and that several species of forest-dwelling mosquitoes also serve as intermediaries. These forest-dwelling mosquitoes do not invade cities, as does *Aedes aegypti;* but jungle travelers, lumbermen, and others who have occasion to visit the forest may be bitten. If, during the incubation period, they are able to reach populated centers, they readily may serve as means of infecting domestic *Aedes* mosquitoes—and the epidemic chain will be reforged.

In 1928, other Rockefeller researchers in Africa, Drs. A. F. Mahaffy and Adrian Stokes, discovered that rhesus monkeys could be infected with yellow fever. Following up on this lead, Dr. Max Theiler and his associates in Rockefeller Foundation's Division of Biological and Medical Research in New York developed two strains of attenuated live yellow fever virus for possible use as vaccines. One, known as the French strain, propagated in mouse brains, is widely used today, especially in Africa. But, because this vaccine occasionally gives rise

314

to serious reactions, Dr. Theiler set up a series of tests employing other tissue cultures. Virus, grown on chick embryos, resulted in a vaccine known as 17D. This vaccine was field tested in Brazil from 1937 to 1940. From 1940 to 1947, the Rockefeller Foundation produced over 28,000,000 doses of 17D vaccine, which it furnished free of charge to health agencies in thirty-three countries, and to the United States military services. In 1951, Dr. Theiler was awarded the Nobel Prize in Medicine in recognition of the vaccines' benefit to mankind.

Thus was yellow fever, scourge of the centuries, conquered in a half century; that is, nearly conquered. It has virtually vanished from the world's major cities; but pools of the virus that defy eradication still lie deep in the world's tropical jungles, passing unnoticed from animal to mosquito to animal, back and forth. The infected mosquitoes will not hesitate to feed on humans that come within their range.

In this day of rapid, world-wide travel, of pushing back of jungle frontiers, of exploding populations, vaccination is the only method available for protection of persons likely to be exposed to the risk of jungle yellow fever, and for protection of people living in communities which may be visited by travelers who have been in the tropics.

WALTER B. CANNON
PHYSIOLOGIC INVESTIGATOR

IT WAS a young student in his first year at Harvard Medical College in 1896 who gave to medicine fundamental research that has been the basis of gastrointestinal diagnostic procedures ever since. Walter Bradford Cannon devised means of employing the newly developed Röntgen ray, or x-ray, to study digestive processes uninhibited by surgical or mechanical intervention. Countless persons, having undergone the temporary discomfort of swallowing a contrast meal containing radiopaque barium sulfate while standing between x-ray apparatus and a fluorescent screen, owe votes of thanks to Dr. Cannon for lives lengthened because of information gained by their physicians from gastrointestinal fluoroscopy. This ingenious young man, whose active career was to parallel the years during which American medical science was gaining increasing international respect, was to become one of the world's great physiologists, and one of his nation's outstanding contributors to science.

Dr. Cannon, who spent a lifetime in research laboratories and in teaching, in his later years expressed his belief that: "Phenomena, no matter how mysterious they may appear to be, have a natural explanation and will yield their secrets to the persistent, ingenious, and cautious efforts of the investigator." His life-work well bore out the truth of a statement by nineteenth-century physicist Joseph Henry: "The seeds of great discoveries are constantly floating around us, but they only take root in minds well prepared to receive them."

Walter Bradford Cannon was born October 19, 1871, in Prairie du Chien, Wisconsin, the son of Colbert H. Cannon and Sarah Denio Cannon. His father was a railroad man, eventually becoming superintendent of transportation for the Great Northern Railroad system. His mother died of pneumonia when Walter was ten years old. On

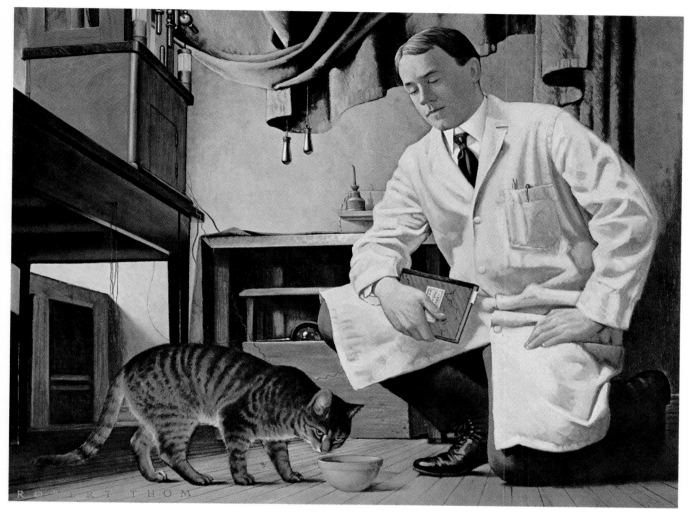

WALTER B. CANNON: PHYSIOLOGIC INVESTIGATOR

While a first-year student at Harvard Medical School, Boston, in 1896, Walter Brad-
ford Cannon (1871-1945) employed newly discovered x-rays to study activities of
digestive organs in animals. Preferring cats, Cannon induced them to eat radiopaque
meals, and followed food through alimentary organs with the aid of a fluoroscopic
screen. Basic studies of digestion, and of effects of emotions on it, led to new under-
standings of food utilization, of transmission of nerve impulses, and of actions of
endocrine glands. Second Professor of Physiology at Harvard, Dr. Cannon earned world-
wide respect as a researcher, as a teacher, and as an ambassador of scientific good will.

her deathbed, she admonished her son: "Walter, be good to the world." It was a legacy he neither forgot nor neglected.

Perhaps, as Cannon has hinted in his writings, the young man's choice of his life's work was influenced by the fact that the place of his birth was near to the site of Fort Crawford, where, fifty years earlier, Dr. William Beaumont had conducted his continuing studies of digestive processes through a fistulous "window" in the abdomen of his patient, Alexis St. Martin. However, it was a woman teacher in a St. Paul high school who advised Cannon to study in the East. So, in 1892, with a cash capital of $180, he entered Harvard College in Cambridge, Massachusetts. From then on, through four years of college and four years of Harvard Medical School in Boston, the young man paid his way with his own earnings. During his last year in medical school, he was invited to conduct courses in comparative anatomy at Harvard College and Radcliffe College. When, in June, 1900, Cannon received his degree in medicine, he accepted an instructorship in physiology at Harvard Medical School. A year after, he married his St. Paul sweetheart, Cornelia James. In 1902, he was named assistant professor; and in 1906, Dr. Cannon was appointed successor to Henry Pickering Bowditch, as George Higginson Professor of Physiology at Harvard—a position which he held for thirty-six years, until his resignation in August, 1942. Dr. Bowditch, who had held the post for thirty-five years, was the first full Professor of Physiology in the United States, and had himself been a student of Carl Ludwig, of Leipzig. Dr. Cannon, with a great deal of affection for his former mentor, often called himself professionally the "son" of Dr. Bowditch, and the "grandson" of Dr. Ludwig. Indeed, the contributions which Dr. Cannon made to advancement of the science of physiology would have earned deep paternal respect from his predecessors.

Professor Bowditch, recognizing potential talent when Walter Cannon volunteered to undertake a research project in addition to his first year medical studies, suggested that he might find a way to utilize the Röntgen ray as a means of studying the process of digestion in animals. Cannon set to work, devising an apparatus in which an animal could be placed above an aperture in a lead-shielded table, under which an x-ray tube was focused. Among his first experiments, Cannon watched the course of a button down a dog's esophagus, and an opaque bolus being swallowed by a goose. While he employed many types of animals, Cannon soon found that cats were most adaptable to his studies. In the main, he employed bismuth subnitrate as a readily dispersible substance opaque to x-rays. Among others, he also tested bismuth oxychloride, and barium sulfate. By mixing these tasteless salts of heavy metals with animals' natural food, for hours at a time Cannon was able to observe natural activities of digestive organs as shadows coursing across a glowing fluorescent screen.

"For centuries, priests and butchers who watched entrails of their sacrificed victims knew as much as physicians about the mechanical factors of digestion," Dr. Cannon wrote. However, traumatic or surgical wounds profoundly alter digestive processes—and as the nineteenth century neared its close, this vital bodily function was little understood either by physicians or laymen.

With his homemade apparatus and skillfully formulated contrast meals, Cannon found that he could observe movements of the alimentary tract without interfering with the animal to any disturbing degree. "By use of the x-rays," Cannon was able to report, "the rate of passage of food through the oesophagus, the speed of gastric peristalsis and rhythm, the oscillating contractions of the small intestine, the peculiar anti-peristalsis of the large intestine, the rapidity of discharge of gastric contents into the duodenum, the time required for material to be carried to the colon, and all the influences external and internal that affect these processes, can be observed continuously for as long a time as the animal remains in a state of peace and contentment . . ." His first report, "The Movements of the Stomach Studied by Means of the Röntgen Rays," was published in the *American Journal of Physiology* in 1898.

With the instinct of a true investigator, Cannon was able to turn one of the early difficulties which he encountered into a bypath of original investigation no less significant than that of his research on digestion. He observed that any change of emotional state in the animal, such as anxiety, distress, or rage, was accompanied by total cessation of movements of the stomach. Additional attention to the effects of emotions on digestive organs led to exploration of the autonomic nervous system which controls these movements. Dr. Cannon became no less a master of this branch of physiology than was he in the physiology of digestion. His findings were published from time to time in professional journals, then summed up in book form in *The Mechanical Factors of Digestion*, published in 1911. Four years later, Dr. Cannon's classic book, *Bodily Changes in Pain, Hunger, Fear and Rage*, was published. In the same year, 1915, he also was able to produce hyperthyroidism experimentally.

Dr. Cannon pursued the dual roles of researcher and teacher throughout his life. As a teacher, he possessed in high degree the characteristics which stimulated students to think for themselves and to embark upon original research. In research activities, as Professor Ralph B. Perry has said, "He was a good prospector—he knew how to locate the veins of rich scientific ore. But he (also) knew how to refine the gold." Though Dr. Cannon did not practice medicine, his strictly scientific code was governed by the code of the physician—his efforts were directed toward cure or relief of human ills.

The demands of World War I interrupted Dr. Cannon's work. He went to Europe with a Harvard medical unit whose duty it became to study and to combat shock. Results of these studies and research stemming therefrom saved lives of many persons wounded in military or in civil pursuits. Twenty-five years later, during World War II, Dr. Cannon was called upon to serve as chairman of the Committee on Shock and Transfusions of the National Research Council.

Following World War I, Dr. Cannon resumed both research and teaching. He was one of the pioneers in study of the autonomic nervous system, isolating at terminals of nerves a chemical product, sympathin, and pointing out its role as mediator of impulses between nerve and muscle. His observations also convinced him that the living body always strives toward a harmonious equilibrium—a state which Dr. Cannon called "homeostasis" in his book, *Wisdom of the Body*, and in other writings.

Dr. Cannon first introduced the word, "homeostasis," into medical vocabulary in the early 1920's; and he explained his ideas by saying:

"The coordinated physiological processes which maintain most of the steady states in the organism are so complex and so peculiar to living beings—involving, as they may, the brain and nerves, the heart, lungs, kidneys and spleen, all working cooperatively—that I suggest a special designation for these states—homeostasis. It means a condition —a condition which may vary—but which is relatively constant.

"Somehow," Dr. Cannon further elaborated, "the unstable stuff of which we are composed has learned the trick of maintaining stability." He reemphasized the word, "learned," for this circumstance, he pointed out, is not a special gift bestowed upon the highest organisms, but is the consequence of a gradual evolution.

Dr. Cannon noted that his idea was not new; it had been discussed by Hippocrates, some 2400 years ago. The great Father of Medicine had called it *vis medicatrix naturae*. He also rightly credited Dr. Claude Bernard of Paris with having been first, in 1878, to have given the idea a more precise analysis. Dr. Bernard called it the *milieu interne*—the internal environment, and stated that free and independent life are dependent upon the fixity of this *milieu interne*.

The views expressed by Bernard and by others before him were theoretical, based upon conjecture and long observation. Those expressed by Dr. Cannon were based upon sound research, which he himself had begun in 1896, and which he continued, either in person, or through brilliant direction of students whom he taught. In six postulates which he first published about 1925, Dr. Cannon elaborated upon his ideas of homeostasis:

1. "In an open system such as our bodies represent, compounded of unstable material and subjected continually to disturbing conditions, constancy is in itself evidence that agencies are acting, or are ready to act, to maintain this constancy.

2. "If a state remains steady, it does so because any tendency toward change is automatically met by increased effectiveness of the factor or factors which resist change.

3. "Any factor which operates to maintain a steady state by action in one direction, does not also act at the same point in the opposite direction.

4. "Homeostatic agents, antagonistic in one region of the body, may be cooperative in another region.

5. "The regulating system which determines a homeostatic state

may comprise a number of cooperating factors brought into action at the same time, or successively.

6. "When a factor is known which can shift a homeostatic state in one direction, it is reasonable to look for automatic control of that factor or for a factor or factors having an opposing effect . . . Homeostasis is not accidental, but is a result of organized government, and search for the governing agencies will result in their discovery."

In his book, *The Wisdom of the Body*, Dr. Cannon poses this question: "If the body can largely care for itself, what is the use of a physician?"

He immediately answered by pointing out that the well-trained physician "is acquainted with the possibilities and limitations of self-regulation and self-repair in the body."

Furthermore, "the physician realizes that he has at his command therapeutic agents with which he can support or replace the physiological or self-protective processes." He cites the examples of the use of insulin in diabetes; of thyroxin in myxedema; antitoxins for bolstering defensive mechanisms; and cold applications to reduce high fever.

"Finally," Dr. Cannon said, "a great service which the physician renders is that of bringing hope and good cheer to his patients. That alone justifies his presence."

The function of adrenal glands and effects of their secretions on the body, especially under conditions of stress or excitement, also were revealed by Dr. Cannon's research. He studied other organs of internal secretion, and especially the genetic, nervous, and psychic problems of sex. He did not hesitate to follow direction of his curiosity toward questions outside physiologic fields. In 1914, he described physical apparatus for determining coagulation time of blood.

Dr. Cannon's interests were not limited by Harvard's campus or by national boundaries. He accepted exchange professorships, in 1929, at the Sorbonne, in Paris, France; and in 1935, at Union Medical College in Peiping, China. More than fifty foreign students, from seventeen different countries, came to his laboratories for advanced study. Leading physiologists of the word were numbered among his friends, and he took an active part in numerous national and international organizations. He was elected to the National Academy of Sciences in 1914, and served as chairman of its Division of Foreign Relations for many

322

years. He also served as chairman of the Committee on Physiology of the National Research Council from its inception in 1916 until his death. As chairman of the American Medical Association's Committee on Protection of Medical Research he did the profession outstanding service in opposing efforts of antivivisectionists to cripple research. At one time he even served on a committee, along with magician Harry Houdini, seeking evidence of supernatural power. His friendship for Pavlov led to acceptance of presidency of the American-Soviet Medical Society upon its organization. He was capable of deep and loyal friendships, readily moved to sympathy and indignation by suffering and injustice. His organization of medical assistance to Spanish loyalists, and to United China Relief, was motivated not by political considerations but by great sympathy for suffering peoples.

Dr. Cannon was a scientific investigator from start to finish. He spent just fifty years at Harvard, as student, instructor, and professor. Although at times he carried a great burden of administrative work, he always kept research projects going, and managed to instill both wisdom and idealism in his students. Dr. Aub states that the advances in clinical research which have characterized this century are due in no small part to his initial inspiration.

Boyhood in Wisconsin and Minnesota had given Dr. Cannon a great love for athletics and for outdoor life. Proof of prowess of Dr. Cannon and his wife at mountain climbing may be found in Montana, where a mountain peak which they were first to scale bears their name. Their family, consisting of a son and four daughters, enjoyed much affection and quiet happiness together. Dr. Cannon was of a simple, straightforward, friendly disposition. His final book, *The Way of an Investigator*, written after his retirement in 1942, is both autobiographical and delightfully discursive on a life of research and scientific discovery.

When, as a young man, Dr. Cannon conducted his extensive studies with x-rays, the dangers attendant with their use were not realized. Fortunately, he had partially shielded his apparatus with lead sheets. However, during the last years of his life, he suffered intensely from acute dermatitis suspected as having been caused by radiation. His life was ended by a malignant lymphoma. He was nearly seventy-four years of age when death came to him, October 1, 1945.

EHRLICH
CHEMOTHERAPY IS LAUNCHED

"WE MUST SEARCH for magic bullets. We must strike the parasites, and the parasites only, if possible, and to do this, we must learn to aim with chemical substances!"

Paul Ehrlich's words were no hollow phrases; he backed them with intensive laboratory experimentation. From his work, and of even more importance, from application by others of the principles which he developed, medicine gained many "magic bullets." The new science of chemotherapy owed its growth largely to stimuli arising from Paul Ehrlich's work in Frankfurt, Germany, during the early years of the twentieth century.

There is hardly a field of medicine that has not benefited from Ehrlich's work. In clinical medicine he contributed studies on blood, and the use of methylene blue in malaria. His methods for staining bacteria were of great importance to bacteriology. His work on immunity made practical the application of Behring's findings; it was Ehrlich who standardized diphtheritic antitoxin, and who recognized the existence and role of toxoids. Finally, Ehrlich's originality and discipline of objective experimentation resulted in synthesis of antisyphilitic drugs and launched the age of chemotherapy.

Paul Ehrlich was born March 14, 1854, in the small town of Strehlen, in Silesia, Germany (now a part of Poland). He was the only son of a well-to-do Jewish family.

At ten years of age, Paul was sent to preparatory school at Breslau, where he became a classmate of Albert Neisser, who in later life was to become discoverer of the gonococcus bacillus. From 1872 to 1878 Ehrlich studied medicine in Strasbourg, Freiburg, and Breslau. Though generally his scholastic work was undistinguished, he continued to experiment in his own way. All of Ehrlich's research developed as offshoots of his preoccupation with one problem: why do different tissues have different affinities to the same dye? In Strasbourg he worked under

324

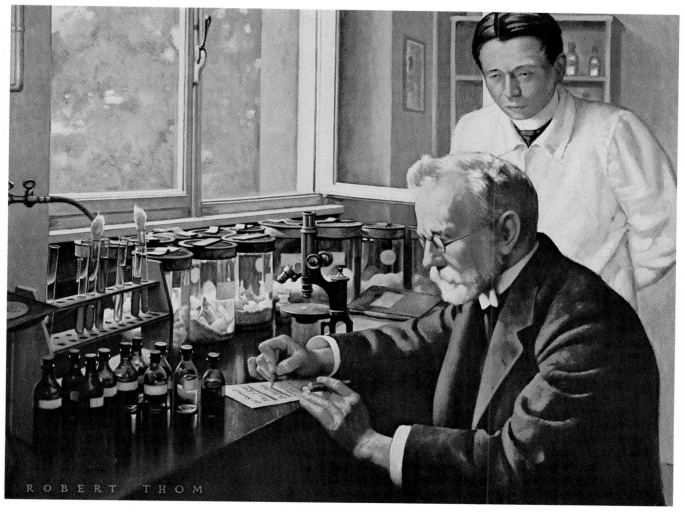

ROBERT THOM

EHRLICH: CHEMOTHERAPY IS LAUNCHED

In his crowded laboratory at Frankfurt's Institute of Experimental Therapy, German research scientist Paul Ehrlich (1854-1915) habitually scrawled work orders to associates with stubby colored pencils on "blocks" of note paper. Dr. Ehrlich and his Japanese assistant, Dr. Sahachiro Hata, announced Salvarsan (606) to the world in 1910 as a "chemical bullet" for treatment of syphilis. Dr. Ehrlich's success with chemical synthesis gave impetus to a new medical science, chemotherapy. Though his greatest achievements were in this field, Dr. Ehrlich contributed to many branches of medicine and shared in a 1908 Nobel Prize for his work on immunology.

the anatomist Waldeyer; in Breslau, under the physiologist Heidenhain and the pathologist Cohnheim. It was the latter's assistant, Ehrlich's older cousin Karl Weigert, who introduced Ehrlich to use of aniline dyes, greatly increasing the range of his research in staining. It was at the Cohnheim laboratory, too, that Ehrlich befriended William H. Welch, later the man most responsible for development of The Johns Hopkins School of Medicine in Baltimore.

While still a student, Ehrlich began to prepare papers for publication on the morphology of blood. This was an outgrowth of his ceaseless preoccupation with dyestuffs—he was able to differentiate the elements of blood by color analysis. This work laid the foundation for modern hematology.

Ehrlich presented his doctoral dissertation in 1878 at the University of Leipzig. The twenty-four-year-old research specialist received his medical degree for a thesis entitled: "Contributions to the Theory and Practice of Histological Staining." In it, Ehrlich laid down a basic principle that was to pervade his work—that pharmacological activity is based on the affinity of molecules of living matter for various chemical substances when brought into relationship with them.

In 1878, Ehrlich became an assistant to Professor von Frerichs at the Second Medical Clinic of Charité Hospital in Berlin. Von Frerichs recognized his talent, and Ehrlich was permitted to continue his research. In the course of ten years he produced more than forty articles, and published his first book on the "Oxygen Requirements of the Organism." He married Hedwig Pinkus in 1883, and received the title of professor, in 1884, at the University of Berlin. This happy decade came to an end with a change in policy which followed the death of von Frerichs. Also, an attack of pulmonary tuberculosis forced Ehrlich to spend parts of 1888 and 1889 recuperating in Egypt.

In 1890, Robert Koch, famous for his work in bacteriology, invited Ehrlich to work with him. Koch had not forgotten Ehrlich's success in 1882 in inventing a staining method for the tubercle bacillus. At Koch's newly founded Institute for Infectious Diseases, in Berlin, Ehrlich entered upon a new phase of his work: bacteriology and immunology. There, too, he began to work with Emil Behring. In 1892, Behring discovered specific immune substances which developed in blood serum of animals infected with diphtheria or with tetanus bacilli. It was Ehrlich, drawing upon his broad experience and his unprecedented experiments, who supplied practical procedures that enabled Behring to develop effective antitoxins.

During the course of his immunologic studies, Ehrlich developed his famous "side-chain" theory of immunity—an idea revealing the close relationship in which the scientist held his ideas of chemistry and of biology. Essentially, Ehrlich believed that "side-chains," produced in profusion by the body during infection (or supplied artificially when antitoxins were injected), unite with toxins released from bacteria, chemically neutralizing them.

In 1896, Ehrlich was named director of the State Institute for Serum Research and Testing at Steglitz. This makeshift institute provided meager facilities, but Ehrlich continued his researches. "As long as I have a water-tap, a flame, and some blotting paper," he told a friend, "I can work just as well in a barn!" Shortly thereafter, through efforts of Dr. Franz Adickes, Lord Mayor of Frankfurt am Main, there was created in that city a large Institute for Experimental Therapy. In 1899, Ehrlich accepted an invitation to become its director. There he was destined to work for the remaining sixteen years of his life, and to make the greatest of his discoveries. For the first time, he had fine laboratories, modern equipment, and capable assistants.

In Frankfurt, though a part of his work had to do with cancer research and with evaluation of serums for the government, Ehrlich's efforts were largely directed toward the field of chemotherapy. Indefatigable in his laboratory work, Ehrlich was original and daring. He had an uncanny way of being able to visualize chemical structures in his mind, even before they had been synthesized. In his own laboratory, there were seeming disarray and disorder, but Ehrlich knew just where to find everything. Of his assistants, however, he demanded strictest adherence to order and to his directions. These he laid out for each person, daily, on his "blocks"—small colored cards, on which were scrawled, with pencils of various colors, brief, cryptic directions or questions. Ehrlich demanded immediate attention to these orders, and daily progress reports from subordinates. Kindly, friendly, almost shy, the small-statured, cigar-smoking director could go into a fury of rage when his instructions were not followed. Chemists unwilling to use methods which he directed, however incredible they seemed, did not remain long at the Institute.

Ehrlich naturally began his studies with his beloved dyes. Methylene blue, with which as a student he had so well demonstrated nerve fibers, proved to have antimalarial properties. By 1904, through continuous chemical variation, he had succeeded in producing a dye known as trypan-red which proved effective against trypanosomes, particularly those causing sleeping sickness.

The side-chain theory continued to intrigue Ehrlich. Behring's anti-toxins, he reasoned, were the first effective specific remedies for infectious diseases. They were natural products, created within the body. Would it be possible to produce a similar effect with chemical compounds? Would it be possible to find chemicals which would kill specific disease-producing microbes before they would seriously harm the cells of the patient? Most research men were pessimistic. But Ehrlich, supported by the knowledge he had gained during immunity studies plus his boundless optimism, set out to find those "magic bullets," as he called them.

The work which Ehrlich was doing in the field of chemotherapy received a big boost in 1906, when the richly endowed Georg Speyer House was built next to his Institute and placed under his direction. In 1908, Ehrlich, together with Elie Metchnikoff of the Pasteur Institute, Paris, shared the Nobel Prize in Medicine "In recognition of his work on immunity."

Continuing his search for "magic bullets" which could be aimed at specific invaders without injury to the body, Ehrlich turned his attention to Atoxyl, an arsenical compound discovered in 1906 by Thomas and Breinl, working in Liverpool, England. Atoxyl had been found to be effective against certain trypanosomes, but at the same time to be highly toxic to optic nerves. Ehrlich disagreed with most contemporary chemists regarding the structural formula of Atoxyl, proved his theory correct, and set his assistants to work on a busy schedule of creating chemical variants—seeking always a compound that would possess maximum killing power against organisms of disease with minimum damage to cells of the host. "Parasitotropic they must be, but not organotropic," Ehrlich continually reminded his associates.

Starting with Atoxyl, Ehrlich and his co-workers created 418 separate compounds built around an arsenic radical and tested each thoroughly on animals before one was found that seemed to fulfill his specifications. No. 418, arsenophenylglycine, proved most effective against tropical diseases caused by trypanosomes. The research continued until, in 1907, compound No. 606 was created—the hydrochloride of dioxy-diamino-arseno-benzene. Ehrlich was optimistic about this compound; but an assistant erroneously reported that it had no effect whatsoever on trypanosomes, and so it was laid aside.

Two events contributed to the advancement of Ehrlich's chemotherapeutic endeavors. In 1905, Professors Fritz R. Schaudinn and Erich Hoffmann had discovered the spirochete, *Treponema pallidum*, to be the cause of syphilis. This pale, corkscrew-shaped organism had wrought immeasurable damage upon the human race for centuries, virtually unchecked by any drug or therapy. Its discoverers believed there was a relationship between spirochetes and trypanosomes, and, because of the far greater significance of the disease, Ehrlich began to study syphilis. Second event was the arrival at the Institute's laboratories, in 1909, of Dr. Sahachiro Hata, a pupil of Ehrlich's friend, Professor Kitasato, bacteriologist of Tokyo. Dr. Hata had been working experimentally with syphilis in rabbits, and had been sent to Frankfurt for further study. His first assignment at the Institute was to test on syphilis-infected animals every compound, old and new, that had been developed in the laboratories. The patient Japanese set about the task with characteristic thoroughness. Eventually, Hata came to compound 606. He reported to Ehrlich that it was by far the most effective and least toxic of all compounds tested against syphilitic infections.

Ehrlich was pleased, but he demanded further tests, hundreds of tests. Hata made them. Then, tests were begun on humans, conducted by cooperating physicians at nearby hospitals. Hundreds more tests were required to determine effective doses, safe doses; to determine whether the relief was permanent, or whether relapses would occur. Meantime, Professor Iversen at the St. Petersburg Hospital for Men reported that 606 completely cured patients with relapsing fever.

Drs. Ehrlich and Hata reported development of 606 and their experiments with the compound to medical men from many countries at the Congress for Internal Medicine, at Wiesbaden, Germany, April 19, 1910. Dr. Schreiber of Magdeburg Hospital gave an account of the first successful treatment of syphilitic patients at his hospital with 606. The announcements had an electrifying effect upon the medical world. Demands and entreaties for the drug poured in on Ehrlich. The name, Salvarsan, was given to compound 606, and it was registered with the patent office. Facilities at Georg Speyer House were put to making the drug in quantity; the Höchst Chemical Works began to build facilities for its manufacture—but for some time demand far exceeded supply. Ehrlich insisted on keeping a close check on any irregularity arising from use of 606. He devised a method for intravenous injection to get away from tissue damage and danger of infection—and then had to educate the medical profession to its use. He continued to search for more and better compounds. Finally, in No. 914, he found what he needed: the drug was not quite so active against the spirochete—but it was far safer, and much less difficult for physicians to administer. No. 914 became Neosalvarsan—and, for three decades, until the introduction of penicillin, Neosalvarsan (neoarsphenamine) and Salvarsan (arsphenamine) remained dominant as remedies for syphilis. In Paris, Ernest Fourneau at the Pasteur Institute applied Ehrlich's techniques to bismuth, creating several antisyphilitic compounds which paralleled and supplemented the arsenicals.

Ehrlich, at last, had created his "magic bullets." Regrettably, his success, while winning him many honors and much fame, also brought attacks. Some were from crackpots, who accused him of trying to poison people. Some were acts of jealousy. Some were anti-Semitic in character. These attacks greatly perturbed the kindly scientist, who wanted only to help the sick. In the scientific field, he could deftly answer any challenge; but these unfounded, unwarranted, unscientific attacks were beyond his understanding. These, together with worries attendant with the beginning of World War I, in August, 1914, undoubtedly contributed to shortening Ehrlich's life. A first stroke, late in 1914, was followed by a second, fatal attack on August 20, 1915. He was buried in the Jewish Cemetery of Frankfurt.

Paul Ehrlich has been variously described by different writers. Some have emphasized his eccentricities, his absent-minded habits, his disregard for conventional order. Some have portrayed him as an unscientific experimenter whose "shots in the dark" luckily hit some marks. But the facts remain: his wealth of ideas, his enthusiasm for biochemistry, his courage to try new avenues and his general creativity, combined with great gifts for organization and for harmonious direction, earned him the title of genius. Medicine has been heir to many "magic bullets" since 1915, created by men who followed in Ehrlich's footsteps in creative chemistry: among them, the antimalarials, the sulfonamides, the antihistamines, the ataraxic drugs.

A modest, kind, faithful man, respected by true scientists and medical men world-wide, beloved not only by his family but by his laboratory assistants, his faithful custodian Kadereit, and his secretary, Martha Marquardt, Paul Ehrlich was one of the greatest figures in medicine in the first half of the twentieth century.

RAMÓN y CAJAL
CHARTING THE NERVOUS SYSTEM

THE STERN fathers at the Latin school in Jaca were agreed: Santiago Ramón y Cajal probably wouldn't amount to much. According to their report, he was a poor student; he didn't use his memory; his flair for art was used more often as an outlet for his resentments than for studious purposes; he seemed stubborn and inflexible: no amount of flogging or denial of suppers would change his ways. So, bruised and half-starved, the boy was returned to his father, a country surgeon who eked out a precarious living in the Spanish Pyrenees village of Ayerbe. The busy doctor was both furious and frustrated. He had hoped his boy would become a physician, too; but perhaps, as teachers predicted, he was destined only to be a tradesman.

From such boyhood experiences came the young man who was destined to become Spain's leading scientist, histologist, neuroanatomist, and a personage revered equally by contemporary scientists, by politicians, by educators, and by peasants.

Santiago had been born eleven years earlier, on May 1, 1852, in Petilla, a tiny village high in the Pyrenees. He was the eldest of the rapidly growing family of Don Justo Ramón Casasús and Doña Antonia Cajal. In the Spanish custom, the boy's surname was compounded of both father's and mother's family names—Ramón y Cajal.

Young Santiago early learned the advantages of solitude to one whose mind runs in channels other than those locally considered conventional. He was interested in the outdoors; in natural history; and, most of all, in art. He devised many unusual pranks to further his interests, much to the consternation of his father and his neighbors. Repeatedly, the boy was placed in formal schools; repeatedly he was turned out of them as a failure. He preferred painting and hiking in the hills. In between courses, as disciplinary measures, his father had him apprenticed once to a barber, and once to a shoemaker. Finally,

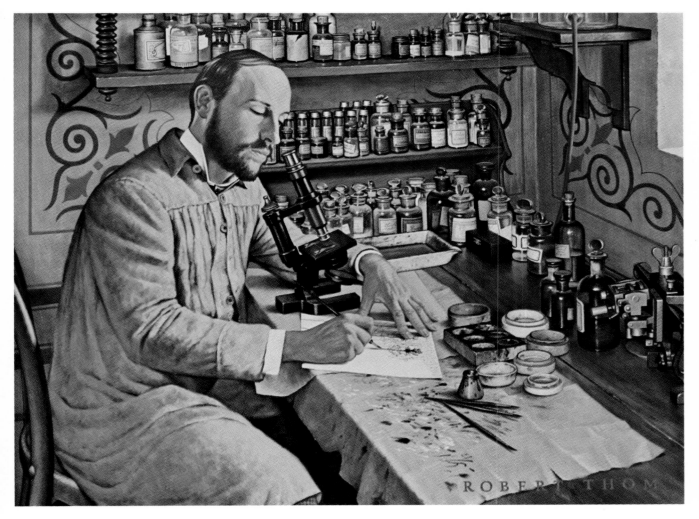

RAMÓN Y CAJAL: CHARTING THE NERVOUS SYSTEM

Boyhood teachers were positive that no good would come from backward, headstrong Santiago Ramón y Cajal (1852-1934), but the country surgeon's son was destined to become Spain's leading medical scientist and a world-renowned neuroanatomist. His contributions to neurology and to psychiatry began in a crowded laboratory in Barcelona. For forty years, Ramón y Cajal combined insatiable scientific curiosity, inventiveness that resulted in new stains for sections under his microscope, intensive observation, and inborn artistic ability, to reveal a wealth of new anatomical and functional facts about the nervous system, and about disorders affecting it. He received the Nobel Prize in Medicine in 1906.

Don Justo sent his son to Zaragoza University and enrolled him in the premedical course.

Fortunately, in the following year, 1869, the elder Ramón received appointment as professor of anatomy on the Faculty of Medicine at Zaragoza. He was at once filled with zeal to train his son as a skilled dissector. Thus, father and son finally found a common interest, and Santiago's artistic abilities at last were compatible with his father's ambitions. Together, they studied the anatomy of bones and bodies in a hidden dissecting room. Santiago sketched with exactness the structures their studies revealed. Proudly, Don Justo thought of publishing his son's sketches and water colors as an atlas of anatomy; but local facilities in graphic arts were not developed sufficiently to assure satisfactory reproductions.

In 1873, Santiago reached his majority, received his degree as licentiate in medicine, and was drafted into the Spanish army. After service in the medical corps during several strategic but nonsanguine Spanish counterrevolutionary campaigns, he was promoted to a rank equivalent to captain, and was assigned to service overseas in rebellious Cuba. He was placed in charge of an inadequately supplied infirmary at Vista Hermosa, on the edge of swamplands. Santiago soon was suffering along with his patients, from a combination of malaria, dysentery, and poor nutrition. By the spring of 1875, when his request for resignation finally was granted, he was a very sick man. In addition to his infirmities, he had been paid but once during his Cuban service.

After a period of recovery at home, Santiago Ramón y Cajal was appointed assistant instructor in anatomy at the Faculty of Medicine, University of Zaragoza. In June, 1877, he went to Madrid to take examinations for his doctorate in medicine. While in Madrid, he had an experience that was to change his life: one of the professors at the University showed him a microscope and some microscopic preparations. Intensely intrigued, Ramón y Cajal spent his savings for a microscope, a microtome, and a few supplies. Thus, in Zaragoza, he possessed the only good microscopic equipment of which the University could boast.

Life was not to be smooth for the young teacher, however. Weakened by malarial attacks, in 1878 Ramón y Cajal experienced symptoms of active tuberculosis. Another long period of convalescence was necessary. In the course of treatment at Panticosa, nursed by his sister Paula, Cajal took to hiking in the mountains, pursuing his hobby of photography. The combination of fresh air, adequate food, and renewed zest for life helped bring about recovery.

Returning to Zaragoza, Ramón y Cajal received an advancement in faculty position, becoming director of the Anatomical Museum. With this assurance of modest security, the young professor married Doña Silveria Fañanás García—much to his family's consternation. Despite their misgivings, the marriage proved beneficial both to the health and the stability of the young professor's career. Señora de Ramón y Cajal encouraged her husband's scientific work while exercising great care over their growing family.

His teaching of anatomy at Zaragoza readily led Ramón y Cajal to develop interest in histology—the study of tissues. His microscope revealed to him secrets of minute structures hidden from the unaided eye. His equipment consisted of his beloved microscope, a few textbooks of doubtful authority, and one or two foreign journals. But to these were added an insatiable curiosity and an ability to concentrate and to work with almost frenzied dedication. His progress in this field is the more amazing in view of the facts: his university appointments up to this time had been undistinguished; he had not met any of the great medical investigators of the day. In his own words, by language and by tradition he was isolated from the main stream of science.

In 1884, Ramón y Cajal was appointed professor of anatomy at the university in Valencia. A cholera epidemic in 1885 diverted his attention temporarily to the study of bacteriology, and his work in this new field attracted some favorable governmental attention. However, he chose to return to the study of histology; and in 1887, he was called to accept the professorship of histology at the University of Barcelona.

In Barcelona, Ramón y Cajal, then 35 years of age, seriously began the work that was to give him distinction and to strengthen his position as a medical researcher. At the beginning, he noted that nearly every published finding on histology was incomplete, and needed further study. This intrigued his curiosity. Also, he had learned from a Valencian neuropsychiatrist, **Dr. Luis Simarro**, of the chrome silver stain for nerve tissues developed by Camillo Golgi, of Pavia, Italy. Dr. Simarro, like many other workers, including, eventually, Golgi himself, had ceased using the method, having found it unreliable. Ramón y Cajal's first important step was to draw upon his experience with photography to make improvements in methods of using Golgi's stain. Then he began a systematic study of the entire nervous system, staining cells and tissues with a clarity which never had been achieved before. Further, he discovered that far better results were obtained by staining nerve cells of specimens from chick embryos, birds, and young animals, before myelin sheaths formed about axis cylinders of nerve cells, hiding them from the revealing stains. To these techniques he added his other great talent: drawing. His skillful illustrations made it possible for him to demonstrate what he saw. He began, rather timidly, to publish his findings and to disagree with the opinions of histologists in other countries. The reaction was skepticism of the validity of his work; and questioning, by some of his own countrymen, as to his audacity in challenging the pronouncements of foreign professors of histology.

To equalize this development, Ramón y Cajal launched upon another phase of his life with intensity equal to his scientific investigation: he joined the German Society of Anatomists; he undertook to learn the German language, so that he could read German medical literature, and communicate in German.

Ramón y Cajal determined to demonstrate his work to his German colleagues. From his meager savings, he took enough to finance attendance, in October, 1889, at a meeting of the German Society of Anatomists at the University of Berlin. Into his bag went the best of his prized microscopic slide specimens and his sketches.

Met only with curiosity and more skepticism, Ramón y Cajal patiently awaited opportunity to demonstrate his findings. First of all, to have a Spaniard among them was regarded by members of the society as without precedent. Spain had no recognized histologists. Further, most of those present were smugly sure of their own concepts. However, the opportunity finally came. With assistance of two or three microscopes,

Ramón y Cajal, in broken French, sought to explain his preparations. It was not long before the few men who had been courteous enough to attend the demonstration had shaken off skepticism and were congratulating their courageous Spanish colleague. How, they asked, had he been able to get such results, when they had experienced only failures? He explained his methods. His demonstrations won Ramón y Cajal the support and lifelong friendship of Albert von Kölliker, dean of German histologists; and through him, of Waldeyer, His, van Gehuchten, Bardeleben, Schwalbe, and the Swedish histologist Retzius. Said Kölliker: "I am glad that the first histologist Spain has produced is a man as distinguished as you, a man worthy of the nobility of science."

Ramón y Cajal's work, now recognized internationally, gained acceptance and appreciation at home. In 1892, he was called to assume the chair of Normal Histology and Pathological Anatomy at the University of Madrid. His new findings received wide publication, and from one country after another came honors. In 1894, he received the highest recognition English scientists could bestow: Sir Michael Foster, secretary of the Royal Society of London, invited him to deliver the Croonian Lecture before that body; and Cambridge University conferred a doctorate upon him.

There was no lack of appreciation of these honors on Ramón y Cajal's part; he chose, however, to regard them as honors accruing to his homeland rather than to him personally. For himself, he asked only to be allowed to continue his work—and life was to grant him another 40 years of productive activity. He was concerned that his work should continue after him; and indeed it did, in the researches of his more renowned students, among whom were del Río Hortega, Nicholas Achucarro, Tello, de Castro, Villaverde, Sánchez, his own son Jorge Ramón y Cajal Fañanás, and his brother Pedro.

The record of scientific work achieved by Ramón y Cajal, during his long, active life is most impressive. In 1888, he increased the applicability of Golgi's stain. In 1903, he worked out his own formula for a silver nitrate stain that demonstrated nerve cells and nerve fibers with clarity. In 1913, he employed a gold sublimate stain for astrocytes that brought another portion of nerve tissue under observation. Subsequently, his pupils carried these studies further with application of a silver carbonate stain. "For the world of the infinitely little," wrote Garrison, "he was better visioned and consequently had better luck from the start than most investigators; and here, his artistic skill with pencil and brush . . . helped."

Among Ramón y Cajal's greater contributions to medical knowledge, and to the fields of neurology and psychiatry, according to Garrison, were elucidation: ". . . of the developmental and structural basis of the dynamics of the neuron; of transmission of impulse; of localization of function; and of degeneration and regeneration in the nervous system . . . His encyclopedic treatises on neurohistology and on degeneration and regeneration in the nervous system are his masterpieces . . ." He published over 250 scientific papers, edited a journal in his field, and wrote a number of books, including the three-volume *Texture of the Nervous System of Man and of the Other Vertebrates* (1897-1904), of which a French edition was issued in 1911; *Degeneration and Regeneration In the Nervous System*, in two volumes (1913-1914); and a two-volume autobiography. These publications have given to medical men and to neurosurgeons an understanding of the cell structure and mode of function of every part of the nervous system, and a better concept of brain structure and of characteristics of brain tumors by which they can be guided in meeting the needs of their patients.

The great scientist was not unaware of the need for balancing the rigors of the laboratory with other interests. His family, grown to include six children, received love and attention. His fascination with photography intrigued him to develop advanced methods, and in 1912 to write a book on color photography. He found much relief and recreation in long walks through Madrid's parks and suburbs; and, in the Spanish custom, nearly every afternoon he visited a favorite café, frequented by his friends, for relaxation and conversation. Out of the philosophic discussions over coffee came an interesting volume of anecdotes and aphorisms, entitled: *Coffee-House Chatter.*

Despite feelings aroused by the Spanish-American War in 1898, Ramón y Cajal was invited to the United States of America the following year to participate in a celebration at Clark University, and to receive an honorary doctorate. In 1900, he received the Moscow prize at the International Medical Congress in Paris; and in 1904, the Helmholtz medal from the Royal Prussian Academy. In 1906, the Royal Caroline Institute of Sweden awarded the Nobel Prize for physiology and medicine jointly to Ramón y Cajal and to Golgi. It was the first time a histologist had been so honored. The medal was presented to him by the Swedish King, Oscar II, at a ceremony in Stockholm. With this recognition came a substantial financial award that was much needed.

In 1922, at age 70, Ramón y Cajal retired from the University of Madrid, closing a 30-year tenure there. But he continued to work, to write, and to guide students from his table in the café. In 1932, a new laboratory was built at government expense and named after him— El Instituto Ramón y Cajal. He was invited to work in it; however, the rooms seemed too grand and the ceilings too lofty; he preferred the cramped little laboratory in his home at Avenida Alfonso XII. Though deafness and feebleness slowed his pace in his last years, according to Penfield, a former student who visited him, Santiago Ramón y Cajal continued to work with a fierce impatience, elaborating a final defense for the first child of his researches, the neuron doctrine. Also, during his last years, he wrote another significant work, entitled: *The World as Seen at Eighty.* Death overtook Ramón y Cajal in his eighty-third year, on October 17, 1934.

An insight into the philosophy that drove him on to greater and greater achievements throughout his life is revealed by Ramón y Cajal's words, in *Coffee-House Chatter:* "When facts are faced squarely, we must admit that it is not so much the thought of our own death that grieves us as the realization that by it we are snatched from the bosom of humanity and thus robbed forever of hope of seeing the unfolding of the heroic struggle constantly being waged between the mind of man and the blind energy of natural forces."

Ramón y Cajal would have liked the Spanish government's final tribute to his memory: it undertook a complete republication of his written works.

HARVEY CUSHING AND NEUROSURGERY

OPERATIONS on the skull provide the oldest evidence of surgical procedures of which there is record. Yet, because of inherent technical difficulties and high mortality risks, surgical conquest of diseases of the brain and nervous system was slow to develop. Not until the twentieth century was there sufficient knowledge of the anatomy and of the functioning of these vital areas to encourage any but the boldest surgeons to invade these tissues; and, with discouraging regularity, their patients were lost. Successful brain surgery and neurosurgery came about only through long study and perfection of exacting, delicate surgical skills. The man who was to lead the way and to place neurosurgery on a sound, scientific footing was Harvey Williams Cushing—an intense, severe man remembered by some of his junior assistants as uncompromising, dictatorial, and indomitable. However, Dr. William H. Welch, "father" of the medical faculty at The Johns Hopkins University, asserted, in 1931, that Dr. Cushing was "undoubtedly the outstanding medical figure in the world." Dr. Franklin S. Newell observed that Dr. Cushing "was an extremely hard man to work with, whether one was over him or under him . . . but when he wanted to be he was one of the most charming people in the world . . ." John F. Fulton, Dr. Cushing's friend, associate, and biographer, describes him thus: "In all he did, Cushing was a perfectionist—on the parallel bars and at tennis, in the experimental laboratory and the operating room where he constantly attempted to extend the horizons of medical science . . . He had the temperament and the sensitive perception of an artist, but he also had the enduring patience of the scientist . . . Along with an unyielding devotion to principle there was warmth and gaiety and humor which lightened the way and proved a source of unending delight to his family and his host of friends." Of him, Elizabeth Thomson wrote: "By devoting his life to neurological surgery and its problems he made operations on the brain of little more hazard than

340

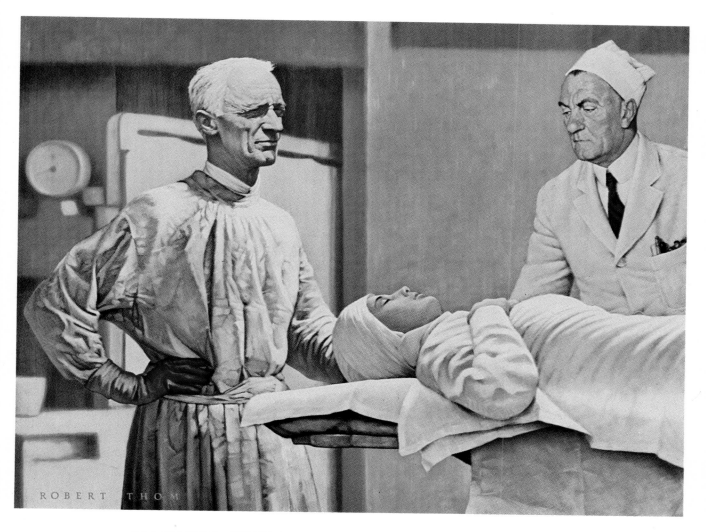

HARVEY CUSHING AND NEUROSURGERY

Surgery on highly sensitive tissues of the brain was seldom attempted, even after anesthesia and asepsis became standard operating room procedures. Not until the early 1900's was the tremendous risk to life reduced by research and by delicate surgical techniques, many of them developed and taught by Ohio-born Dr. Harvey W. Cushing, at Johns Hopkins, at Harvard, and at Yale. Dr. Cushing removed 2,000 brain tumors; developed a "school" of students from many lands who put up with his pungent personality in order to learn his methods. Adolph Watzka, surgical orderly, for many years was his constant operating room companion.

those involving the abdomen . . ." and, "By example he taught that a physician is obligated to consider more than a diseased organ, more even than the whole man—he must view the man in his world."

Surgery as a discipline of medicine had advanced but slowly over the centuries, as knowledge of anatomy and of pathology increased. Speed and dexterity were prime operational skills prior to the introduction of anesthesia by Dr. Morton in 1846; and after that, although operations increased tenfold, there were only limited improvements either in the technique of surgery or in the management of wounds. Dangers and complications of infection inevitably arose. Introduction of antisepsis by Joseph Lister in 1865 paved the way, and adoption a decade later of aseptic techniques for surgery and for care of wounds laid the foundations for tremendous advances in surgery. More and more of the body's organs, such as the intestines, the thyroid, and the ovaries, once considered beyond the range of the scalpel, came under the jurisdiction of the surgeon.

Still another discovery, however, was essential to the development of neurosurgery: the demonstration by Fritsch and Hitzig, in 1870, of the electrical excitability of the cortex of a dog's brain. A whole new field of physiologic investigation was opened as researchers sought to learn which parts of the brain and spinal cord controlled specific organs and body functions. Late in the nineteenth century a number of investigators, many of them British, began exploration of the brain. Sir Charles Sherrington used anthropoid apes for study. Sir William Macewen started removal of brain tumors in 1879, and Sir Victor Horsley followed in 1887. It was Dr. Horsley, a man of great courage, who introduced the curved scalp flap to conserve blood supply, who developed bone wax to control bleeding, and who was first to remove a spinal cord tumor. The work in Spain of Santiago Ramón y Cajal in charting the nervous system also contributed greatly to the development of neurosurgery. It was to this field of brilliant surgical pioneering and development that young Dr. Cushing was introduced as the nineteenth century ended.

Harvey Cushing was born in Cleveland, Ohio, April 8, 1869, the son, grandson, and great-grandson of physicians. His grandfather, Erastus Cushing, had come to the Western Reserve state of Ohio

342

from Massachusetts in 1835. His father, Henry Kirke Cushing, a graduate of the Medical Department of the University of Pennsylvania, practiced in Cleveland most of his life. Dr. Kirke and Betsey Williams Cushing had ten children, seven of whom reached maturity. Of these, Harvey was the youngest. He and his brother, Edward, were destined to carry on the family's medical traditions.

Harvey entered Yale University in 1887, graduating in 1891. That fall, he went to Boston and entered Harvard Medical School. At one point, a death which occurred while he was administering an anesthetic depressed him to the point where he nearly abandoned medical studies. He overcame this shock by developing a system for charting respiration and pulse during operations. Later, he added blood pressure to this record. These were definite contributions to the technique of anesthesia, and to safety for patients undergoing operations. Also, during his final year in medical school, he had opportunity to work with Dr. J. W. Elliot, who had studied with Dr. Horsley in London. Observation of Dr. Elliot's operations for brain tumors undoubtedly stimulated the young student in choice of his life's specialty.

Graduated from Harvard with the degrees of M.D. and A.M., *cum laude*, in June, 1895, Dr. Cushing entered on a year of internship at Massachusetts General Hospital. It was in December of 1895 that Wilhelm Conrad Röntgen discovered x-rays; and Dr. Cushing was active among those who first tried out the new apparatus at the Boston hospital.

In the fall of 1896, Dr. Cushing went to Baltimore, Maryland, to become a surgical resident under Dr. William S. Halsted, director of surgical service at The Johns Hopkins Hospital. Dr Halsted was then the most outstanding American surgeon, and the newly opened Johns Hopkins Medical School and Hospital were teeming with activity. Dr. Cushing's drive and ability fitted in well at The Hopkins, but his personality contributed to difficulties. Neither he nor Halsted readily understood one another during this period, although in later life they achieved a mutual respect. During his initial period of four years at The Hopkins, Dr. Cushing laid the foundations for close friendships with Dr. William Osler and Dr. Welch. His native artistic ability received stimulus from friendship with Max Broedel, The Hopkins' great medical artist. Dr. Cushing also began to make a name for himself for his studies of the gall bladder, his surgical work in repairing intestines perforated during typhoid, and his splenectomies. It was at The Hopkins, too, that he did his first gasserian ganglion resection to relieve the intolerable pain of trigeminal neuralgia.

In June, 1900, Dr. Cushing sailed for Europe. Having made up his mind that neurosurgery was to be his field (despite the fact that it hardly existed as a specialty), he sought out Dr. Horsley in London. He also visited the Hunterian Museum, and many hospitals in London and in Paris. In Berne, Switzerland, he found a pleasant and profitable association with the surgeon, Theodor Kocher, and the physiologist, Hugo Kronecker. In their laboratories he carried on experiments concerning the relation of blood pressure to pulse and to intracranial pressure. Later, he visited Italy, then spent a month in Liverpool with Dr. Sherrington, where he assisted in craniotomies on anthropoids.

Returning to The Hopkins in 1901, Dr. Cushing endeavored to launch his career in neurosurgery. Despite scarcity of suitable neurological patients, and appalling mortality rates following operations, Dr. Cushing struggled on toward his objective.

One of Dr. Cushing's contributions to The Hopkins was establishment of the Hunterian Laboratory, in 1905. Named for John Hunter, famous London anatomist, the laboratory became a center for teaching and research in surgery.

In June, 1902, Dr. Cushing married the sweetheart of his youth, Katharine Crowell, and they settled in a house next door to the Oslers, who were to become lifelong friends. The Cushings were to have five children, for whom the doctor had great love, but little time; he drove himself and his associates without mercy. The fact that so many of his patients were doomed added much to his load of care.

From his father, Harvey Cushing had learned to find relaxation in collecting books. This hobby received a great impetus during his friendship with Dr. Osler.

Early in his work on brain surgery, Dr. Cushing found that improvement of existing techniques was imperative. He owed his successes to painstaking attention to detail and constant striving for improvement. Particularly difficult was the problem of control of bleeding. In 1904,

Dr. Cushing developed a cranial tourniquet that proved very helpful. In 1908, he began to study and to operate on the pituitary gland, which is deeply buried in the skull and closely associated with the brain and with bodily functions. In 1912, he published a book, *The Pituitary Body and Its Disorders*, which documented fifty operations. This gland and tumors affecting it were to hold his attention for the rest of his life; and a specific pituitary disease, first described by him in 1932, has been called Cushing's syndrome.

Dr. Cushing's style of research has been described as intuitive. Once he had settled upon an idea, the objective of his investigations was to prove the correctness of his theory. Many times he was successful, research proving his ideas to be sound. At other times, he had difficulty in abandoning an idea, despite proof of its error.

During his stay at The Hopkins, which lasted until 1912, Dr. Cushing had many invitations to take professorships and other posts at leading medical schools and hospitals; but he had one objective in mind: Harvard. Finally, when plans were under way for construction of Peter Bent Brigham Hospital in Boston, Dr. Cushing was offered the post of chief of surgery at the hospital, and one of the professorships in surgery at his alma mater, Harvard Medical School. These he accepted. Among the rules for the new teaching service, in the passage of which Dr. Cushing had a part, was that of compulsory retirement at age 63—a ruling he was later to regret.

World War I interrupted Dr. Cushing's work in Boston. From 1915 to 1919, he served in France, first with the British, and later with the American Expeditionary Force. Very lively excerpts from his wartime diaries were published many years later, in 1935. During the war, the vascular disease in his legs, which was to plague him the rest of his life, manifested itself.

After the war, Dr. Cushing resumed teaching and neurosurgery, pioneering in the field of brain surgery. His careful study of patients, before operation as well as after, and development of extremely delicate techniques, resulted in greater successes, bolder operations, and reduction of danger of mortality. He was responsible for development of many new procedures, instruments, and safety measures that saved patients' lives and returned an increasing proportion of them to useful pursuits. During the last fifteen years of his service in Boston, he attracted men from all over the world who came to observe or for periods of service in his clinic. He also established the Harvard Experimental Surgical Laboratory, an institution similar to the Hunterian Laboratory at The Hopkins. An important step forward was Dr. Cushing's introduction of electrosurgery to neurological operations in 1926. In that same year, too, Dr. Cushing received the Pulitzer prize for his two-volume work: *The Life of Sir William Osler*. A high light of the Cushings' family life was the marriage of their daughter, Betsey, to James Roosevelt, in 1930. This was to bring Dr. Cushing and Governor Franklin D. Roosevelt into close communication; and during Roosevelt's early years of the Presidency, Dr. Cushing served on a number of important governmental advisory committees.

In 1931, Dr. Cushing operated for the two thousandth time for a verified brain tumor—an unprecedented record of accomplishment. In 1932, with Percival Bailey, he reported on this series of two thousand tumors in a book: *Intracranial Tumors*. That year, too, he published *The Pituitary Body and Hypothalamus*. His great classic, *Meningiomas*, written jointly with Dr. Louise Eisenhardt, was published in 1938.

During the course of his career, Dr. Cushing had made many trips abroad and had developed friendships with most of the world's leading neurologists. He had given lectures on many important occasions, had received many honors and honorary memberships in medical organizations of other nations, and had received a score or more of honorary doctorate degrees from great universities.

The rule covering compulsory retirement, which Dr. Cushing had helped formulate, caught up with him in 1932—a situation to which he adjusted with some difficulty. His successor was Dr. Elliott Cutler, a former pupil. The fact that he was not invited to continue to serve as a sort of senior consultant hurt Dr. Cushing deeply.

The following year, 1933, upon the urging of a number of friends, and particularly, of Dr. John F. Fulton, then Professor of Physiology, Dr. Cushing accepted appointment as Sterling Professor of Neurology at Yale University. Dr. Louise Eisenhardt, who had started with Dr. Cushing as a secretary and later studied medicine, joined him at New

Haven, bringing from Boston Dr. Cushing's collection of specimens of brain tumors. Together, they established a unique institution: the Brain Tumor Registry.

Over the years, Dr. Cushing's interest in books on medical history, particularly the works of Vesalius, had increased. He had pursued book collecting enthusiastically, along with his friends, Dr. Arnold Klebs, of Nyon, Switzerland, and Dr. Fulton. He joined with them in an agreement that their collections should be combined and be presented to the Medical School at Yale. Dr. Cushing set about to put his own books and papers in order, and to influence Yale to provide suitable housing for the contemplated medical history library.

In December, 1937, Dr. Cushing again retired and became Emeritus Professor, but continued to busy himself with his library project. Though his vascular difficulties prevented him from travel, honors continued to come to him. On April 8, 1939, the Harvey Cushing Society paid tribute to him on his seventieth birthday at a meeting in New Haven. Friends from many countries attended. In June, 1939, he received an honor which he deemed most significant: he became the first surgeon, and the sixth person in 250 years, to have been elected to honorary fellowship in the Royal College of Physicians of London. A month later, he was gratified to learn that Yale University had appropriated $600,000 for a medical library, one wing of which was to be devoted to medical history.

Death came to Dr. Cushing, October 7, 1939, following a heart attack. In his will, he bequeathed his library to Yale, naming Dr. Fulton his "literary executor." He also bequeathed funds for cataloging and putting his collection into shape for easy reference. In 1946, Dr. Fulton published an extensive biography of Dr. Cushing.

Final rites for Dr. Cushing were held in New Haven, October 9, after which his earthly journey ended where it began—his ashes were taken back to Cleveland and placed beside those of his mother, father, and the sister and brothers who had preceded him.

But Dr. Cushing's neurosurgical work was not at an end. A truly great teacher, he turned it over to his pupils, and their pupils, who carry it forward in clinics and operating rooms the world over.

JOSEPH GOLDBERGER
DIETARY DEFICIENCY AND DISEASE

THE TALL, slim doctor with the piercing eyes was making rounds of the orphanage with his young assistant. In orderly lines of twos, children were marching by. Suddenly, a small boy broke from the line, ran to the tall doctor and grabbed him about the legs. Looking up from a face shining with shy admiration, the boy said: "Are you the man giving us all the good things to eat?"

"Yes," said the doctor, a rare smile illuminating his face, "do you like them?"

"Oh, indeed we do. I hope you won't stop!"

The smile lingered briefly as an attendant shooed the small boy back into line. Then the customary seriousness returned, and the flashing eyes continued their rapid, restless survey of the surroundings. Particularly, Dr. Goldberger studied the faces of the little folk. Why must they suffer these unsightly pellagrous lesions, and all the accompanying discomforts? Why had pellagra visited over half the children in the orphanage, year after year, during the seventeen years the institution had been in existence? Would the new diets he had prescribed cure the afflicted? Would they prevent a recurrence of pellagra next spring?

Dr. Goldberger's mind impatiently demanded answers, but his scientific training warned that only time would tell. Meantime, there were so many things to attend to. Dr. Waring could manage studies at the orphanages; he'd have to see how Dr. Willets was getting along at the State Sanitarium. Then, there was the appointment with the Governor...

That was the way Dr. Joseph Goldberger, surgeon in the United States Public Health Service, went about his work. By this time, 1914, Dr. Goldberger was a veteran; his record as an investigator in matters of health and sanitation was well established. When a particularly knotty problem demanding immediate action faced the Surgeon General, it was likely that Dr. Goldberger would be hurried on the mission. Now,

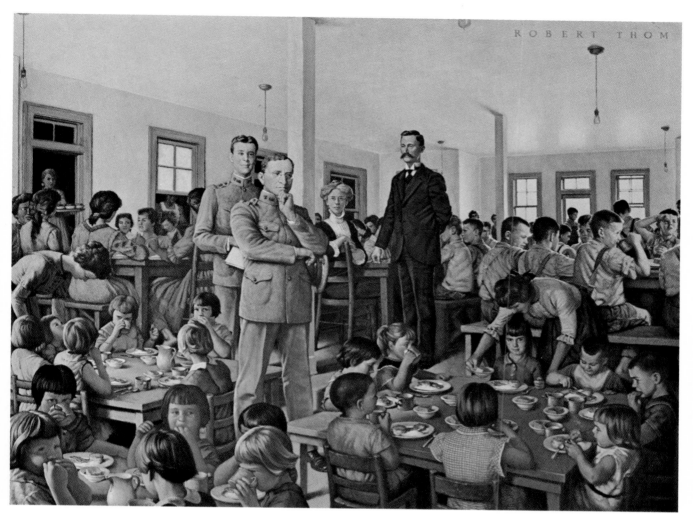

GOLDBERGER: DIETARY DEFICIENCY AND DISEASE

When Dr. Joseph Goldberger, Surgeon, United States Public Health Service, and his assistant, Dr. C. H. Waring, began studies of pellagra at the Baptist Orphanage near Jackson, Mississippi, in 1914, they faced puzzling questions: why were adults, older children, and the very young, free of the disease? Why, every year, did it strike children aged three to twelve? Dr. Goldberger ruled out infection or toxic foods as causes. With cooperation of Director J. R. Carter and House Mother "Miss Ida," the doctors added fresh meat, eggs, and milk to diets. Pellagra disappeared. By bold experiments, Dr. Goldberger proved dietary deficiency the cause of pellagra; pointed other researchers toward discovery of essential nutrients, now called vitamins, required to maintain health.

there was the problem of pellagra. If anybody could find the answers, Goldberger could.

Dr. Goldberger did find the answers to the causes and cure for pellagra; proved them beyond doubt in the face of powerful opposition from some of his medical colleagues; and thereby he helped put on solid footing the foundations for scientific study of vitamins and nutrition.

Diseases which are now known to have been caused by nutritional deficiencies were observed and described in the writings of Hippocrates and of Pliny. Beriberi has been known in the Orient for three thousand years. James Lind, in 1757, recognized that scurvy could be cured or prevented by juices of citrus fruits. Pellagra had first been studied comprehensively in 1730 by Gaspar Casal, physician of Oviedo, Spain; and its name, first used by Frapolli, in 1771, derived from the Italian words, *pelle agra*, meaning "rough skin." It came to notice in Spain and in Italy after introduction of corn from the New World as a food product. Pellagra was first described in North America in 1864, although undoubtedly it had been widespread long before. By the first decades of the twentieth century, it had become a serious and baffling problem in southern United States. Did it arise, as some physicians believed, from a powerful, unknown toxin, perhaps in corn? Or, was it caused by infectious microorganisms, as other physicians believed? The affliction defied the usual patterns of infections: it was a disease commonly associated with poverty; unlike infections, it struck more often in rural regions than in crowded cities; it was particularly serious among inmates of institutions, such as orphanages, prisons, or asylums —yet it never was noted among attendants or administrative staffs, even though their work brought them in close contact with patients.

Modern knowledge of the entire field of nutritional deficiencies stems from the work of Casimir Funk, who, in 1911, described the isolation from rice polishings of an active substance that would cure beriberi. His work was preceded by that of a group of Dutch medical officers in the East Indies: Eijkman, in 1897, established that beriberi among prisoners could be cured and prevented by adding rice polishings to their diet; his successor, Grijns, postulated the then revolutionary idea that the disease was due to a nutritional deficiency, and not to toxicity or infection. Funk, believing the substance he had isolated had characteristics of the chemical family known as amines suggested the term, "vitamine," and went on to develop the theory of deficiency diseases, and of existence of dietary factors specific for the cure of each: the "antiberiberi vitamine," the "antiscurvy vitamine," and the like.

Meantime, pellagra had become so widespread in the cotton-growing areas in southern United States that it was seriously affecting the economy. Cotton producers put pressure upon Senators and Congressmen from the South; and they, in turn, put pressure on the United States Public Health Service to do something about pellagra. Although an able staff from the Public Health Service already had spent five years studying the disease, and every conceivable clue had been traced down —none had led to a satisfactory answer. So, early in 1914, Surgeon General Rupert Blue ordered Dr. Goldberger to leave Detroit's diphtheria problems in the hands of an assistant and take over investigations of pellagra in the cotton country.

Indeed, Dr. Goldberger was well fitted for his new assignment. He had already proved to be an able clinician, a good bacteriologist, an epidemiologist, and a parasitologist, as well as an excellent investigator.

Joseph Goldberger was born July 16, 1874, on a peasant tenant farm near Giralt, Austria-Hungary (now a part of Czechoslovakia). Crop failures plagued the peasants, and fascinating tales came back from relatives in the New World. In 1881, when Joseph was seven, father Samuel and mother Sarah Goldberger decided to make the break: they converted all their resources to cash and sailed for New York. They settled on the lower East side, and the family's eight children were sent to school. Samuel peddled on the Bowery until they could open a little grocery store. Joseph and his brothers were delivery boys; but Joseph usually had a book under his coat. He haunted libraries and second-hand book stalls. At home, his upbringing was strictly Jewish orthodox; at school, his companions were of every race and creed.

At sixteen, Joseph entered the course of civil engineering at New York City College, standing fifth in his class of six hundred at the end of his second year. However, his friend, Pat Murray, who had entered Bellevue Hospital Medical College, persuaded Joseph to accompany him to hear Dr. Austin Flint, Jr., deliver a medical lecture. To the consternation of his family, Joseph transferred to medicine, entering the Bellevue school. In 1895, he graduated second in his class, and stood at the top of the list for appointment as an intern at Bellevue Hospital. There he demonstrated a remarkable aptitude for precise, accurate detail in reports.

The lower East side offered little opportunity for a young physician, so Dr. Goldberger entered practice in Wilkes Barre, Pennsylvania. Two years there convinced him that private practice was not his field. There was money to be made—but no adventure. To Joseph, money without adventure had no appeal. Dr. Goldberger was never to be entirely free of petty financial worries—but adventure he found indeed.

After unsuccessfully trying to join the Navy as the Spanish American War began, Dr. Goldberger entered the Public Health Service in 1899, as an assistant surgeon. His first assignment at Reedy Island, Delaware, brought him under the influence of Farrar Richardson, who gave Goldberger sound instruction and free rein to improve on routine inspection methods then in use. In 1902, Surgeon General Walter Wyman sent Dr. Goldberger to Tampico, Mexico, to study yellow fever. Within five years, spent in Tampico and in New Orleans, Dr. Goldberger became one of the world's authorities on yellow fever—a disease of which he himself nearly died.

In 1906, Dr. Goldberger dealt his family another shock: he announced his intent to marry a pretty Gentile girl—Mary Farrar, daughter of a prominent New Orleans family and niece of Farrar Richardson. The Farrar family, no less than the Goldbergers, had serious misgivings—but neither the stubborn doctor nor his equally determined fiancée would be swayed. They were married April 19, 1906. Mary's life was to be no bed of roses, for Dr. Goldberger's protracted assignments away from home, his constant exposure to danger, and his poor scale of pay, gave rise to many anxieties. His first son was but thirty-six hours old when Dr. Goldberger was assigned to Brownsville, Texas, to study dengue fever—and he suffered a severe attack of the disease before his work there was finished. Apart from these problems, theirs was a happy marriage, blessed by three sons and a daughter.

Dr. Goldberger was to spend several years in laboratories in Washington, D. C., and at Woods Hole, Massachusetts, becoming an expert on helminthology. In 1909, his acute powers as a "health detective" were spectacularly demonstrated. A disease, first described by Schamberg in 1901, had appeared in epidemic form every spring in Philadelphia, manifesting itself as a temporarily disfiguring and acutely itching skin disease. Assigned to try to track down the responsible agent, Dr. Goldberger went to Philadelphia. Within forty-eight hours, he had eliminated the possibility of germ infection; had determined that the disease was caused by vermin; and had isolated specimens of the villain —the tiny acarine mite (*Pediculoides ventricosus*) which was carried to its victims in mattresses filled with fresh wheat straw. Sterilization of mattresses ended this source of human discomfort.

At Woods Hole, Dr. Goldberger formed a friendship with Dr. H. T. Ricketts, of the University of Chicago, who had done work on Rocky Mountain spotted fever. Later, in 1909, the two were to meet again in Mexico City, working on typhus. Dr. C. J. H. Nicolle, a French physician working in Tunis, had been first to describe transmission of typhus by the body louse. Dr. Goldberger's work confirmed this; and further, he demonstrated that the head louse could transmit typhus. His work also proved that typhus and Rocky Mountain spotted fever, both insect-borne, were separate diseases. Dr. Goldberger nearly paid for his knowledge with his life, in 1910, but he recovered from a typhus infection resulting from a laboratory accident. A few months later, Dr. Ricketts was not so fortunate: he died of typhus.

Dr. Goldberger was involved in a number of other assignments, including research on measles, in 1910. He was first to demonstrate that monkeys could be infected with measles, opening the way to new knowledge of infectious diseases. In 1913, he was sent to Detroit, Michigan, to study a diphtheria epidemic that was seemingly out of control. Despite serious political opposition, the stern and courageous Public Health Surgeon soon got to the bottom of a problem of official neglect, demonstrated the danger of diphtheria carriers, and instituted methods for their detection and control. It was from this triumph that

Dr. Goldberger, with considerable personal misgivings, headed south to the cotton fields and pellagra.

Knowing little about the disease he was to study, Dr. Goldberger set out to learn all he could. He went to cotton-mill towns; to the cotton fields; to the hills and valleys. He found hundreds of people afflicted with skin lesions, weakness, digestive upsets, diarrhea, and mental disturbances—typical signs of pellagra. Many insane patients had been sent to institutions by pellagra; others had contracted pellagra after institutionalization.

Of particular interest to Dr. Goldberger were two orphanages near Jackson, Mississippi. There, mass studies could be made. The Methodist and the Baptist orphanages were less than a mile apart. Despite good institutional care, reasonably good buildings, and, by the day's standards, nutritious meals, more than half of the children could be expected to suffer one or more attacks of pellagra each year. The suffering on the little faces haunted the doctor, despite his steely outward demeanor.

In his characteristic way, Dr. Goldberger cut across the confusion of custom and of literature and arrived at basic conclusions quickly: it seemed unlikely that pellagra was infectious, because it did not afflict all persons in a group, even though they might live in intimate association, as did orphanage personnel and children; it did not appear to be a toxin, because adults and children ate many of the same foods. It was strange that it seldom afflicted adults at these institutions; stranger still, it seemed to be confined almost exclusively to one age group: those children between three and twelve years of age. In this group, the percentage of pellagra was extremely high.

With his assistant, Dr. C. H. Waring, Dr. Goldberger studied the orphanage, the orphans, the management, the buildings, the sanitary facilities, the soil, the surroundings, the diets, and the habits of all persons associated with the institutions.

It was not long before the inquiring mind of the medical detective began to visualize patterns in the puzzle. Although the children's diet was adequate caloriewise, adults received considerably more meat and protein foods. The little children, during their first two years, received plenty of milk; but after that age, the children's diet was largely carbohydrate: corn bread, grits, cane syrup, and molasses. They received meat only once a week; and vegetables of high protein content, such as peas and beans, were seldom served, especially in the early spring.

Dr. Goldberger's sharp eyes detected another interesting thing: the children over twelve frequently supplemented their institutional diet by "swiping" extra foods which they craved. Among this age group, pellagra was less common. But the group between infancy and puberty had to live on the food they were served; they suffered most.

The Public Health doctors conferred with administrations and boards. These were sympathetic, but felt that they could not afford to meet Dr. Goldberger's suggestions for supplementary foods. Not to be thwarted, Goldberger turned to the Public Health Service: would it grant an appropriation to provide the foods needed for the test? He received an affirmative answer from Washington about the middle of September. The superintendent of the orphanage, Dr. J. R. Carter, and "Miss Ida," the House Mother (who actually was Mrs. Carter), were very cooperative. The children began to get meat four times a week; eggs daily; milk regularly; and the corn foods, while not eliminated, were reduced and supplemented by oatmeal, peas, beans, and other vegetables.

Soon, Drs. Goldberger and Waring noticed, signs of pellagra on little faces and bodies began to disappear. Apparently they were winning against pellagra. But could they prevent recurrence the following spring, 1915? Only time would tell.

Meantime, with the aid of another assistant, Dr. David G. Willets, Dr. Goldberger launched another study—this time with a control group—at the Georgia State Sanitarium at Milledgeville. At this asylum, two wards, one of colored women, and one of white women, were turned over to the Public Health officers for their test. Apart from the change in diet and increased watchfulness over individual feeding, no change in habitual routine was made. Of the seventy-two patients, equally divided among Negro and white, eighteen had previous histories of at least two attacks of pellagra.

During the period of observation—December 31, 1914, to October 1,

1915, none of the group receiving special diets presented recognizable evidence of a recurrence of pellagra.

Of the control group (the other inmates of the asylum) who received the customary institutional diet—about the usual number, or forty-seven per cent, experienced recurrence of pellagra!

Dr. Goldberger was sure, now, that he could cure pellagra, and that he could prevent it. But he was equally certain that many of his colleagues—those championing the infection or the toxin theory—would remain unconvinced. Now, he wanted to see if he could produce pellagra by dietary control, as well as prevent it. But, who would be so courageous as to risk such a test? Dr. Goldberger had a bold idea.

Dr. E. H. Galloway, head of the State Board of Health in Mississippi, had been very sympathetic and helpful to Dr. Goldberger. Dr. Galloway also was a close friend of Governor Earl Brewer. Dr. Goldberger asked permission to lay his plan before the Governor. It was startling—but, having satisfied himself as to the legal aspects and as to the medical safety of the plan, the Governor gave it his stamp of approval.

At the Mississippi State Penitentiary, eight miles from Jackson, Dr. Goldberger and his assistant, Dr. G. A. Wheeler, presented their plan: they wanted twelve healthy, white, adult male volunteers for a six-month restricted diet test. (These men, it was felt, would be least likely to be susceptible to pellagra under normal conditions.) The volunteers would be segregated as to quarters and meals, but otherwise would be treated substantially as were other prisoners. If they became ill, they would receive the best of care. At the end of the test period, each would receive a pardon from the Governor.

There were plenty of volunteers, and a dozen men soon were selected. From February 4 to April 19, 1915, the men were kept under observation without any change in diet. None showed evidence of pellagra. Then, the diet was changed. The volunteers were fed biscuits, mush, grits, gravy, syrup, sweet potatoes, rice, collards—all items common to the diet of the region—but no meat, milk, beans, or peas. The rest of the prison population, receiving normal diet, were the "controls."

One volunteer had to be released for medical reasons in July; but eleven finished the test. Little of note occurred for five long, agonizing months—April 19 to September 12—but then, pellagrous dermatitis began to show up. By October 1, 1915—the end of the test period—six of the eleven volunteers exhibited pellagrous lesions. The diagnoses were confirmed by Dr. Galloway and by several other expert physicians. Dr. Goldberger was elated. He had proved not only that pellagra could be prevented or cured by diet, but also that it could be produced by dietary deficiency.

The balance of Dr. Goldberger's life was devoted to study of pellagra, the foods that were somehow deficient, and the relative values of those foods that would prevent the disease. He was quick to point out that poverty was one of the greatest factors contributing to pellagra—impoverished persons ofttimes could not afford to buy the foods needed to protect them against the ailment. Other persons, out of habit, chose to avoid foods that would have protected them.

Some medical men, however, still took issue with Dr. Goldberger and the Public Health Service. They clung to the infection theory. So, Dr. Goldberger, to leave no stone unturned, launched another series of experiments—drastic, revolting, but nonetheless conclusive. Using a group of sixteen volunteers, including himself and his wife, he set out to try to pass pellagra from one person to another. He injected blood of pellagra patients into the volunteers; he introduced nose and throat swabbings from pellagrins into the orifices of volunteers. He collected urine and feces from pellagrous patients, and scales from their skins, and rolled these with bread dough into pills which the stouthearted volunteers swallowed. Though the experiments were repeated time and again, not a one of the sixteen volunteers developed the slightest symptom of pellagra. The published results of these tests quieted all but die-hard opposition.

Dr. Goldberger found that brewer's yeast, of all foodstuffs, contained the highest percentage of pellagra-preventive substance, which he called the P-P factor. With more time, likely Goldberger would have discovered the chemical nature of the P-P factor—but time was not allotted him. It remained for other men to discover what came to be called vitamin B; and still others to discover vitamin B to be a complex; and in the course of the next three decades, to break the vitamin B complex down into at least eleven different substances—including B_1, or thiamin, the antiberiberi vitamin; B_2, or riboflavin; niacin, or niacinamide, the antipellagra factor; B_6, or pyridoxine; B_{12}, or cyanocobalamin, the antipernicious anemia vitamin; and folic acid, biotin, pantothenic acid, as well as other factors thus far less understood. The list of names of researchers who have contributed to Medicine's knowledge of vitamins —those compounds which the human body cannot synthesize for itself but which are vitally essential to body well-being and to life—would fill a directory of distinguished scientists.

A rare form of cancer finally began to slow down Dr. Goldberger's work. He had to give up his beloved research, and he died January 17, 1929.

Dr. Goldberger's ashes were taken to Haines Point, above the Potomac River. After a simple ceremony conducted by Rabbi Abram Simon, Dr. McCoy, carrying out Dr. Goldberger's wishes, strewed the ashes to winds that swept them over the surface of the river he had loved.

WORLD EVENTS AND MEDICAL HISTORY

Dates, persons, and events of significance to the evolution of Medicine include:

1942	Collection of blood donations begun by Red Cross in U.S.A. for treating battle casualties. Fore-runner of blood bank system.
1942	Atomic energy released and controlled in first nuclear chain reaction.
1942	First jet aircraft tested at Muroc, California.
1942	Opening of Alcan Highway.
1942	Food and gasoline rationing in U.S.
1943	Penicillin production gets under way.
1943	Selman A. Waksman announced discovery of streptomycin.
1943	Cell smear method used to detect uterine cancer.
1943	ACTH isolated from the anterior pituitary gland.
1943	Nobel prize awarded to Dam and Doisy for their research on vitamin K.
1944	First operation for asphyxia livida.
1944	Synthesis of quinine.
1944	Negorski performed first resuscitation following clinical death.
1944	Nobel prize awarded to Erlanger and Gasser for their discoveries in neurologic research.
1945	Promin® (sodium glucosulfone) effective against leprosy, made available by Parke-Davis.
1945	Walter Bradford Cannon died.
1945	Fleming, Florey, and Chain jointly awarded Nobel prize.
1945	Alfred Blalock, Helen Taussig, (U.S.) devised "blue baby" operation.
1945	First atomic bomb explosion.
1945	End of World War II, April 6.
1945	World-wide antimalarial campaign with DDT.
1945	First session of the U.N.
1946	Thiamin and folic acid used in treatment for pernicious anemia.
1946	Nobel prize awarded to H. J. Müller for his research on x-ray mutations.
1946	Paris conference clash between U. S. and U.S.S.R. marks beginning of "cold war."
1946	Penicillin produced synthetically.
1947	Parke-Davis research team announced discovery of Chloromycetin® (chloramphenicol).
1947	Rocket aircraft (Bell X-1) developed in U.S.A. with speeds up to 1500 m.p.h.
1947	Nobel prizes awarded to C. Cori, G. Cori, and B. Houssay for their studies on metabolism of glycogen and sugar.
1948	B. M. Duggar (Lederle) announced discovery of aureomycin.
1948	Rickes and Smith described vitamin B_{12} (cyanocobalamin).
1948	Sidney Farber found antagonists to folic acid alleviate leukemia.
1948	Charles Bailey (U.S.) improved heart surgery.
1948	World Health Organization founded.
1948	Kinsey report on *Sexual Behavior of the Human Male*.
1948	200-inch telescope installed in Mount Palomar Observatory.
1948	Therapeutic properties of cortisone recognized.
1948	Berlin Air Lift.
1948	Nobel prize awarded to Müller for his discovery of DDT.
1949	Betatron used in cancer therapy.
1949	Two-stage rocket (250 miles high).
1949	North Atlantic Treaty Organization founded in Washington, D.C.
1949	Dedication of permanent U.N. site in New York City.
1949	Nobel prize awarded to Hess and Moniz for their studies on physiology and surgery of the brain.
1950	Team of Pfizer researchers announced discovery of terramycin.
1950	Beginning of Korean conflict.
1950	Intensified interest in geriatric medicine due to longer life expectancy.
1950	A.M.A. launched vigorous program opposing socialized medicine.
1950	Müller developed the electron field microscope.
1950	Nobel prize awarded to Hench, Kendall and Reichstein for their studies on treatment of rheumatoid arthritis with cortisone and ACTH.
1951	Ludwig Gross showed virus transmission of leukemia in mice.
1951	André-Thomas developed the heart-lung machine.
1951	Operation with vegetative blockade by Laborit.
1951	International Pharmacopoeia of the World Health Organization.

BANTING, BEST, AND DIABETES

THE NIGHT of July 30, 1921, was hot, humid, uncomfortable—a summer condition well known to natives of Toronto, the metropolis that sprawls northward from the Canadian shore of Lake Ontario. The air was stifling in the laboratory under the eaves of the medical building on the campus of the University of Toronto. As midnight approached, two young workers fought drowsiness and discomfort; impatience, too, as they checked the slow creep of the clock's hand. At 12:15 a.m., they aroused their patient—a diabetic dog. They took blood and urine samples, and injected another 5 cc. of precious pancreatic extract from a vial floating in a bowl of ice. Patiently they made routine tests.

Then came the thrill for which they had dreamed so many long weeks—there was no sugar in the dog's urine; its blood sugar had been halved. No longer were Charles Best and Dr. Frederick Banting sleepy. They looked at one another incredulously for a moment; then, as comprehension of their findings grew, grins turned to shouts of triumph. The staid laboratory walls looked down upon a strange scene—two research men dancing about for joy. Banting and Best had reached their first goal: they had stopped the almost inexorable death march of diabetes.

Frederick G. Banting, 29-year-old surgeon, and his associate, 22-year-old Charles Best, had come a long way on the path of research since the morning in May, 1921, when they began collaboration in the medical library of the Department of Physiology at the University of Toronto. However, they still had a long way to go to prove their findings beyond doubt; and to develop their discovery from a laboratory curiosity to a practical therapeutic tool. Yet, fate of millions of diabetic persons depended on what they did that hot July night—and during the days and nights that followed.

Few great medical advances have developed from less auspicious beginnings than the discovery of insulin. The literature that Banting and Best reviewed before starting their laboratory work showed that

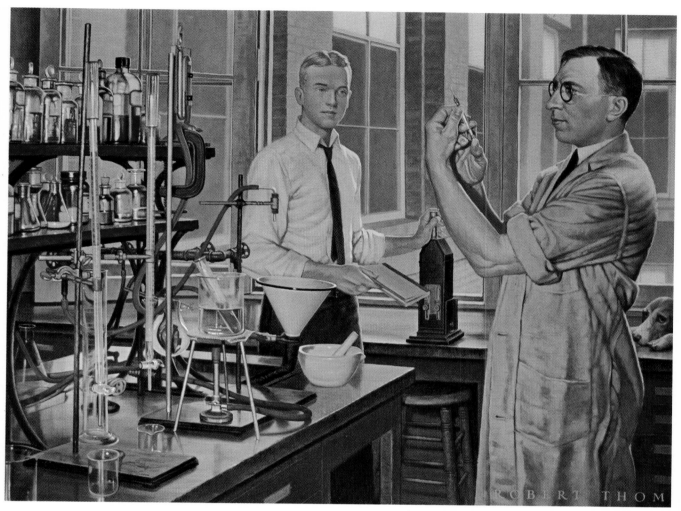

BANTING, BEST, AND DIABETES

During the summer of 1921, Charles H. Best, youthful biologist, and Dr. Frederick G. Banting experimented in laboratories loaned by Professor J. J. R. Macleod of the Physiology Department, University of Toronto. The inexperienced Canadian investigators found what trained research men before them had missed—an extract of the pancreas that controlled the high blood sugar of diabetes mellitus. Proved and reproved on laboratory animals, their extract was first tried on a human diabetic in February, 1922. Best developed mass production methods while studying for his medical degree. Banting and Best's discovery of insulin gave hope of life to millions of diabetics who otherwise would have been doomed.

results of research during the previous century were uniformly negative. The men themselves had little research training or experience. The department head who made laboratory space available to them for a few summer weeks was positive that they were wasting time. Further, their financial resources were barely sufficient for subsistence. Their only assets were courage, determination—and an idea.

Dr. Banting, in whose mind the idea originated, was born November 14, 1891, near the small country town of Alliston, some sixty miles north of Toronto. He grew up on his father's farm, was educated locally, sought to follow his parents' wishes by studying for the ministry. This proved an unhappy choice, however, and Banting switched to study of medicine at the University of Toronto. His medical education was hurried by the advent of World War I, and Banting, fresh from medical school, went overseas as an officer of the Fifteenth General Hospital Unit of the Canadian Army Medical Corps. In France, he had ample opportunity to gain surgical experience—and was wounded only six weeks before the end of the war.

Returned to Canada following recuperation, Dr. Banting joined the orthopedic department of the Toronto Hospital for Sick Children for a period of experience, then accepted an instructorship in orthopedic surgery at the University of Western Ontario, in London. Here, too, he opened a modest office as an orthopedic surgeon, and awaited patients. Few came to his door. Having considerable time to think, Dr. Banting's keen mind sought employment. He became a frequenter of the medical library, avidly reading results of the latest developments in the profession.

The spark that set off the quest for insulin was an article by Dr. Moses Barron, of the University of Minnesota, in the October, 1920, issue of *Surgery, Gynecology and Obstetrics*. Dr. Banting, preparing for a lecture on functions of the pancreas, read the article, and marked a paragraph. The paper commented on the work of Minkowski and von Mering, and suggested that, had their experiments been carried further, a substance secreted by the pancreas might have been found; and, perhaps, such a substance might alleviate *diabetes mellitus*.

That night, Banting reviewed the article in his mind. Also, he thought back to his childhood, when he had watched a bright, active girl playmate wither and die of diabetes. Sleepless, Banting found his notebook,

362

and scribbled: "Ligate the pancreatic ducts of dogs. Wait six to eight weeks for degeneration. Remove the residue and extract."

Discussing the idea with his faculty associates during the next few days, Banting found some encouragement; but all were convinced that facilities of the University of Western Ontario were inadequate for carrying on such a series of experiments. They recommended that Banting consult with Professor John James Rickard Macleod, head of the physiology department of the University of Toronto, regarded as an outstanding authority on carbohydrate metabolism.

Thus began the first of many discouraging trials for Dr. Banting: two trips to Toronto in his battered auto netted only polite but firm turndowns. Professor Macleod cited to Dr. Banting literature on the pancreas over the centuries, and his own opinion that the organ secreted no such chemical as Banting hoped to find. Furthermore, he pointed out none too gently, predecessors in pancreatic investigation had the advantage of extensive research training—of which Banting had none. However, the Scotch professor met up with conviction and stubbornness as strong as his own; and when, on his third visit, Dr. Banting came armed with pleas for consideration voiced by a number of Professor Macleod's own associates, the Professor gave ground and agreed that Banting might have some test animals and take over a temporarily unused laboratory for eight weeks during the summer—while Professor Macleod would be vacationing in his native Scotland. Recognizing that Banting had little knowledge of the chemical aspects of the problem, Professor Macleod inquired of his final year class in physiology and biochemistry whether some student would like to volunteer to help a young surgeon with some experiments relative to diabetes. Charles Best, about to graduate, and with no fixed plans for the summer, thought this an opportunity to gain experience in biochemistry.

The second member of the team, Best, was born of Canadian parentage in 1899, the son of a physician who lived in West Pembroke, a small village on the United States side of the Maine-New Brunswick border, but who took all his patients to a hospital at St. Stephen, New Brunswick. As soon as he was old enough to accompany his father, Charley Best was assisting at surgical operations frequently performed on kitchen tables in northern Maine and in New Brunswick. He, too, had a background of interest in diabetes, having seen a favorite aunt die of the affliction. Anna Best, trained as a nurse at Massachusetts General Hospital in Boston, had been a patient of Dr. Elliott P. Joslin, who was to become an eminent authority on treatment of diabetes.

His education at Toronto University interrupted by World War I, Best had returned after the armistice to courses in physiology and biochemistry, and had written his final examinations in this course only the day before he and Banting began their work as a team. Banting, with hardly funds to support himself, was unable to offer Best any stipend; however, they quickly formed bonds of friendship and of motivation that carried them through the trying weeks of the summer.

On the morning of May 17, 1921, the two young men began their first task—study of the literature concerning the pancreas. They found that diabetes was known to ancient Egyptians, Hindus, Chinese, and Greeks; and that classification of diabetes as an endocrine disturbance was supported by work of Minkowski and von Mering, who in 1889 produced diabetes in dogs by removing pancreases; and Langnesse had concluded that it was not absence of the total gland, but only of that portion known as the islands of Langerhans, that led to the disease. Apart from these reports, the literature was far from encouraging; it recorded a half century of failures to find an antidiabetic substance. However, the team refused to be discouraged. Soon they were hard at work seeking proof of Banting's theory. As W. R. Feasby has written, "The theory was wrong, but it drove them to make the experiments which resulted in the production of insulin—something that experienced researchers had failed to do."

The second task facing the team was to put their laboratory in order. A small room under the eaves of the Medical Building, it had not been used for some time, so walls and floor had to be thoroughly scrubbed. There were no assistants—Best and Banting had to do the job themselves. Soon, however, the test dogs were installed in the animal room next door, and surgical operations began. Banting, with Best assisting, tied off the pancreatic ducts of several of the animals, employing anesthetics and the finest of surgical procedures. Best, with Banting as assistant, carried out numerous biochemical tests on blood and urine. Patiently, they waited out the six-week period thought necessary for tissues that produced digestive enzymes to degenerate. Then—if their theory was right—the special pancreatic tissues, known as the islands of Langerhans, would still remain. In absence of the destructive digestive enzymes, they hoped to be able to find the unknown substance that would lower sugar content of the blood. Meantime, the dogs had to be fed, exercised, and their cages cleaned. There was no one but themselves to do the job. Most of such work fell upon young Charley Best.

With six of their allotted eight weeks gone, Banting and Best reopened abdomens of their test animals. What a disappointment awaited them! Their catgut sutures had given way, and healthy pancreases greeted them. Six weeks' time lost! They began again, tying off the glands with another suture material. Again they waited through six hot summer weeks.

Already, Banting and Best had overrun their allotted time; but Dr. Macleod was still in Scotland. As the end of July approached, they made a dog diabetic by removal of its pancreas. Again, test dogs were examined. This time, the hoped-for results were there: the acinar cells, the portion of the pancreas that produces digestive enzymes, had atrophied; the islands of Langerhans were healthy. The shriveled pancreas was removed and ground up with sand in a chilled mortar; this material was suspended in Ringer's solution— a saline liquid—and filtered. The temperatures were kept as low as possible to discourage unwanted digestive activity by any remaining enzymes. Such was the source of the solution that was injected into the diabetic dog, that night of July 30. Blood chemistry and urine tests indicated, for the first time, that Banting and Best were on the right track. The high blood sugar, resulting from absence of body insulin, was reduced.

For the next few weeks, Banting and Best worked day and night. There were more disappointments: test animals became infected and died; there was no measure of the strength of their extract; they ran out of the precious extract and had to see their diabetic animal die. They called their mysterious extract "isletin," named for the isles of

Langerhans; later on, they were persuaded to adopt the more easily pronounced term, "insulin."

As September approached, the research team repeated and repeated their experiments until they were absolutely certain that their mysterious substance would prevent death of diabetic dogs. As Feasby points out, "It is quite fair to state that they made their experiments and their discovery completely as a result of the hypothesis put forward by Banting, with the equipment and animals allowed them by Macleod and with their own efforts, unaided by any other person or assistant. The reactions to the discoveries made by the two young men during the summer months were various. The most significant was that of the Professor (who had been away all summer). It must be remembered that he was a professor of the old European school, that the head of the department was the Director, with a capital 'D'. He very much doubted that these two young inexperienced workers had been able to discover anything that had been overlooked by experienced workers in European and American universities for twenty years. Therefore, he asked them to repeat their experiments. On many occasions they obtained the same satisfactory results. At this stage there developed a conflict of personalities which resulted in unhappy days for all concerned."

Having proved that a successful extract could be produced, the team began looking for more practical sources of insulin. At first, pancreas from fetal calves was used—they knew that insulin-producing cells developed in the embryonic pancreas before those cells secreting digestive enzymes. This source proved successful, but limited. Then Best found that insulin could be extracted successfully from adult beef pancreas by utilizing acidified alcohol as the solvent.

Late in 1921, there was no longer doubt that a substance had been discovered that would control diabetes. Even Professor Macleod was convinced. Papers were presented to the Physiological Journal Club in Toronto; to the American Physiological Society, in New Haven, Connecticut, between Christmas and New Year's, 1921; and, in February, 1922, to the Toronto Academy of Medicine. Shortly afterward, newspapers carried the story, creating new problems. Pressure built up, demanding insulin to save the lives of thousands of diabetics around the world—but thus far there were only laboratory quantities of crude material available. Professor Macleod arranged for Professor J. B. Collip to join the team to assist in chemical procedures.

Insulin had yet to be tried on a human. Dr. Banting decided that first trials should be conducted in Toronto. A twelve-year-old boy, Leonard Thompson, at the Toronto General Hospital, was near death from diabetes. Banting released some of the extract that he and Best had made from adult beef pancreas, and which they first tested upon themselves for toxicity. It was given to the boy by his physician, Dr. Walter Campbell. The effect of the treatment on the boy was dramatic. He made a steady recovery; and, with the aid of insulin, was to live for several years, until death resulted from a motorcycle accident.

In February, 1922, another crisis arose: the method for preparing insulin failed. Differences of opinion developed. Professor Collip left to take up other duties. Dr. Banting opened an office in Toronto for clinical practice. Charles Best was appointed director of insulin production at the Connaught Laboratories, a pharmaceutical manufacturing plant born of wartime need and operated by the University of Toronto. Working harder than ever before, Best was able to develop techniques by which ever-increasing amounts of insulin could be produced.

This was the end of the partnership between Charles Best and Dr. Frederick Banting, although they remained the best of friends during Banting's lifetime. However, Banting continued to feel bitterness toward Macleod, whom he felt had tried to take the credit for the discovery from him and Best. As Best later expressed it, there soon developed considerable pressure, "exerted by senior and more experienced investigators, who had not invested an hour's work before the discovery but who were now more than anxious to appropriate a share of it."

"At every opportunity," Feasby pointed out, "Dr. Banting sought to give Charles Best credit equal to his own in the partnership of discovery. To Banting, it seemed ironic that the Nobel Prize of 1923 was awarded jointly to himself and Macleod. He promptly announced that he would split his share of the prize money with Best. Not to be outdone, Macleod shared his with Collip."

Early in 1922, Eli Lilly & Company, of Indianapolis, Indiana, expressed interest in the production of insulin. Lilly scientists worked closely with Best and with Sir Henry Dale and his colleagues of the National Institute for Medical Research in London, England. Within a year, insulin was being manufactured or distributed world-wide.

Much remained to be done, however. A way to measure insulin's strength had to be devised, and standardized. Clinicians had to work out dosages to fit various degrees of requirements of diabetic patients. Dietary regimens compatible with insulin treatment had to be developed. Ways to combat hypoglycemia—too low blood sugar level, the opposite of diabetes—had to be developed to counteract accidental insulin overdosage. Patients had to be taught how to care for themselves; how to assure themselves of a proper diet; how to administer insulin to themselves. Clinicians were kept busy, and they got considerable assistance from diabetic physicians, who, granted new opportunity to live, were able to analyze and interpret their own reactions to the new drug. Banting was among the foremost of the clinicians, as was Boston's Dr. Joslin, who years before had helplessly witnessed the death of Charley Best's diabetic aunt.

Problems of control of the new lifesaving hormone also arose. Dr. Banting and Charles Best refused to profit directly from their discovery. They finally acceded to requests and applied for patents on the discovery of insulin, with the understanding that the University of Toronto would accept the patents and arrange for their proper administration. For this purpose, the Insulin Committee of the Governors of the University of Toronto was established, in 1923. An Insulin Committee Laboratory was organized for the purpose of assaying all batches of insulin preparations prior to distribution in Canada and the United States. In 1925, the Insulin Committee joined with the Health Organization of the League of Nations in establishing a specially prepared dry sample of insulin to serve as an international standard by which to regulate the world's supply.

On the production side of insulin, advances came rapidly. Charles Best combined research and management of insulin production with the study of medicine, graduating in medicine in 1925. He then spent several years in London in Dr. Dale's research laboratories, and received a degree of Doctor of Science from the University of London. Upon his return to Toronto, in 1928, Dr. Best became head of the University of Toronto's newly formed Department of Physiological Hygiene, and Associate Director of Connaught Laboratories. When Professor Macleod retired from his Chair of Physiology at the University, Dr. Best succeeded him.

For Dr. Banting, many honors from near and far were to follow the Nobel Prize. Perhaps most satisfying of all to him was the establishment, in 1923, of the Banting and Best Department of Medical Research at the University of Toronto. He was appointed the first director. In 1925, the Banting Research Foundation was established. In 1934, he was knighted by the British King. Dr. Banting's life was no bed of roses, however. He had to make innumerable speeches—and each of them was a trial. He fought continuing duels with newspaper reporters. As an avocation, Banting developed his latent artistic ability. In 1939, he married Henrietta Ball, with whom he was to have a happy but short companionship.

World War II made its demands upon Dr. Banting. He reentered the army, and soon had rank of Major. He was assigned as a liaison officer between the Canadian National Research Council and its counterparts in the United States and in Britain. Tragically, while he was on one of these military missions, the plane in which he was riding crashed in a storm over Newfoundland, and Banting died of injuries, February 22, 1941.

The war also brought new demands upon Dr. Best. Connaught Laboratories again was called upon to serve military medical needs. In 1940, Dr. Best joined a Naval Medical Research Unit, and was responsible for a number of advances in military medical techniques. After Dr. Banting's death, Dr. Best was requested to resign his posts with Connaught Laboratories and with the School of Hygiene, and to assume direction of the Banting and Best Department of Medical Research in addition to being Professor of Physiology.

In 1954, the Charles H. Best Institute was constructed beside the Banting Institute on Toronto's College Street. In 1961, a new wing was added. The two institutes were joined by an overhead passageway, so that, symbolically, the research efforts begun by the two young partners of 1921 continue to go on, under the direction of Dr. Best. From research conducted in these twin institutes have come many additions to medicine's fund of knowledge, not only about diabetes, but concerning other critical problems. Dr. Best finds time for consultation on major medical problems with scientists in many countries, in addition to his duties at the University of Toronto.

Many advances have been made in production and administration of insulin since Dr. Best's work made commercial quantities available. Researchers in many nations made significant contributions of benefit to diabetics. Today, insulin is available in six forms, each having different advantages and periods of effective action. In addition, oral anti-diabetic drugs have been developed which are of value in treating some, but not all, diabetic patients. Though four decades have passed since the initial discovery, neither the action of insulin nor of oral anti-diabetic agents is fully understood; nor has the cause of the affliction been determined. Recent studies indicate that diabetes may be a symptom of a more extensive systemic upset than mere failure of the islets of Langerhans.

Though answers to these problems can only come from future research, millions of diabetics today owe thanks for their lives to Drs. Banting and Best. Dr. Feasby has pointedly summed up evidence about insulin: "Without Banting, there would have been no attempt; without Best, there would have been no discovery . . ."

WORLD EVENTS AND MEDICAL HISTORY

Dates, persons, and events of significance to the evolution of Medicine include:

1951   Nobel prize awarded to Max Theiler for his work on yellow fever.

1951   Effect of fluoride on development of dental caries discovered.

1952   Reserpine, blood pressure lowering drug, discovered.

1952   First open-heart operation by Baily.

1952   First hydrogen bomb explosion (Bikini).

1952   Restoration of Western European manufacturing facilities nearly complete (Marshall Plan).

1952   Peaceful uses of atomic energy encouraged by U.S.

1952   Nobel prize awarded to S. Waksman for his discovery of streptomycin.

1953   Nobel prize awarded to Krebs and Lipmann for their studies in carbohydrate metabolism and on coenzyme A.

1954   Launching of the first atomic-powered submarine *Nautilus*.

1954   Enders, Robbins and Weller shared Nobel prize for their work on tissue culture of poliomyelitis virus.

1955   Sir Alexander Fleming died.

1955   Poliomyelitis vaccine (Jonas Salk, U.S.) introduced.

1955   Nobel prizes awarded du Vigneaud and Theorell for their studies on the chemical synthesis of oxytocin, and on the oxygen transport system in living tissues.

1955   Canadian Academy of the History of Pharmacy founded.

1956   Research on the peaceful uses of nuclear fissionable material. Development of nuclear power stations.

1956   Weizäcker established the foundation for psychosomatic therapy.

1956   Nobel prize awarded to Forssmann, Cournand and Richards for their work on cardiac catheterization.

1957   First space satellite (Sputnik I).

1957   Nobel prizes awarded to Todd and Bovet for their studies on nucleotide coenzyme and on antihistamines and muscle relaxants.

1958   Nobel prizes awarded to Sanger for his work on synthesizing insulin and to Beadle, Tatum and Lederberg for their genetic research.

1959   Ochoa and Kornberg shared the Nobel prize for their work on synthesizing nucleic acids by means of enzymes.

1959   Polonski described the function of desoxyribonucleic acid on cellular mechanisms.

1959   Further research on seasonal and climatic factors in disease.

1959   Beginning of space medicine, physiologic problems, radiation protection.

1960   Introduction of the "laser."

1960   Nobel prize awarded to Burnet and Medawar for their studies on acquired immunity.

1961   First manned satellite (Gagarin).

1961   Nobel prize awarded to von Békésy for his research on sound wave stimulation of the cochlea.

1962   Nobel prize awarded to Francis Crick for his work in molecular biology.

1963   Research on nucleic acids in connection with viruses and cancer cells.

1963   Further improvements in electrodiagnostics (chronaximetry, encephalography, electrocardiography and cardioscopy).

1963   New developments in experimental pharmacology, drug, and irradiation therapy.

1963   New and improved surgical instruments: high performance endoscope; machine for suturing of blood vessels and intestines; high-frequency sound implements for coagulating and checking hemorrhage; laser rays used in skin grafting, cataract operations, tumor and cancer operations.

1963   Improvements in obstetrics: development of vacuum extractor and administration of oxytocics and analgetic agents reduces incidence of operative trauma.

1963   Improvements in psychiatry: great advances through fever and shock therapy; psychopharmacals replace leukotomy.

1963   Nobel prize awarded to Hodgkins, Huxley and Eccles for their work in neurologic research.

THE ERA OF ANTIBIOTICS

ONE OF the most significant and dramatic advances in medicine during the first half of the twentieth century came with the introduction and use of antibiotic medicines (substances produced with the aid of microorganisms which are antagonistic to the growth of certain other organisms). Perhaps more than any other group of drugs, antibiotics changed the pattern of treatment of infectious diseases and gave hope of longer life and better living to countless millions of people.

Introduction of antibiotics to medicine in the early 1940's was truly an international event: the discovery of penicillin in London had been announced in 1929 by the Scottish bacteriologist, Alexander Fleming. Ten years later, Howard W. Florey, from Australia, Ernst B. Chain, from Germany, and their English associates at Oxford University extracted penicillin from mold broth, and tested it. First in animals, then in men, they found the mold extract almost unbelievably active against certain infective organisms, yet remarkably low in toxicity toward living cells. It was the work at Oxford that gave penicillin to the world. However, it took the know-how and the resources of governmental and pharmaceutical establishments in the United States, cooperating with British scientists, to convert laborious, low-yield laboratory procedures to the high-yield, massive quantity production needed to fulfill the medical demands of World War II.

Sudden and spectacular though the introduction of the antibiotic era may have seemed to the public, behind it lay more than a half century of experimentation by many men and women in many countries. In fact, introduction of penicillin, and of the many other medically useful antibiotics which followed, was made possible by the merging of two quiet streams of scientific investigation that had been progressing, step by laborious step, for many decades.

One stream, research in chemotherapy (the creation and employment of chemical compounds for specific therapeutic uses), had been organized into some semblance of scientific pattern by the German

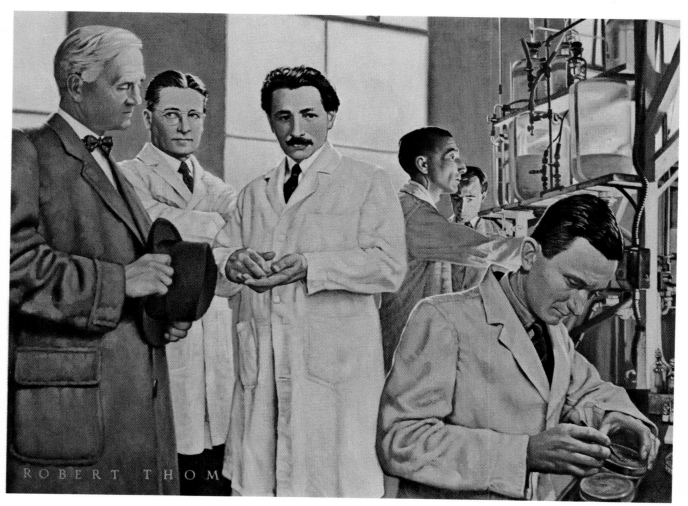

ROBERT THOM

THE ERA OF ANTIBIOTICS

When Dr. Alexander Fleming, British bacteriologist who had discovered penicillin in 1928, heard in 1940 that Drs. Florey, Chain, and their "team" had isolated the antibiotic and had found it successful when tested on mice for efficacy and toxicity, at the Sir William Dunn School of Pathology, Oxford, he decided to visit them and see their work. The three men shared a Nobel Prize in Medicine in 1945. Cooperation of British and United States scientists, governments, and institutions developed mass production methods for penicillin; met wartime needs; launched new research. Antibiotics brought about a revolution in the practice of medicine. In the laboratory are: Drs. Fleming, Howard W. Florey, Ernst B. Chain, A. G. Sanders, E. P. Abraham, and Norman G. Heatley.

physician and chemist, Paul Ehrlich, and his followers, around the turn of the century.

The other stream of observations of antibiotic phenomena began with notes recorded by the Scot, Dr. Joseph Lister, in 1871, and by French chemists Louis Pasteur and Jules F. Joubert, in 1877.

Not until these two streams of investigation met and merged in the 1940's were the people of the world privileged to receive benefits of the newly recognized class of antibiotic therapeutic agents. The vast significance of this revolution in medicine cannot yet be measured; it can be grasped only when placed in perspective with the tragico-ironic likelihood that the microbial and chemical sources from which these lifesaving drugs were finally created have been present in and upon the good earth as long as man has lived upon it. Only in the second quarter of the twentieth century did man's powers of observation and of scientific understanding, and the requisite technology, develop to the point where he could recognize the potentials of antibiotic phenomena and direct them to his advantage.

Pasteur's demonstrations that microbes can be a cause of disease; Lister's proof of the value of antiseptics to combat them; and Ehrlich's development of synthetic chemicals to seek out specific germs and kill them, all had contributed to high hopes for the role of chemotherapy in the battle against disease. Yet, in the two decades following 1910, no single drug having significant activity against the most widespread class of disease-producing microorganisms—the bacteria—had been developed. Disappointedly, medical men and laymen had begun to regard chemotherapy as an impractical dream. However, the synthesis of prontosil in Germany by Gerhard Domagk in 1935, and demonstration the same year in France by M. and Mme. Tréfouël, Nitti, and Bovet that prontosil's antibacterial action was due to its sulfanilamide fraction, changed the picture. A new wave of optimism carried chemotherapy back into fashion. Hundreds of sulfa compounds were synthesized, studied for activity and toxicity, and those found safe and effective entered the armamentarium of the medical profession.

This return of interest to chemical substances soon led chemists to look further afield for sources of new compounds. They began combing the reports of earlier scientific workers for ideas . . . ideas that by further

374

work might be carried to more successful conclusions. Among the literature reviewed was the half-forgotten paper about penicillin published in 1929 by Dr. Fleming.

The antibiotic activity which Fleming had observed and studied was not new in principle. For countless years a home-remedy practice in many lands had been to use moldy bread as a poultice. The Mayans had used a mold from corn for intestinal troubles. Manassein and Polotebnow had treated wounds with molds in 1871, the year Lister had noted his observations. Metchnikoff, like Pasteur, had described the process of antibiosis; and it had been given its name by Vuillemin in 1889. Ten years later, Emmerich and his collaborators had isolated a bactericidal substance, pyocyanase. Gosio in 1896, and Gratia and Dath in 1925, had worked with Penicillium molds. Twort in 1915 and d'Herelle in 1917 had reported on bacteriophages. In the interim, many other researchers had contributed to the growing literature on the subject.

Dr. Alexander Fleming discovered penicillin independently and accidentally, in 1928. He observed that a mold which invaded a culture of staphylococci in a petri dish had prevented growth of the bacteria over a considerable area. Dr. Fleming, working in the Inoculation Department of St. Mary's Hospital in London, had the curiosity to cultivate the mold on broth, to make an extract, and to test it. To his amazement, it arrested the growth of many gram-positive bacteria (staphylococci, streptococci, pneumococci) and of the bacilli that cause diphtheria. He named the impure broth "penicillin" for convenience, and announced that it was far more powerful than carbolic acid or other antiseptics, yet it could be applied undiluted to body surfaces. The broth, he reported, was "non-toxic to animals in enormous doses" and nonirritant. It did not interfere with the function of leukocytes in blood, as did most antiseptics. Finally, he suggested that "It may be an efficient antiseptic for application to, or injection into, areas infected with penicillin-sensitive microbes."

Some attempts have been made to depreciate Fleming's discovery, and to convey the impression that he did nothing further after he had reported his findings. However, as Pasteur wrote: "Fortune favors the prepared mind." That the Scottish physician was well prepared there is no doubt: as a medical student in London, he took top honors; as a bacteriologist in Sir Almroth Wright's crowded laboratory at St. Mary's Medical School, London, he made excellent contributions to research in the field of immunization; as a medical officer in World War I, he had great opportunity to observe the shortcomings of known antiseptics in treatment of massive wounds. Following the war, he conducted extensive investigations concerning lysozyme, the bactericidal protective substance found in many body tissues, especially in tears. He sought to extract lysozyme in pure form, but was disappointed.

As to the mold which produced penicillin, Maurois has pointed out: "Pure chance deposited this substance on his bench. But, had he not been waiting for fifteen years, he would not have recognized the unknown visitor for what it was."

The myth that Fleming abandoned penicillin after 1929 has no factual foundation. Though his paper in 1929 attracted little attention, Fleming continued to experiment with the substance, to talk about penicillin, to write papers on it, and to endeavor to interest chemists in extracting it. Not a chemist himself, Fleming had little success. Chemists Harold Raistrick and P. W. Clutterbuck, and bacteriologist R. Lovell, at the London School of Hygiene and Tropical Medicine, attempted to extract pure penicillin—but the substance proved unstable, and disappeared during their processes. Then, the advent of the sulfa drugs drew attention away from most other efforts, until it became obvious that the sulfas, too, had some limitations and undesirable side effects.

Meantime, R. J. Dubos had described the antibiotic tyrothricin in 1939. He had extracted it from a culture of *Bacillus brevis*, found it made up of two constituents, gramicidin and tyrocidine. The product was an effective antibacterial, but, disappointingly, proved quite toxic, and could be used only for limited local application.

Meantime, too, destiny was shaping another phase of the approach to antibiotics. Howard Florey, born in Adelaide, Australia, in 1898, studied medicine in his native land and came to Oxford on a Rhodes scholarship. In 1925, the Rockefeller Foundation sent him to the United States to gain experience in a number of laboratories. Upon return to England, Dr. Florey heard about the work Fleming had been doing on lysozyme and took an interest in it. In 1935, Dr. Florey was appointed to the Chair of Pathology at the Sir William Dunn School in Oxford. This position afforded Dr. Florey excellent opportunities to direct and coordinate research teams, as the school housed laboratories for pathology and bacteriology under one roof—and Dr. Florey was competent in each of these subjects.

Shortly after taking over his professorial duties, Dr. Florey invited Dr. Ernst B. Chain to organize a biochemical department. Dr. Chain was born in Berlin in 1906, of a Russian father and a German mother. At the Friedrich-Wilhelms University in Berlin, Chain specialized in biochemistry and physiology, receiving his degree shortly before the Nazis came into power. Of Jewish faith, Dr. Chain emigrated to England in 1933, working at the Cambridge School of Biochemistry until he joined Florey in 1935.

Work on the mode of action of lysozyme at the Sir William Dunn School of Pathology led Dr. Chain to systematically investigate older literature having to do with bacteriolytic agents. In the course of numerous discussions of lysozyme, Florey and Chain decided to undertake jointly a systematic investigation of some of the antibacterial substances produced by microorganisms. They applied for help to the Natural Sciences Division of the Rockefeller Foundation, in November, 1939.

"The first investigations decided upon at Oxford included a study of penicillin because its relative instability indicated that it might have interesting chemical properties, and because it was stated to be active against the staphylococcus, against which no other effective remedy was known at the time," the research team at Oxford reported in *Antibiotics*. Chain and Falk had begun work on a culture of Fleming's strain of *Penicillium notatum* in 1938; however, it was not until late in 1939 that work on penicillin was taken up vigorously by Florey, Chain, and Heatley.

The crude testing methods first employed were improved; various culture media were tried to increase the yield of penicillin; and freeze-drying in vacuum made possible extraction of penicillin in small amounts without loss of activity. The brown powder containing the sodium salt of penicillin proved to be remarkably active—1 in 500,000 dilutions proved effective against staphylococci. (It was to be found out later that this brown residue contained only about 1 per cent of penicillin).

Gradually, a small store of the impure penicillin was gathered—enough for trial on mice. The first test was made May 25, 1940. Mice were infected with a virulent strain of hemolytic streptococcus. Two groups were injected with penicillin; one group of controls was unprotected. All the control mice were dead after sixteen hours; the penicillin-protected mice survived. Other tests on mice, conducted a few days later, confirmed these results.

Imperfect as they were, the mouse tests stimulated hope for penicillin. Dr. Heatley devoted his attention to production of penicillin. A. D. Gardner and J. Orr-Ewing took up bacteriologic investigations; Dr. Florey and M. A. Jennings undertook pharmacologic and biologic investigations. Dr. Chain, with A. G. Sanders and E. P. Abraham, collaborated on chemical and biochemical aspects. When the stage of clinical trial was reached, Dr. H. W. Florey, his wife, Dr. M. E. Florey, and C. M. Fletcher, were responsible. This group formed the nucleus of what came to be called the "Oxford team." Later, several other scientists joined the effort.

Another complication now entered the penicillin picture: World War II. This added to the difficulty of obtaining supplies and apparatus. However, the need for improved medicines to care for war wounded stimulated researchers to greater efforts—even though bombs were falling on Britain almost nightly.

Penicillin as a Chemotherapeutic Agent was the title of the first paper to come from the Sir William Dunn School of Pathology. Published in *The Lancet*, August 24, 1940, it caught the eye of Dr. Fleming. He had never stopped hoping that some day penicillin would be concentrated and purified—and the article was a happy surprise. He had not known of the work going on at Oxford. He determined to see for himself. Dr. Fleming went to Oxford, on September 2, 1940, and called on Drs. Florey and Chain in their laboratory. To Chain, it was indeed a surprise—he had thought that Fleming was dead! Dr. Fleming was in touch with the Oxford group from time to time thereafter; but it was the work of the team at Oxford that developed penicillin production to practicality.

Efforts to produce penicillin in larger quantities presented many problems. The mold would only grow on shallow layers of fluid. Wartime demands made it difficult to secure needed apparatus. At first, old-time circular bedpans were pressed into service; later, flat ceramic bottles were used. Extraction apparatus was ingeniously constructed out of available odds and ends, not the least useful of which were milk churns.

First clinical trials of penicillin began in 1941. The first patients to be treated were severely ill, and usual methods of treatment had failed. On February 12, an Oxford policeman, dying of septicemia, was given penicillin intravenously at intervals. Within twenty-four hours, he showed marked improvement, and continued to progress for five days—until the supply of penicillin was exhausted. Then the patient relapsed and died. As supplies of penicillin increased, and as experience was gained with dosages and with length of treatment time, lives of several patients, considered moribund before they received penicillin, were saved. To stretch the pitifully small supplies, at times penicillin was reextracted from the urine of patients who had received the drug.

Laboratory production facilities for penicillin were inadequate, even for clinical testing; and, because of wartime pressures, English pharmaceutical firms felt it impossible to invest the time and equipment needed to perfect mass production. Therefore, in 1941, Drs. Florey and Heatley embarked for the United States, which was not yet at war. Arriving just before the Fourth of July holiday, they were guests of Dr. John F. Fulton, professor of history of medicine at Yale University. Dr. Fulton put them in touch with Dr. Ross Harrison, chairman of the National Research Council, who advised them to talk to Dr. Charles Thom, of the Bureau of Plant Industry (who years before had identified Fleming's mold as *Penicillium notatum*). Dr. Thom took them to Dr. Percy A. Wells of the Department of Agriculture. After learning of the problem, Dr. Wells sent Drs. Florey and Heatley to the Northern Regional Research Laboratory of the Department of Agriculture at Peoria, Illinois. The problem of producing more penicillin was put to the director of the laboratory, Dr. Orville E. May, and to the director of the fermentation division, Dr. Robert D. Coghill, on July 14. Dr. Coghill suggested that perhaps the deep-tank fermentation methods then used to produce gluconic acid might be applied to penicillin production.

Dr. Heatley remained at Peoria for several months, cooperating in development of production improvements. Dr. Florey visited a number of drug firms in the United States and Canada, attempting to interest them in penicillin production, and consulted with governmental agencies. His old friend, Dr. A. N. Richards, had become chairman of the Committee on Medical Research of the United States office of Scientific Research and Development. Dr. Richards helped materially in stimulating research activity. A number of United States pharmaceutical firms began production of penicillin, among whom were Merck & Company, E. R. Squibb & Sons, Charles Pfizer & Company, Bristol Laboratories, Abbott Laboratories, Winthrop Chemical Company, Eli Lilly & Company, the Upjohn Company, Cutter Laboratories, and Parke, Davis & Company.

Several advances came from the laboratories in Peoria. First, corn steep liquor was added to the culture medium—and the output of penicillin was stepped up twenty times. Substitution of lactose for glucose further improved the output. A search for better molds was undertaken, and from a rotting cantaloupe found in a Peoria market there was cultured out a species of *Penicillium chrysogenum* that improved yields of penicillin still further. Artificial mutations made the progeny of this strain even more fruitful.

In addition to the work at Peoria, United States pharmaceutical manufacturers began intensive application of mycologic experience gained in other fields—brewing, manufacture of citric acid, and other chemicals—to the penicillin problem. Entry of the United States into the war, December 7, 1941, added further stimulation to the effort. Techniques were developed to produce enormous quantities of the drug by deep-tank fermentation. The government took control of distribution of the entire penicillin output, assuring its availability for war needs, and for the most urgent civilian needs. Of the tremendous growth of penicillin production, it has been said that, actually, in 1941, there was not sufficient penicillin in the United States to treat a single case; in 1942 there were probably insufficient quantities to treat 100 cases; but, by September, 1943, there was enough to satisfy the demands of the Armed Forces of the country and those of its allies as well.

There was constant interchange of information between government scientists of both nations. As mass production methods developed, English firms, including Boots Pure Drug Company, British Drug Houses, Glaxco Laboratories, May & Baker, and Burroughs & Well-come, began large-scale production.

Research further revealed that there were several types of penicillin produced by the molds. Chemical methods of refinement replaced the impure brown amorphous powders with pure, crystalline salts. Penicillin F became most popular in England, while Penicillin G became standard in the United States.

When Fleming announced his work on lysozyme, in 1921, his listeners were barely polite. When he announced his findings on penicillin, in 1929, there was no show of enthusiasm. Nor was there any for another ten years. After Florey and Chain announced their work, and penicillin began to become generally available, honors showered upon all of them. Florey was elected a Fellow in the Royal Society in 1941; Fleming was elected in 1943. Each was made a Knight Bachelor by the King of England in 1944. Chain also was elected to the Royal Society. In December, 1945, Fleming, Chain, and Florey were jointly awarded the Nobel Prize for Medicine. Honors and honorary degrees were showered upon all three.

Dr. Fleming became professor of Bacteriology at St. Mary's; was named first, Rector, then Chancellor, of Edinburgh University; and, upon Sir Almroth Wright's retirement, Principal of the Wright-Fleming Institute. He died in 1955, and was buried in a crypt at St. Paul's, in London. Dr. Florey retired as Professor and Director of the Sir William Dunn School of Pathology in 1962, and is now Provost of The Queen's College, at Oxford. Dr. Chain in 1949 became Head of the International Research Centre for General Biochemistry and Chemical Microbiology at the Institute of Public Health of the Italian

State, in Rome; and in 1961 was appointed Professor of Biochemistry at the Imperial College of Science and Technology, in London.

The impetus given to the search for new antibiotics during and since World War II has resulted in investigation of thousands of organisms, and reports of hundreds of antimicrobial substances. Tested carefully in research laboratories, by far the majority of them have been discarded—but from time to time, new antibiotics appear, and useful varieties of older ones are developed, to take their place among the weapons available to physicians in the constant fight against disease. The main classes include the penicillins, streptomycin and other oligosaccharides, erythromycin and other macrolides, the polypeptides, the tetracyclines, and chloramphenicol.

A strain of *Streptomyces griseus* capable of producing a new antibiotic, streptomycin, was first isolated in 1943, in the laboratories of Rutgers University under the direction of Dr. Selman A. Waksman. Its clinical importance was soon well established, and its usefulness, particularly against the tuberculosis organism, generally recognized. It, too, has undergone intensive research, and a number of variants have been developed by several manufacturers, though none has surpassed the parent compound.

Among the tetracyclines are aureomycin, announced by B. M. Duggar of Lederle Laboratories Division of American Cyanamid Company, in 1948; and terramycin, announced by a team of eleven scientists at Charles Pfizer & Company, in 1950. Somewhat similar in chemical construction, aureomycin and terramycin both have a broad spectrum of sensitive organisms. Newer forms of the tetracyclines have proved more efficient, with fewer undesirable actions.

One of the most dramatic chapters in antibiotic history concerns chloramphenicol, the first of the broad-spectrum antibiotics, pharmaceutical formulations of which are marketed by Parke, Davis & Company under the trademark Chloromycetin.® Chloramphenicol, which was reported in 1947, was obtained from culture fluids of a species of actinomycete isolated from a sample of soil collected from a mulched field near Caracas, Venezuela—one of the more than 6,000 soil samples examined in a screening program by Dr. Paul R. Burkholder of Yale University. This actinomycete was one of many such organisms passed on to the laboratories of Parke, Davis & Company for further evaluation under the cooperative program.

A team of research scientists, including mycologists, biochemists, organic chemists, physicists, and many others, grew this organism under various experimental conditions, and eventually isolated the pure, biologically active substance. Then the research teams divided. One group studied methods of growing the mold on a large scale submerged in aerated nutrient media in fermentation tanks. Another set out to translate the laboratory methods of isolation of crystalline chloramphenicol into pilot-plant terms preliminary to determining mass-production methods. A third team intensified studies of the effect of the new antibiotic against a wide range of bacteria, viruses, rickettsiae, fungi, and protozoa. Still another team tested effects of the drug on animals. Chemists sought to determine the chemical structure of the unknown compound.

The chemists were successful in determining the chemical structure of chloramphenicol and subsequently in devising practical methods for creating the unique molecule from simple chemicals by synthetic means. Thus the identical chloramphenicol molecule could be made either by fermentation and extraction procedures or wholly by chemical synthesis. It was the first antibiotic to have been successfully produced on an industrial scale by chemical methods.

Meantime, the new antibiotic showed some remarkable properties. It was the first to reveal an effectiveness against a wide range of microorganisms—a truly broad-spectrum antibiotic. It overlapped parts of the spectra of penicillin and streptomycin, and also proved valuable against a number of other bacteria and rickettsiae, untouched by previously available medicine.

Equally dramatic was the clinical evaluation of chloramphenicol. Among the microorganisms against which the drug showed particular activity was that of typhus fever. It is interesting that this untried antibiotic, produced by using an organism native to the soil of South America, should be particularly indicated for a disease which had periodically scourged that area of the world since history began.

It fell to the lot of Dr. Eugene H. Payne of the Parke-Davis Department of Clinical Investigation to try out the new drug on living patients. Epidemic typhus was raging in Bolivia, and Dr. Payne headed for La Paz with the world's total supply of chloramphenicol—less than half a pound. He administered Chloromycetin capsules to twenty-two typhus patients, all of whom recovered—including one man whose death certificate already had been signed, and awaited only notation as to time. The certificate was not used.

Shortly before, Dr. Joseph E. Smadel, of Walter Reed Hospital, had received a small sample of chloramphenicol from Parke-Davis, and had confirmed in his laboratory the antirickettsial activity previously observed at Parke-Davis. Later, during the winter of 1947-1948, a team of U. S. Army medical men, led by Drs. Smadel and Theodore E. Woodward, tested the drug against scrub typhus at Kuala Lumpur, Malaya. Again it proved a lifesaver for typhus victims—and also, uniquely, for those suffering from typhoid fever. Before long, many other diseases fell to chloramphenicol, and the new drug took its place among the highly useful members of the spectacularly successful antibiotic family of therapeutic agents.

As antibiotics came into wide usage, other problems arose that demanded attention of physicians, of hospitals, and of research laboratories. These problems were associated with development of resistant strains of disease-causing organisms. This led to careful restudies of antibiotics and preparation of new varieties of some classes of the drugs. New penicillin forms have overcome some of the limitations experienced when this antibiotic came into wide use. Newer forms of the tetracyclines have proved more efficient, with fewer undesirable actions.

Although no antibiotic product has proved to be entirely free of side effects, or of dangerous reactions when given to persons who prove to be abnormally sensitive to them, the relatively few people thus affected by antibiotics are outnumbered by countless millions of patients whose health has benefited, or whose lives have been saved, by judicious prescription of antibiotic drugs by their attending physicians.

The world has an almost inexhaustible biotic reservoir from which antibiotic substances may be sought. At least 50,000 kinds of molds are known; and the antibiotic-producing potentialities of this and other natural groups are far from exhausted. Research teams in pharmaceutical laboratories around the world have turned their attention less toward numbers of new antibiotics, and more toward antibiotics which have a qualitative selectivity for specific groups of disease-causing organisms as yet not controlled.

No single individual, laboratory, branch of science, nation, institution, or corporation can claim credit for the historical developments that made antibiotics readily available and accepted therapeutic agents. However, as Fleming once pointed out, "The spores didn't just stand up on the agar and say, 'I produce an antibiotic, you know.'" Fulton once wrote that "credit for the introduction of penicillin as a therapeutic agent . . . goes to those who first isolated penicillin and gave clear-cut proof of its clinical usefulness . . ." But Fourneau commented sagely that: "The chemist gives birth to the drug, but the doctor supports its first steps."

One must agree with Dr. Waksman that it is still too early to write a closing chapter on antibiotics. They are too recent in origin and their development has been too spectacular to allow historical evaluation of them. Many problems, too, still await solution.

A new chapter in the history of science and of medicine is being written before our eyes.

MEDICINE TODAY AND TOMORROW

MEDICINE is a paradox: it is ancient; yet ever new. Its practice is an art; yet that art must be grounded on solid foundations of science, of practicality, and of the needs of the patient. It is one of the most important fields of scientific discipline; yet in practice it must employ and apply essential knowledge gleaned from many other fields of science. Medicine's practitioners have at their command the epitomization of knowledge and discovery gained over fifty centuries; yet, they face a great wall of unknown factors as formidable as any faced by their predecessors—challenging, baffling, yet urgently demanding solution because of needs of a humanity faced with speeded-up living processes that outdistance man's ability to adjust.

In his primitive state, man tried to explain the rigors and uncertainties of his surroundings by imagining himself a toy of the gods. He sought relief by attempts to propitiate the unknown. Today, with tools of many sciences at hand, man seeks to grasp reality and to surround himself with the comforts and conveniences that he and his fellows have wrought, and to push on to new horizons. His knowledge and his skills give him visions of goals undreamed a few decades ago; and confidence to move boldly toward these objectives. This confidence bolsters him and carries him forward—until illness and distress strike him. Then, modern man reacts much in the same manner as did his ancestors: he seeks help, turning to men of religion and of medicine, reaching out for someone in whom he can have faith and who may be able to help restore his health and his confidence in himself.

Never before in the world's history have its people had the advantage of medicines and medical services equal to those available today. The knowledge gained by countless generations of dedicated medical men is at the command of today's physician, and through him, is brought

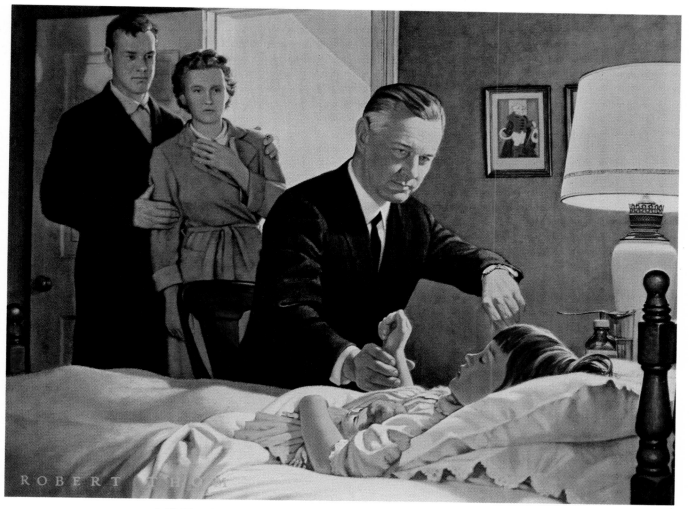

ROBERT THOM

MEDICINE TODAY AND TOMORROW

Medicine is ancient, yet ever new. The scientific discoveries and advances resulting from work of countless thousands of dedicated medical men throughout fifty centuries are at the command of today's physician, and through him, brought to focus upon the needs of sick patients. Never before in the world's history have its people had the medical advantages available today. Physicians, research scientists, specialists in production and distribution, are collaborating in a constant effort to improve medical service and to make available better diagnoses, better treatment, and better medicines for a better world.

to focus upon the needs of the individual patient at the bedside, in the laboratory, in the consultation room, and in the hospital.

During no period in history has man experienced such rapid and revolutionary advances in medicine and in opportunity for improved health as during the twentieth century; and the accelerated pace of scientific research holds promise of still greater advances in the years ahead.

As the twentieth century opened, the great gains of the nineteenth century were being consolidated and perfected: anesthesia and asepsis were becoming better understood, as were the medical potentials of x-rays. Together, they combined to make possible tremendous advances in surgery. The field of biological medicines—vaccines to prevent diseases and antitoxins to combat them—was expanding rapidly. Chemotherapy, which had already developed basic analgesics such as aspirin and phenacetin, was on the verge of blossoming to full potential.

Early in the century, dependence on drugs of vegetable origin—largest source of medicines then available to practicing physicians—began to wane as scientific advances improved the whole field of drug therapy. While many valuable drugs still in use were originally derived from vegetable sources (ephedrine, reserpine), disappearance of many medicines of doubtful value was hastened by the contributions of chemotherapy. Given impetus by Ehrlich's creation of the arsphenamines as specifics for syphilis, chemists brought forth a number of new classes of medicines—anesthetics, barbiturates, and antimalarials. However, research in chemotherapy did not hit its full stride until, about 1937, sulfanilamide and its chemical relatives entered the physician's armamentarium. Following upon the sulfas came the antibiotics—an entirely new concept in development of drugs. Demonstration that hitherto deadly diseases could be treated successfully with these new medicines reestablished confidence in chemotherapy and initiated a tremendous advance in industrial medicinal and chemical research. Laboratories increased their scientific manpower by a hundredfold. There resulted a tremendous speedup of discovery and development of new compounds useful to medicine.

Meantime, research was bearing fruit in other areas. The use of hormones in medicine, first by employing thyroid extract, in 1891, for treatment of myxedema, followed by the discovery of epinephrine, first made available by Parke-Davis, which marketed its Adrenalin® brand in 1900, led to examination of other glandular functions. From one phase of this study came the theory that in 1921 led Banting and Best to the discovery of insulin, which prolonged and saved lives of millions of diabetics. From hormone research there also developed study of the complex chemistry of steroids, opening another new source of compounds useful to medicine.

The study of vitamin deficiencies got under way with the work of many men in many countries, encouraged by the findings of Eijkman and his associates in the Far East, of Casimir Funk, in 1911, and of Joseph Goldberger in 1914, in the United States. These scientific studies led not only to better understanding of causes and treatment of vitamin deficiencies, but to improved nutritional practices. New food products, and new methods of preparing and preserving natural vitamin content of foods, as well as fortification of foods with additives, have gone a long way in prevention of deficiency diseases that once plagued a large sector of the population. Pellagra, beriberi, and rickets have largely disappeared in world areas where preventive nutritional measures are understood and practiced.

Need for improved sulfa drugs stimulated chemists to make thousands of experiments with synthetic compounds, many of which led them to previously unexplored bypaths. From these experiments came compounds that opened several new areas of endeavor. Promin® (sodium glucosulfone), the first synthetic drug to prove truly effective in arresting leprosy, resulted from the new intense interest in synthetic compounds. Out of research studies of sulfa derivatives have come a group of oral diuretic compounds; and of oral antidiabetic drugs that supplement and sometimes replace injections of insulin. Other areas of chemotherapeutic development include the psychic energizers; the tranquilizers; the antihistamines; the anticoagulants; and a group of compounds that hold promise of leading to control of certain types of tumors. Paralleling development of synthetic medicinal compounds has been that of improved insecticides. While new medicines can cure many insect-borne diseases, far more progress toward elimination of these problems, especially of malaria and of yellow fever, has been made through preventive measures. Spraying of swamplands, of huts and homes, and of individuals with DDT or compounds that developed from this field of research, has resulted in great savings economically in many world areas, as well as prevention of human misery and incapacitation. Research into use of recently discovered compounds in animal feeds has added to production and to improvement of meat and poultry food products. Improved agricultural fertilizers have increased yields and quality of food crops. All of these auxiliary results of scientific research have made indirect but important contributions to human health.

Developments no less spectacular and important to the patients whom medical men serve have come from other fields.

Great improvements have been made in anesthetics, both injectable and inhalant types. Understanding of importance of electrolyte balance in body fluids has made possible advances in surgery and has improved patients' likelihood of rapid recovery. Physicomedical developments, such as the artificial lung, the artificial kidney, and the artificial heart, have greatly extended the surgeon's field of operation. Tissue banks, making possible such procedures as corneal transplants, replacement of arteries, of bones, and other parts of the body, have enabled medical men to restore to useful lives patients who otherwise would have been cripples. Recognition of importance of fractions of the blood, and of how to utilize these substances, extended lives of still another group of patients.

Bold explorations into brain surgery, better diagnosis of mental diseases, advances in psychiatry, and employment of tranquilizers and psychic energizers, all have contributed greatly to restoring afflicted persons to normalcy, and to reduction of population of mental care institutions.

Heart surgery—going far beyond procedures thought possible a decade or two ago—has corrected many lesions, congenital or chronic, and given chance of useful life to persons otherwise doomed to death or crippling. Mechanical developments, such as artificial heart valves, and electronic equipment that will stimulate or regulate performance

390

of abnormal hearts, also have contributed tremendously to welfare and comfort of many people.

Application of new knowledge of radiation, and especially adaptation to medical use of products of the atomic age, have further extended lives of persons suffering from lesions beyond reach of surgery.

These developments of the twentieth century not only have revolutionized the therapeutic practice of the medical profession; they have had an impact upon the lives of every person in the civilized world:

Approximately a quarter century has been added to the life expectancy of persons born in the 1960's, as compared with those born in the 1900's.

Millions of people are living today who would have died from infectious diseases under conditions existing during the first quarter of this century.

The death rate of mothers during childbirth has declined ninety per cent, and infant mortality has been greatly reduced during this century.

Deaths from influenza have been cut ninety per cent in twenty-five years; deaths from tuberculosis and from rheumatic fever are down more than eighty per cent.

Due to extension of the work begun on vaccines and biological medicines just before the turn of the century, diphtheria and smallpox have nearly disappeared; typhoid and tetanus are seldom encountered in settled communities; and the threat of polio has been largely diminished.

Ninety per cent of the drugs which physicians prescribe today were unknown twenty-five years ago.

There have been many changes in the practice of medicine, too. Specialization has increased, with disciplines and boards to govern each group. While the old-style "family doctor" has largely disappeared, general practitioners have organized courses for postgraduate education that assure continuation of high standards of family care in neighborhoods and in smaller centers of population. Furthermore, they are not allowing educators to overlook the future need for general physicians.

The rise of prepaid hospital, surgical, and medical care also has had its impact upon medical men and their patients. Further experience with these comparatively new services undoubtedly will solve their "growing pains" problems and bring about standards beneficial to all concerned.

As improved methods of medical care and better medicines have become available and the average life expectancy of people has been lengthened, new problems have arisen for patients, for physicians, for other health professions, and for research workers. Lowering of death rates from infectious diseases has resulted in more persons reaching the older age brackets, and consequent medical focus on groups of diseases that were not so frequently seen in the past. The degenerative diseases, particularly those affecting the circulatory system, mental processes, and various forms of cancer, now rank among the foremost afflictions demanding the skills of physicians, surgeons, and researchers.

In addition, psychosomatic considerations are demanding more and more of the attention of medical men, as their patients are affected by the pressures and stresses of modern working and living. To this may be added the concern which physicians share with sociologists and engineers for the sociopsychological aspects of the rising rate of accidental injuries, particularly those influenced by the hazards of mass and rapid transportation.

Future research in the various scientific fields related to medicine may be expected to bring about breakthroughs in new areas that will be of benefit to the people of the world. Research having to do with preventive medicine, chemotherapy, antibiotics, and hormones, shows great future promise. The intensive search for agents—biological as well as chemical—effective against cancer undoubtedly will uncover means of combating various forms of this dread killer.

What will the space age, just ahead, mean to medicine? No one can tell—but in all likelihood, citizens of the twenty-first century will be able to look back upon medicine of our day with much of the same combination of superiority, humor and pity as that with which we are likely to regard the practices and remedies of nineteenth-century physicians. However, it must be realized that such feelings of superiority or humor are not justified; we owe a great deal of gratitude to the physicians of the nineteenth century for the contributions which they made. Among these nineteenth-century advances, one has only to consider recognition that germs are a cause of disease; advances in understanding of anatomy and of cellular pathology; discovery of the principles of anesthesia and of asepsis; of bacteriology, and of biological medicines; of physical devices, such as the ophthalmoscope, the otoscope, the stethoscope, and x-rays. Literally, physicians and scientists of today stand upon the shoulders of those stalwarts of yesterday. It seems certain that, as more scientific and technological advances are made, they will contribute, directly or indirectly, to products and procedures that will increase the effectiveness of the physician's therapy, and extend the operative field of the surgeon.

Indeed, the future will bring changes in the practice of medicine and of surgery, in hospital care, in relationships with patients. A more sophisticated people will demand services in keeping with their advancing world. However, whatever the age or stage of world affairs, there will be men and women, educated, experienced, dedicated, and imbued with compassion, ready to offer help to persons who need their medical ministrations.

However highly placed or lowly may be the individual's position in the future socioeconomic scheme—when his child cries out in the night, racked with pain and fever, the first thought will be: "Call the doctor!" When he or she personally falls ill—age-old instincts of fear and of self-preservation will cut through the veneer of sophistication and turn the ailing one's mind to the question that has been heard across the centuries:

"Doctor, I'm sick. What can you do for me?"

ACKNOWLEDGMENTS

ACKNOWLEDGMENT of most helpful assistance, and sincere thanks, are extended to the many persons, experts in their fields, who have assisted in the development and authentication of these stories, and of the pictures which accompany them. Particular thanks are due Erwin H. Ackerknecht, M.D., Professor and Director of the Institute of the History of Medicine and Biology, University of Zurich, Switzerland, whose advice, assistance, and criticism, have guided the author-artist team throughout the project, and without which the task would have been almost insurmountable.

This project also was dependent in large measure upon the interest, support, and cooperation extended it by Parke-Davis personnel. Among those who contributed advice, encouragement, and assistance were: President Harry J. Loynd; Vice Presidents Carl Johnson, Graydon L. Walker, W. R. Jeeves, George Rieveschl, Jr., and C. D. Smith; Drs. J. P. Gray, H. E. Carnes, and J. E. Gajewski; Ralph G. Sickels, Walter L. Griffith, Arthur N. Sorenson, George Donat, Barnard Thompson, D. W. Gilmore, Miss Clara Banfield, Miss G. Losie, and Mrs. J. M. Lotze. International research and travel were facilitated by the cooperation of Messrs. L. O. Smith, J. R. Archer, Jules Snoijink, William Norcia, and Drs. Gerhard H. Matejka, F. Macdonald, and H. W. Pearson.

Other persons who gave freely of their time, knowledge, advice, and assistance in connection with various subjects, include the following:

Medicine in Ancient Egypt

William C. Hayes, Curator of Egyptian Art, The Metropolitan Museum of Art, New York City.

Cyril Aldred, Assistant Keeper of the Royal Scottish Museum, Edinburgh, Scotland.

The Code of Hammurabi

Dr. Leo Oppenheim, Professor of Assyriology, The Oriental Institute, University of Chicago, Chicago, Illinois.

Thomas N. Hakim, Detroit, Michigan.

American-Syrian-Lebanon Association, Detroit, Michigan.

Trephining in Ancient Peru

Dr. Junius Bird, Associate Curator of Archaeology, American Museum of Natural History, New York City.

Donald Collier, Jr., Curator, South American Archaeology and Ethnology, Chicago Natural History Museum, Chicago, Illinois.

Dr. Bertha Dutton, Curator of Anthropology and Ethnology, Museum of New Mexico, Santa Fe, New Mexico.

Primitive Medicine

Kenneth E. Foster, Curator, Museum of Navaho Ceremonial Art, Santa Fe, New Mexico.

Dr. Bertha Dutton, Curator of Anthropology and Ethnology, Museum of New Mexico, Santa Fe, New Mexico.

394

John Candelario, Santa Fe, New Mexico.

Mrs. F. J. Newcomb, Albuquerque, New Mexico.

M. L. Woodard, Gallup, New Mexico.

William Norton, Pinedale, New Mexico.

Leland C. Wyman, Ph.D., Professor of Biology, College of Liberal Arts, Boston University, Boston, Massachusetts.

The Temples and Cult of Asclepius

Dr. Ludwig Edelstein, Professor of Humanistic Studies, Johns Hopkins University, Baltimore, Maryland.

Dr. John Young, Professor of Archaeology, Johns Hopkins University, Baltimore, Maryland.

The Metropolitan Museum of Art, New York.

Dr. Elias Zioghas, personal secretary to the Archbishop, Greek Archdiocese of North and South America, New York City.

Arthur Dore, public relations, Greek Archdiocese of North and South America, New York City.

Basil Vasiliades, Patriarchy of Instanbul, Greek Archdiocese of North and South America, New York City.

Suśruta—Surgeon of Old India

H. Dayal, Chargé d'Affaires, Embassy of India, Washington, D.C.

D. K. Hingorani, Educational Attaché, Embassy of India, Washington, D.C.

Amiya Chakravarty, Professor of Comparative Religions, School of Theology, Boston University.

Kohiro Tomita, Curator of Asiatic Art, Museum of Fine Arts, Boston, Massachusetts.

Robert Austin, Armed Forces Medical Library, Washington, D.C.

Walter H. Maurer, Division of Orientalia, Library of Congress, Washington, D.C.

Hippocrates: Medicine Becomes a Science

Dr. Ludwig Edelstein, Professor of Humanistic Studies, Johns Hopkins University, Baltimore, Maryland.

Dr. John Young, Professor of Archaeology, Johns Hopkins University, Baltimore, Maryland.

The Metropolitan Museum of Art, New York.

Dr. Elias Zioghas, personal secretary to the Archbishop, Greek Archdiocese of North and South America, New York City.

Arthur Dore, public relations, Greek Archdiocese of North and South America, New York City.

Basil Vasiliades, Patriarchy of Instanbul, Greek Archdiocese of North and South America, New York City.

Galen, Influence for 45 Generations

Professor Adalberto Pazzini, Director of the Institute of the History of Medicine, University of Rome, Italy.

Dr. Alberto Lodispoto, University of Rome, Italy.

Dietrich von Bothmer, Associate Curator, Greek and Roman Department, Metropolitan Museum of Art, New York City.

Rhazes and Arabic Medicine

Dr. Ali Amini, Ambassador of Iran, Washington, D.C.

Mahoud Mir-Fakhrai, Minister of Iran, Washington, D.C.

Ahmad Minai, Press Attaché, Iranian Embassy, Washington, D.C.

Ibrahim V. Pourhadi, Reference Librarian, Division of Orientalia, Library of Congress, Washington, D.C.

Dr. Maurice S. Dimand, Curator, Department of Near Eastern Art, Metropolitan Museum of Art, New York City.

Hannah E. McAllister, Associate Curator, Department of Near Eastern Art, Metropolitan Museum of Art, New York City.

Medieval Hospitals

Jean Beliard, Secretary of the French Ministry of Foreign Affairs, Paris, France.

Gaston Papeloux, Cabinet of the Secretary of State for Arts and Letters, Paris, France.

Professor René Hazard, M.D., Faculté de Médecine, University of Paris, France.

Ralph Setton, Ph.D., National Center for Scientific Research, Paris, France.

Louis Latour, Curator of the Museum, Hôtel-Dieu, Beaune, France.

Sister Roussel, pharmacist, Hôtel-Dieu, Beaune, France.

Professor Adalberto Pazzini, Director of the Institute of the History of Medicine, University of Rome, Italy.

Dr. Alberto Lodispoto, University of Rome, Italy.

F. N. L. Poynter, Librarian, The Wellcome Historical Medical Library, London, England.

Henry R. Carstens, M.D., Springfield, Massachusetts.

Don E. Francke, D.Sc., Editor, the American Journal of Hospital Pharmacy, Ann Arbor, Michigan.

Roberta Leigh, New York.

Rev. Thomas J. Clynes, Pastor, Holy Ghost Church, Detroit, Michigan.

Carmen Stewart, Detroit, Michigan.

Paracelsus—Stormy Petrel of Medicine

Roy W. Hill, Ciba, Ltd., Basel, Switzerland.

Dr. Werner E. Raths, Ciba, Ltd., Basel, Switzerland.

Dr. E. Lang, Ciba, Ltd., Basel, Switzerland.

Dr. H. Buess, Ciba, Ltd., Basel, Switzerland.

Roger Larose, Ciba, Ltd., Montreal, Canada.

Dr. Phil A. Lutz, Curator of the Swiss Museum of Pharmaceutical History, Basel, Switzerland.

Dr. Rudolf Sachtleben, Keeper of the Chemistry Department, Deutsches Museum, Munich, Germany.

F. N. L. Poynter, Librarian, The Wellcome Historical Medical Library, London, England.

George B. Griffenhagen, Curator, Division of Medical Sciences, Smithsonian Institution, Washington, D. C.

Robert P. Multhauf, Curator, Department of Science and Technology, Smithsonian Institution, Washington, D.C.

Vesalius—and the Anatomy of Man

Dr. Sergio Bruzzo, Secretary to the Rettore Magnifico, University of Padua, Italy.

Dr. Umberto Carretta, College of Pharmacy, University of Padua, Italy.

Dr. Carlo A. Benassi, College of Pharmacy, University of Padua, Italy.

Dr. Ferruccio D'Angeli, College of Pharmacy, University of Padua, Italy.

Dr. Glauco De Bertoli, Assistant Instructor of the History of Medicine, University of Padua, Italy.

Signora Lea Greselin, Librarian, Biblioteca Pinali, University of Padua, Italy.

Gordon H. Scott, Ph.D., Dean, College of Medicine, Wayne State University, Detroit, Michigan.

Plinn F. Morse, M.D., Head, Department of Pathology, Harper Hospital, Detroit, Michigan.

Ambroise Paré: Surgery Acquires Stature

Jean Beliard, Secretary of the French Ministry of Foreign Affairs, Paris, France.

Gaston Papeloux, Cabinet of the Secretary of State for Arts and Letters, Paris, France.

Professor René Hazard, M.D., Faculté de Médecine, University of Paris, France.

Paul Lechat, M.D., Faculté de Médecine, Paris, France.

Ralph Setton, Ph.D., National Center for Scientific Research, Paris, France.

Dr. Maurice Genty, Librarian, Académie de Médecine, Paris, France.

Musée Carnavalet, Paris, France.

Musée de l'Armée, Paris, France.

Harvey and the Circulation of the Blood

L. M. Payne, Assistant Librarian, Royal College of Physicians, London, England.

Philip Wade, Librarian, Royal Society of Medicine, London, England.

E. Ashworth Underwood, Director, The Wellcome Historical Medical Museum, London, England.

F. N. L. Poynter, Librarian, The Wellcome Historical Medical Library, London, England.

C. H. Gibbs-Smith, Keeper of Museum Extension Services, Victoria and Albert Museum, London, England.

G. F. Wingfield-Digby, Keeper of Textiles, Victoria and Albert Museum, London, England.

M. B. Blumstein, Research Assistant, Victoria and Albert Museum, London, England.

Dr. Louis B. Wright, Director, the Folger Shakespearean Library, Washington, D.C.

Professor Charles Morgan, Meade Arts Building, Amherst College, Amherst, Massachusetts.

Leeuwenhoek and the "Little Animals"

Dr. D. A. Wittop Koning, pharmacist, Amsterdam, Holland.

Dr. Maria Rooseboom, Directress, National Museum for the History of Science, Leyden, Holland.

P. van der Star, Conservator, National Museum for the History of Science, Leyden, Holland.

J. van der Werff, Director, the Huis Lambert van Meerten Museum, Delft, Holland.

J. Lanen, Director, Netherlands Foundation for Educational Films, The Hague, Holland.

J. Kramer, Netherlands Foundation for Educational Films, The Hague, Holland.

R. van der Linden, Netherlands Foundation for Educational Films, The Hague, Holland.

Sydenham:
Proponent of Clinical Medicine

Philip Wade, Librarian, Royal Society of Medicine, London, England.

E. Ashworth Underwood, Director, The Wellcome Historical Medical Museum, London, England.

F. N. L. Poynter, Librarian, The Wellcome Historical Medical Library, London, England.

C. H. Gibbs-Smith, Keeper of Museum Extension Services, Victoria and Albert Museum, London, England.

G. F. Wingfield-Digby, Keeper of Textiles, Victoria and Albert Museum, London, England.

M. B. Blumstein, Research Assistant, Victoria and Albert Museum, London, England.

Delves Molesworthy, Victoria and Albert Museum, London, England.

National Portrait Gallery, London, England.

National Trust for Places of Historic or Natural Beauty, London, England.

Country Life Magazine, London, England.

Connoisseur Books, Rainbird MacLean, Ltd., London, England.

Thorne Rooms collection, The Art Institute of Chicago, Illinois.

Governor's Mansion, Williamsburg, Virginia.

Rare Book Room of the Library of the New York Academy of Medicine, New York.

Detroit Institute of Arts, Detroit, Michigan.

National Gallery of Canada, Ottawa, Ontario.

James Lind: Conqueror of Scurvy

Philip Wade, Librarian, Royal Society of Medicine, London, England.

E. Ashworth Underwood, Director, The Wellcome Historical Medical Museum, London, England.

F. N. L. Poynter, Librarian, The Wellcome Historical Medical Library, London, England.

F. E. G. Carr, Director, National Maritime Museum, Greenwich, London, England.

Edward H. H. Archibald, Curator of Oil Paintings, National Maritime Museum, Greenwich, London, England.

J. Munday, Librarian, National Maritime Museum, Greenwich, London, England.

Instructor Captain T. E. Jackson, R.N. (ret.) Curator, the Victory Museum, Portsmouth, England.

C. H. Gibbs-Smith, Keeper of Museum Extension Services, Victoria and Albert Museum, London, England.

G. F. Wingfield-Digby, Keeper of Textiles, Victoria and Albert Museum, London, England.

M. B. Blumstein, Research Assistant, Victoria and Albert Museum, London, England.

Morgagni and Pathologic Anatomy

Professor Loris Premuda, M.D., Director, Institute of the History of Medicine, University of Padua, Italy.

Franco DiCianni, M.D., Assistant Director, Institute of the History of Medicine, University of Padua, Italy.

Baldo Viterbo, M.D., Professor of Legal Medicine, University of Padua, Italy.

Ferruccio D'Angeli, Ph.D., Professor of Chemistry, University of Padua, Italy.

Signora Lea Greselin, Librarian, Biblioteca Pinali, University of Padua, Italy.

Lavoisier:
Oxygen, Combustion, and Respiration

Jean Beliard, Secretary of the French Ministry of Foreign Affairs, Paris, France.

Gaston Papeloux, Cabinet of the Secretary of State for Arts and Letters, Paris, France.

Professor René Hazard, M.D., Faculté de Médecine, University of Paris, France.

Paul Lechat, M.D., Faculté de Médecine, Paris, France.

Ralph Setton, Ph.D., National Center for Scientific Research, Paris, France.

Musée des Arts Décoratifs, Paris, France.

Musée Carnavalet, Paris, France.

Musée des Arts et Métiers, Paris, France.

Rudolf Sachtleben, Ph.D., Keeper of the Chemistry Department, Deutsches Museum, Munich, Germany.

Denis I. Duveen, Duveen Historical Library, Long Island City, New York.

Herbert S. Klickstein, M.D., Philadelphia, Pennsylvania.

John Hunter:
Founder of Scientific Surgery

W. R. LeFanu, Librarian, The Royal College of Surgeons, London, England.

Jessie Dobson, Curator of the Anatomical Museum, The Royal College of Surgeons, London, England.

E. Ashworth Underwood, Director, The Wellcome Historical Medical Museum, London, England.

F. N. L. Poynter, Librarian, The Wellcome Historical Medical Library, London, England.

Philip Wade, Librarian, The Royal Society of Medicine, London, England.

C. H. Gibbs-Smith, Keeper of Museum Extension Services, Victoria and Albert Museum, London, England.

G. F. Wingfield-Digby, Keeper of Textiles, Victoria and Albert Museum, London, England.

M. B. Blumstein, Research Assistant, Victoria and Albert Museum, London, England.

Benjamin Rush:
Physician, Pedant, Patriot

J. H. Powell, M.D., Philadelphia, Pennsylvania.

Alexander Rush, M.D., Philadelphia, Pennsylvania.

William Barber, Jr., of Woodford Mansion, Philadelphia, Pennsylvania.

Horace H. Jayne, Philadelphia Museum of Art, Philadelphia, Pennsylvania.

The Pennsylvania Hospital, Philadelphia, Pennsylvania.

Mrs. T. Charlton Henry, Chestnut Hill, Pennsylvania.

Frick Collection, New York City.

Pinel Unchains the Insane

Jean Beliard, Secretary of the French Ministry of Foreign Affairs, Paris, France.

Gaston Papeloux, Cabinet of the Secretary of State for Arts and Letters, Paris, France.

Professor René Hazard, M.D., Faculté de Médecine, University of Paris, France.

Paul Lechat, M.D., Faculté de Médecine, Paris, France.

Ralph Setton, Ph.D., National Center for Scientific Research, Paris, France.

Audie Mangeot, Chief Pharmacist, La Salpêtrière, Paris, France.

Professor Th. Alajouanine, La Salpêtrière, Paris, France.

Dr. Maurice Genty, Librarian, Académie de Médecine, Paris, France.

Pharmacie Centrale, Paris, France.

Musée des Arts Décoratifs, Paris, France.

Musée Carnavalet, Paris, France.

Jenner: Smallpox is Stemmed

Canon John Fisher, the Vicarage, Berkeley, England.

W. R. LeFanu, Librarian, The Royal College of Surgeons, London, England.

Jessie Dobson, Curator of the Anatomical Museum, The Royal College of Surgeons, London, England.

Philip Wade, Librarian, The Royal Society of Medicine, London, England.

E. Ashworth Underwood, Director, The Wellcome Historical Medical Museum, London, England.

F. N. L. Poynter, Librarian, The Wellcome Historical Medical Library, London, England.

C. H. Gibbs-Smith, Keeper of Museum Extension Services, Victoria and Albert Museum, London, England.

G. F. Wingfield-Digby, Keeper of Textiles, Victoria and Albert Museum, London, England.

M. B. Blumstein, Research Assistant, Victoria and Albert Museum, London, England.

Laennec and the Stethoscope

Léon Binet, M.D., President of the Académie de Médecine, Paris, France.

Jean-Pierre Kernéis, M.D., Professor of Pathologic Anatomy at the Faculté de Médecine, Nantes, France.

Ralph Setton, Ph.D., National Center for Scientific Research, Paris, France.

Conquerors of Pain

E. Michael White, Assistant Director, Massachusetts General Hospital, Boston, Massachusetts.

Henry Knowles Beecher, M.D., Chief of Anesthesia Service, Massachusetts General Hospital, Boston, Massachusetts.

Mrs. W. W. Ford, Historian, Department of Anesthesia, Massachusetts General Hospital, Boston, Massachusetts.

Edward Delos Churchill, M.D., Chief of General Surgical Services, Massachusetts General Hospital, Boston, Massachusetts.

Cora F. Holbrook, Archivist, Massachusetts General Hospital, Boston, Massachusetts.

Henry R. Viets, M.D., Curator, Boston Medical Library, Boston, Massachusetts.

Kenneth L. Waters, Ph.D., Dean, School of Pharmacy, University of Georgia, Athens, Georgia.

F. N. L. Poynter, Librarian, The Wellcome Historical Medical Library, London, England.

G. R. Paterson, Associate Professor of Pharmaceutical Chemistry, Faculty of Pharmacy, University of Toronto, Ontario, Canada.

Semmelweis: Defender of Motherhood

Leopold Schönbauer, M.D., Director, Allgemeines Krankenhaus, Vienna, Austria.

Universitatsdozent Marlene Jantsch, M.D., Institute for the History of Medicine, University of Vienna, Austria.

Erna Lesky, M.D., Ph.D., Director of the Institute of the History of Medicine, University of Vienna, Austria.

F. N. L. Poynter, Librarian, The Wellcome Historical Medical Library, London, England.

Irving I. Edgar, M.D., F.A.C.P., Detroit, Michigan.

Founding of The American Medical Association

Kenneth W. Prescott, Ph.D., Managing Director, The Academy of Natural Sciences of Philadelphia, Pennsylvania.

Horace G. Richards, Ph.D., Chairman, Department of Geology and Paleontology, The Academy of Natural Sciences of Philadelphia, Pennsylvania.

Dr. Venia T. Phillips, Manuscript Librarian, The Academy of Natural Sciences of Philadelphia, Pennsylvania.

College of Physicians of Philadelphia, Pennsylvania.

The National Library of Medicine, Washington, D.C.

The New York Academy of Medicine, New York City.

Leo E. Brown, Director, Communications Division, The American Medical Association, Chicago, Illinois.

John L. Bach, Director, Press Relations, The American Medical Association, Chicago, Illinois.

David L. Cowen, Chairman, Department of History and Political Science, University College, Rutgers University, New Brunswick, New Jersey.

Dr. James H. C. Martens, Professor of Geology, Rutgers University, New Brunswick, New Jersey.

Virchow and Cellular Pathology

Professor Robert Herrlinger, M.D., Ph.D., Director of the Institute of the History of Medicine, University of Würzburg, Germany.

Irving I. Edgar, M.D., F.A.C.P., Detroit, Michigan.

Helmholtz: Physicist-Physician

Professor Robert Herrlinger, M.D., Ph.D., Director of the Institute of the History of Medicine, University of Würzburg, Germany.

William Munich, M.D., University of Würzburg, Germany.

Professor Johannes Steudel, M.D., Director, Institute of the History of Medicine, University of Bonn, Germany.

Rudolf Sachtleben, Ph.D., Keeper of the Chemistry Department, Deutsches Museum, Munich, Germany.

Ludwig Kraft, Oberamtmann, Münchner Stadtmuseum, Munich, Germany.

Professor Gernot Rath, M.D., Chairman of the Department of the History of Medicine, University of Wisconsin Medical School, Madison, Wisconsin.

Henry A. Dunlap, M.D., Ophthalmologist, Jennings Hospital, Detroit, Michigan.

J. Marion Sims: Gynecologic Surgeon

W. A. Dozier, Jr., Executive Secretary, The Medical Association of the State of Alabama, Montgomery, Alabama.

W. V. Wallace, Executive Assistant, The Medical Association of the State of Alabama, Montgomery, Alabama.

James Pratt Marr, M.D., F.A.C.S., Attending Surgeon, Woman's Hospital, New York.

Claude Bernard:
Explorer of Physiologic Frontiers

Léon Binet, M.D., President of the Académie de Médecine, Paris, France.

Staff of the Collège de France, Paris, France.

Professor P. Huard, Paris, France.

Ralph Setton, Ph.D., National Center for Scientific Research, Paris, France.

Pasteur:
The Chemist Who Transformed Medicine

Léon Binet, M.D., President of the Académie de Médecine, Paris, France.

Staff of the Ecole Normale, Paris, France.

Jacques Trefouël, Directeur, Institut Pasteur, Paris, France.

Mlle. D. Wrotnowska, Conservateur, Musée Pasteur, Paris, France.

Ralph Setton, Ph.D., National Center for Scientific Research, Paris, France.

Lister Introduces Antisepsis

A. L. Goodall, M.D., Consultant Surgeon and Honorary Lecturer in Surgery, Glasgow University, Glasgow, Scotland.

J. Killoch Anderson, M.D., Medical Superintendent, Glasgow Royal Infirmary, Glasgow, Scotland.

Professor T. Symington, M.D., and W. P. Duguid, M.D., the Pathological Institute; Miss Court Brown, Matron, and members of the staff, Glasgow Royal Infirmary, Glasgow, Scotland.

E. Ashworth Underwood, Director, The Wellcome Historical Medical Museum, London, England.

F. N. L. Poynter, Librarian, The Wellcome Historical Medical Library, London, England.

Charcot: Master of Neurology

Professor Th. Alajouanine, La Salpêtrière, Paris, France.

Audie Mangeot, Chief Pharmacist, La Salpêtrière, Paris, France.

Ralph Setton, Ph.D., National Center for Scientific Research, Paris, France.

The Hopkins:
A Revolution in Medical Education

Staff members of The Johns Hopkins Medical Institutions, including:

William A. Miller, Jr., Director of Public Relations, Johns Hopkins Medical Institutions.

Alan M. Chesney, M.D., Dean Emeritus of the Medical Faculty.

Milton S. Eisenhower, President of the University.

Thomas B. Turner, M.D., Dean of the Medical Faculty.

Russell A. Nelson, M.D., Director of the Hospital.

Oswei Temkin, M.D., Editor, Bulletin of the History of Medicine, and William H. Welch Professor of the History of Medicine, Baltimore, Maryland.

Janet Koudelka, Curator, Rare Books and Archives, Welch Medical Library, Baltimore, Maryland.

Eugenia Calvert Holland, Assistant Curator, The Maryland Historical Society, Baltimore, Maryland.

Röntgen:
Invisible Rays That Save Lives

Professor Robert Herrlinger, M.D., Ph.D., Director of the Institute of the History of Medicine, University of Würzburg, Germany.

Dr. Heinrich Schröer, Physiologisches Institut, University of Würzburg, Germany.

Diplom-Physiker Helmut Schmiedel, Deutsches Museum, Munich, Germany.

The Conquest of Yellow Fever

Staff members, Walter Reed General Hospital, Washington, D.C.

John L. Lentz, Young & Rubicam, Inc., New York.

Walter B. Cannon:
Physiologic Investigator

C. Sidney Burwell, M.D., Special Consultant to the Dean of the Faculty of Medicine, Harvard Medical School, Boston, Massachusetts.

Eugene M. Landis, M.D., George Higginson Professor of Physiology, Harvard Medical School, Boston, Massachusetts.

Ehrlich:
Chemotherapy Is Launched

Dr. Walter Artelt, Professor of the History of Medicine, University of Frankfurt, West Germany.

Professor Dr. Richard Prigge, Director, Paul Ehrlich Institute, Frankfurt am Main, West Germany.

Professor Dr. Edith Heischkel-Artelt, Director, History of Medicine, University of Mainz, West Germany.

Sir Henry Hallet Dale, M.D., Chairman Emeritus, The Wellcome Trust, London, England.

E. Ashworth Underwood, Director, The Wellcome Historical Medical Museum, London, England.

F. N. L. Poynter, Librarian, The Wellcome Historical Medical Library, London, England.

David L. Cowen, Chairman, Department of History and Political Science, University College, Rutgers University, New Brunswick, New Jersey.

Ramón y Cajal: Charting The Nervous System

Dr. Julián Sanz Ibáñez, Director, Consejo Superior de Investigaciones Científicas, Instituto Santiago Ramón y Cajal, Madrid, Spain.

Dr. Antonio Portolés, Instituto Jaime Ferrán, Madrid, Spain.

Dr. Julio Pardo Canalís, Profesor de la Historia de la Medicina, Escuela de Sanidad del Ejército del Aire, Madrid, Spain.

El Real Academia de Medicina, Madrid, Spain.

Dr. Jorge Ramón y Cajal Fañanás, Madrid, Spain.

Profesor José Soler Roig, Catedrático de Cirugía Ortopédica, Hospital San Pablo, Barcelona, Spain.

El Real Academia de Medicina, Barcelona, Spain.

Marcelino Galatas, Vice President and General Manager, Laboratorios Parke-Davis, S.A.E., Madrid, Spain.

Eduardo Castaño C., Vice President, Laboratorios Parke-Davis, S.A.E., Madrid, Spain.

Arturo L. Roberts, M.D., Editor, Therapeutic Notes, Overseas Division, Parke, Davis & Company, Detroit, Michigan.

Harvey Cushing and Neurosurgery

C. Sidney Burwell, M.D., Special Consultant to the Dean of the Faculty of Medicine, Harvard Medical School, Boston, Massachusetts.

Francis C. Newton, M.D., Emeritus Professor of Clinical Surgery, Harvard Medical School, Boston, Massachusetts.

Miss Madeline E. Stanton, Librarian, Historical Collections, Medical Library, Yale University, New Haven, Connecticut.

Goldberger: Dietary Deficiency and Disease

Jesse L. Boyd, Executive Secretary, Mississippi Baptist Historical Commission, Clinton, Mississippi.

Wheeler C. Cathey, Jackson, Mississippi.

Mrs. J. R. Carter, Magnolia, Mississippi.

Mrs. Marjorie Luther, Reference Librarian, National Institutes of Health, Bethesda, Maryland.

Reverend J. H. Morrow, Jr., The Methodist Home, Jackson, Mississippi.

Paul N. Nunnery, Superintendent, The Baptist Children's Village, Jackson, Mississippi.

Robert P. Parsons, M.D., Carmel, California.

David E. Patterson, Wesson, Mississippi.

J. W. Terrell, Sr., Pass Christian, Mississippi.

Col. E. Todd, Director of the Museum, West Point Academy, West Point, New York.

Mrs. C. H. Waring, Gulfport, Mississippi.

Banting, Best, and Diabetes

Charles H. Best, M.D., Director and Professor of the Banting and Best Department of Medical Research, and Professor and Head of the Department of Physiology, University of Toronto, Ontario, Canada.

Sir Henry Hallet Dale, M.D., Chairman Emeritus, The Wellcome Trust, London, England.

W. R. Feasby, M.D., Lecturer on the History of Medicine, Banting and Best Department of Medical Research, and Medical Director of Seccombe House, Toronto, Canada.

Linda Mahon, secretary to Dr. Best, Toronto, Ontario, Canada.

Donald Meredith, Manager, Trade and Guest Relations, The Upjohn Company, Kalamazoo, Michigan.

The Era of Antibiotics

Ernst B. Chain, Ph.D., Professor of Biochemistry, Imperial College of Science and Technology, London, England.

Professor Howard W. Florey, M.D., Provost, The Queen's College, Oxford, England.

REFERENCES

MANY SOURCES of information, both published and unpublished, have contributed to the factual background for stories and paintings in this series. Due acknowledgment and thanks are extended to authors and sources. Persons interested in further information on the subjects covered, or in background information, may find these sources worthy of consultation. Except for general references, sources are listed under the subject headings used in this book.

General References

The following sources of general information concerning the History of Medicine have proved to be of great value:

Ackerknecht, E. H., *A Short History of Medicine*. New York, Ronald Press Co., 1955.

Castiglioni, A., *A History of Medicine*. New York, Alfred A. Knopf, 1947.

Encyclopaedia Britannica. Chicago, 1958.

Garrison, Fielding H., *An Introduction to the History of Medicine*, Ed. 4. Philadelphia, W. B. Saunders Co., 1929.

Major, Ralph H., *A History of Medicine*, 2 vols. Springfield, Illinois, Charles C Thomas, 1954.

Medicine In Ancient Egypt

Breasted, James H., *The Edwin Smith Surgical Papyrus*, 2 vols. Chicago, University of Chicago Press, 1930.

Gordon, B. L., *Medicine Throughout Antiquity*. Philadelphia, F. A. Davis Co., 1949.

Ranke, Hermann, *Medicine and Surgery in Ancient Egypt*. Studies in the History of Sciences. Philadelphia, University of Pennsylvania Press, 1941.

Sigerist, Henry E., *The Great Doctors*. New York, W. W. Norton & Co., 1933.

Sigerist, Henry E., *A History of Medicine*, Vol. 1. New York, Oxford University Press, 1955.

Walker, Kenneth, *The Story of Medicine*. New York, Oxford University Press, 1955.

The Code of Hammurabi

Chiera, Edward, *They Wrote On Clay*. Chicago, University of Chicago Press, 1938.

Edwards, Charles, *The Hammurabi Code*. London, 1921.

Gordon, B. L., *Medicine Throughout Antiquity*. Philadelphia, F. A. Davis Co., 1949.

Sigerist, Henry E., *A History of Medicine*, Vol. 1. New York, Oxford University Press, 1955.

Walker, Kenneth, *The Story of Medicine*. New York, Oxford University Press, 1955.

Trephining In Ancient Peru

Bird, Junius, *Paracas Fabric and Nazca Needlework*. Washington, D. C., National Publishing Co., 1954.

Cachot, Rebeca Carrion, *Paracas Cultural Elements*. Lima, Peru, Corporacion Nacional de Turismo, 1949.

Hrdlicka, Ales, *Trepanation Among Prehistoric People*. Ciba Symposia, Vol. 1, No. 6, 1939.

Muñiz, M. A., and McGee, W. J., *Primitive Trephining in Peru*. Report, Bureau of American Ethnology, Smithsonian Institution, 1895.

Stewart, T. D., *Significance of Osteitis in Ancient Peruvian Trephining*. Bulletin of the History of Medicine, Vol. 30, No. 4, 293-320, July-August, 1956.

Wakefield, E. G., and Dellinger, S. C., *Possible Reasons for Trephining the Skull in the Past*. Ciba Symposia, Vol. 1, No. 6, 1939.

Primitive Medicine

Dutton, Bertha P., *New Mexico Indians*. Santa Fe, New Mexico Association of Indian Affairs, 1955.

Kluckhohn, Clyde, and Leighton, Dorothea, *The Navaho*. Boston, Harvard University Press, 1946.

Matthews, Washington, *The Mountain Chant: A Navajo Ceremony*. Fifth Annual Report of the Bureau of Ethnology, 1883-84, Washington, D. C., Gov't Printing Office, 1887.

Reichard, Gladys M., *Navaho Religion*, 2 vols. Bollingen Series XVIII, 1950.

Rivers, W. H. R., *Medicine, Magic, and Religion.* New York, Harcourt, 1924.

Sigerist, Henry E., *A History of Medicine*, Vol. 1. New York, Oxford University Press, 1955.

Underhill, Ruth M., *The Navajos.* Norman, The University of Oklahoma Press, 1956.

Wyman, Leland C., *The Religion of the Navajo Indians.* Pub. in Forgotten Religions, Philosophical Library, 1949.

Wyman, Leland C., and Harris, Stuart K., *Navaho Indian Medical Ethnobotany.* University of New Mexico Bulletin No. 366, 1941.

Wyman, Leland C., *The Sandpaintings of the Kayenta Navaho.* University of New Mexico Publications in Anthropology No. 7, 1952.

Wyman, Leland C., *Psychotherapy of the Navaho.* Tomorrow Magazine, Vol. 4, No. 3, 1956.

The Temples and Cult of Asclepius

Edelstein, Emma J., and Ludwig, *Asclepius*, Vol. 2. Baltimore, Johns Hopkins Press, 1945.

Gordon, B. L., *Medicine Throughout Antiquity.* Philadelphia, F. A. Davis Co., 1949.

Suśrutu—Surgeon of Old India

Barnett, L. D., *Antiquities of India.* New York, G. P. Putnam's Sons, 1914.

Gordon, B. L., *Medicine Throughout Antiquity.* Philadelphia, F. A. Davis Co., 1949.

Jolly, Julius, *Indian Medicine*, translated into English by C. B. Kashikar. Poona, 1951.

Keith, Arthur Berriedale, *A History of Sanskrit Literature.* Oxford at the Clarendon Press, 1928.

Kunja Lal, Bhishagratna, *The Sushruta Saṁhitā.* Calcutta, J. N. Bose, 1907.

Maurer, Walter H., *A Note on the Origin and History of the Fables of Bidpai.* Unpublished article.

Macdonell, A. A., *India's Past.* Oxford at the Clarendon Press, 1927.

Mukhopādyāya, Girīndranāth, *The Surgical Instruments of the Hindus*, Vol. 1. Calcutta University, 1913.

Muthu, D. C., *The Antiquity of Hindu Medicine.* London, Balliere, Tindall & Cox, 1927.

Zimmer, Henry R., *Hindu Medicine.* Baltimore, Johns Hopkins Press, 1948.

Hipprocates: Medicine Becomes a Science

Gordon, B. L., *Medicine Throughout Antiquity.* Philadelphia, F. A. Davis Co., 1949.

Hamilton, W., *History of Medicine and Surgery.* London, 1831.

Hippocrates, *On the Sacred Disease*, in *Works*, translated by Francis Adams. London, 1849.

Galen, Influence for 45 Generations

Brockbank, William, *Ancient Therapeutic Arts.* London, William Heinemann, 1954.

Green, Robert M., *A Translation of Galen's Hygiene.* Springfield, Illinois, Charles C Thomas, 1951.

Lehmann, Phyllis W., *Roman Wall Paintings from Boscoreale.* Cambridge, Massachusetts, The Archaeological Institute of America, 1953.

Neuburger, Max, *History of Medicine*, Vol. 1. London, Oxford University Press, 1910.

Robinson, V., *Pathfinders in Medicine.* New York, Medical Life Press, 1929.

Sarton, George, *Galen of Pergamon.* Lawrence, Kansas, University of Kansas Press, 1954.

Rhazes and Arabic Medicine

Neuburger, Max, *History of Medicine*, Vol. 1. London, Oxford University Press, 1910.

Robinson, V., *Pathfinders in Medicine.* New York, Medical Life Press, 1929.

Medieval Hospitals

Carstens, Henry R., *The History of Hospitals, with Special Reference to Some of the World's Oldest Institutions.* Annals of Internal Medicine, Vol. 10, 670-682, 1937.

Clay, Rotha Mary, *Medical Hospitals of England.* London, 1909.

Evans-Howard, *Romance of the British Voluntary Hospital Movement.* London, 1930.

Gordon, Benjamin Lee, *Medicine Throughout Antiquity.* Philadelphia, F. A. Davis Co., 1949.

Neuburger, Max, *History of Medicine*, Vol 1. London, Oxford University Press, 1910.

Riesman, David, *The Story of Medicine in the Middle Ages.* New York, Paul B. Hoeber, Inc., 1936.

Stein, Henri, *L'Hôtel-Dieu de Beaune.* Paris, Henri Laurens, 1933.

Walker, Kenneth, *The Story of Medicine.* New York, Oxford University Press, 1955.

Anonymous, *Une Visite à L'Hôtel-Dieu de Beaune*. Beaune, France, Héry & Granjon, 1956.

Anonymous, *Hospitals Throughout the Centuries*. Journal of the American Hospital Association, Vol. 30, June 1, 1956.

Catholic Encyclopedia. New York, Catholic Encyclopedia Press, 1922.

Paracelsus—Stormy Petrel of Medicine

Multhauf, Robert, *Medical Chemistry and "The Paracelsians."* Bulletin of the History of Medicine, Vol. 28, No. 2, 1954.

Multhauf, Robert, *The Significance of Distillation in Renaissance Medical Chemistry*. Bulletin of the History of Medicine, Vol. 30, No. 4, 1956.

Pachter, Henry M., *Paracelsus, Magic into Science*. New York, Henry Schuman, 1951.

Riesman, David, *The Story of Medicine in the Middle Ages*. New York, Paul B. Hoeber, Inc., 1936.

Robinson, V., *Pathfinders in Medicine*. New York, Medical Life Press, 1929.

Vesalius—and the Anatomy of Man

Cushing, H. W., *A Bio-bibliography of Andreas Vesalius*. New York, Schuman's, 1943.

Lind, L. R., *The Epitome of Andreas Vesalius*. New York, The Macmillan Co., 1949.

Robinson, V., *Pathfinders in Medicine*. New York, Medical Life Press, 1929.

Saunders, J. B. deC., and O'Malley, Charles D., *The Illustrations from the Works of Andreas Vesalius of Brussels*. Cleveland, Ohio, The World Publishing Co., 1950.

**Ambroise Paré:
Surgery Acquires Stature**

Packard, Francis R., *Life and Times of Ambroise Paré*. New York, Paul B. Hoeber, Inc., 1926.

Robinson, V., *Pathfinders in Medicine*. New York, Medical Life Press, 1929.

Walker, Kenneth, *The Story of Medicine*. New York, Oxford University Press, 1955.

Harvey and the Circulation of the Blood

Anonymous, *William Harvey, Tercentenary Commemoration*. Washington, D.C., U.S. Department of Health, Education, and Welfare, 1957.

Farr, Frederic J., *A Short History of the Royal College of Physicians in London*. Handwritten manuscript in the library of the College, 1883.

Keele, K. D., *William Harvey: The Man and the College of Physicians*, in Medical History, Vol. 1, No. 3. London, Wm. Dawson & Sons Ltd., 1957.

Leake, Chauncey D., *Anatomical Studies on the Motion of the Heart and Blood*, English translation. Springfield, Illinois, Charles C Thomas, 1928.

Martí-Ibáñez, Félix, *Padua and London—A Harveian Tale of Two Cities*, in International Record of Medicine. New York, MD Publications, Inc., 1957.

Power, D'Arcy, *William Harvey*. London, T. Fisher Unwin, 1897.

Singer, Charles, *The Discovery of the Circulation of the Blood*. London, Wm. Dawson & Sons Ltd., 1956.

Wright, A. Dickson, *Dr. William Harvey*. The New Scientist. London, 1957.

Leeuwenhoek and the "Little Animals"

Dobell, Clifford, *Antony van Leeuwenhoek and His "Little Animals."* London, Staples Press Ltd., 1932.

Rooseboom, Maria, *Microscopium*. Leyden, Holland, National Museum for the History of Science, 1956.

**Sydenham:
Proponent of Clinical Medicine**

Connoisseur *Concise Encyclopedia of Antiques*. London, Rainbird MacLean, Ltd., 1954.

Fastnedge, Ralph, *English Furniture Styles from 1500 to 1830*. London, Penguin Books, Ltd., 1955.

Frid, J. I., *Some Aspects of Gout*. Hamilton, Ontario, McGregor Clinic Bulletin, Vol. 19, No. 2, April, 1958.

Payne, J. F., *Thomas Sydenham*. London, T. Fisher Unwin, 1900.

Rolleston, Sir Humphry, *Sydenham: Father of Clinical Medicine in Britain*. British Medical Journal, Vol. 2, No. 3333, 917-919, Nov. 15, 1924.

Willett, C., and Cunnington, P., *Handbook of English Costume in the 17th Century*. London, Faber & Faber, Ltd., 1954.

James Lind: Conqueror of Scurvy

Ackerknecht, E. H., *Naval Surgery from 1500 to 1800*. Ciba Symposia, Vol. 4, Nos. 9-10, 1394-1404, Dec. 1942-Jan. 1943.

King, Lester S., *The Medical World of the Eighteenth Century*. Chicago, The University of Chicago Press, 1958.

Roddis, Louis H., *James Lind, Founder of Nautical Medicine*. London, Wm. Heinemann, Ltd., 1951.

Stewart, C. P., and Guthrie, Douglas, *Lind's Treatise on Scurvy*. Edinburgh, University Press, 1953.

Surgeons of the Sea. MD Medical Newsmagazine, Vol. 2, No. 6, 125-129, June, 1958.

Morgagni and Pathologic Anatomy

Benassi, Enrico, *Giambattista Morgagni, Consulti Medici*. Bologna, L. Capelli, 1935.

Jarco, Saul, *Giovanni Battista Morgagni, His Interests, Ideas and Achievements*. Bulletin of the History of Medicine, Vol. 22, No. 5, Sept.-Oct., 1948.

Premuda, Loris, and Cremonini, Luciano, *Morgagni Minore*. Acta Medicae Historiae Patavina, Vol. 2, 21-92, 1955-56.

Richardson, Sir Benjamin Ward, *John Baptist Morgagni, M.D., F.R.S., and the Birth of Pathology*. Asclepiad, 5:147-173, 1888.

Sigerist, Henry E., *The Great Doctors*. New York, W. W. Norton & Co., 1933.

Stefanutti, U., *L'Università di Padova nella Storia della Medicina*. Milano, Rassegna Medica, Vol. 36, No. 1, Jan.-Feb., 1959.

Walsh, James J., *Morgagni, the Father of Pathology*. The Messenger, Vol. 37, No. 2, 113-128, Feb., 1902.

Lavoisier:
Oxygen, Combustion, and Respiration

Duveen, Denis I., *Antoine Laurent Lavoisier and the French Revolution*. Journal of Chemical Education, Vol. 31, 60-65, February, 1954.

Duveen, Denis I., *Lavoisier*. Scientific American, Vol. 194, No. 5, 84-94, May, 1956.

Duveen, Denis I., and Klickstein, Herbert S., *Antoine Laurent Lavoisier's Contributions to Medicine and Public Health*. Bulletin of the History of Medicine, Vol. 29, No. 2, 164-179, March-April, 1955.

Encyclopaedia Britannica, Vol. 13, 777-778. Chicago, Encyclopaedia Britannica, Inc., 1958.

McKie, Douglas, *Antoine Lavoisier, Scientist, Economist, Social Reformer*. New York, Henry Schuman, Inc., 1952.

John Hunter:
Founder of Scientific Surgery

Gray, E. A., *John Hunter and Veterinary Medicine*. Medical History, Vol. 1, No. 1, 38-50, Jan., 1957.

Paget, Stephen, *John Hunter, Man of Science and Surgeon*. London, T. Fisher Unwin, 1897.

Peachey, G. C., *A Memoir of William and John Hunter*. Plymouth, William Brendon & Son, Ltd., 1924.

Robinson, Victor, *Pathfinders in Medicine*. New York, Medical Review of Reviews, 1912.

Thomas, K. B., *John Hunter and An Amputation Under Analgesia in 1784*. Medical History, Vol. 2, No. 1, 53-56, Jan., 1958.

Benjamin Rush:
Physician, Pedant, Patriot

Blanton, Wyndham B., *Medicine in Virginia in the Eighteenth Century*. Richmond, Garret and Massie, 1931.

Corner, George W., *The Autobiography of Benjamin Rush*. Princeton, Princeton University Press, 1948.

Flexner, J. T., *Doctors On Horseback*. New York, The Viking Press, 1937.

Goodman, N. G., *Benjamin Rush, Physician and Citizen*. Philadelphia, University of Pennsylvania Press, 1934.

Powell, J. H., *Bring Out Your Dead*. Philadelphia, University of Pennsylvania Press, 1949.

Richardson, Sir Benjamin Ward, *The American Sydenham, Benjamin Rush, M.D.*, in Disciples of Aesculapius, Vol. 1. London, Hutchinson & Co., 1900.

Smithcors, J. F., *The Contributions of Benjamin Rush to Veterinary Medicine*. Journal of the History of Medicine and Allied Sciences, Vol. 12, No. 1, January, 1957.

Pinel Unchains the Insane

Ackerknecht, E. H., *A Short History of Psychiatry*, translated from the German by Sulammith Wolff. New York, Hafner Publishing Co., 1959.

Bixler, E. S., *A Forerunner of Psychiatric Nursing, Joan-Baptiste Pussin*. Annals of Medical History, new series, Vol. 8, 518-519, 1936.

Bromberg, W., *Man Above Humanity: A History of Psychotherapy*. Philadelphia, J. B. Lippincott Co., 1954.

Kavka, J., *Pinel's Conception of the Psychopathic State*. Bulletin of the History of Medicine, Vol. 23, 461-468, Sept.-Oct., 1949.

Lewis, A., *Philippe Pinel and the English*. Proceedings of the Royal Society of Medicine, Vol. 48, 581-586, 1955.

Packard, F. R., *The Centenary of the Death of Pinel*. Annals of Medical History, Vol. 9, 103-104, 1927.

Riese, Walther, *Philippe Pinel.* Journal of Nervous and Mental Disease, Vol. 114, No. 4, 313-323, Oct., 1951.

Walk, A., *Pioneers in Psychiatry.* The Lancet (London), Vol. 1, No. 6861, 461, 1955.

Zilboorg, Gregory, and Henry, George W., *A History of Medical Psychology.* New York, W. W. Norton & Co., 1941.

Jenner: Smallpox is Stemmed

Camac, C. N. B., *Epoch-making Contributions to Medicine, Surgery, and the Allied Sciences.* Philadelphia, W. B. Saunders Co., 1909.

Diefenbach, W. C. L., *The Beginning of Vaccination.* The Merck Report, Vol. 64, No. 4, October, 1955.

LeFanu, W. R., *A Bio-Bibliography of Edward Jenner.* London, Harvey and Blythe, 1951.

Mellanby, E., *Jenner and His Impact on Medical Science.* British Medical Journal, Vol. 1, 921-926, May 28, 1949.

Robinson, V., *Pathfinders in Medicine.* New York, Medical Life Press, 1929.

Taylor, B., *Edward Jenner, Conqueror of Smallpox.* London, Macmillan and Co., 1950.

Underwood, E. A., *Edward Jenner, the Man and His Work.* British Medical Journal, Vol. 1, 881-884, May 21, 1949.

Van Itallie, P. H., "*So the Lord Smote Them with Smallpox.*" Pulse of Pharmacy, Vol. 9, No. 1, 1955.

Waterhouse, Benjamin, *A Prospect of Exterminating the Smallpox.* Cambridge, William Hillard, 1800.

Laennec and the Stethoscope

Binet, Léon, *Médecins, Biologistes et Chirurgiens.* Paris, Segep, 1954.

Binet, Léon, *Laennec à l'Hôpital.* Histoire de la Médecine, Vol. 8, No. 4, April, 1958.

Camac, C. N. B., *Epoch-making Contributions to Medicine, Surgery, and the Allied Sciences.* Philadelphia, W. B. Saunders Co., 1909.

Richardson, Sir Benjamin Ward, *Disciples of Aesculapius,* Vol. 1. London, Hutchinson & Co., 1900.

Robinson, Victor, *Pathfinders in Medicine.* New York, Medical Review of Reviews, 1912.

Sigerist, Henry E., *The Great Doctors.* New York, W. W. Norton & Co., 1933.

The First Stethoscope. Therapeutic Notes, Vol. 60, No. 2, February, 1953.

Webb, Gerald B., *René Théophile Hyacinthe Laennec, A Memoir.* New York, Hoeber, 1928.

Conquerors of Pain

Archer, W. Harry, *Life and Letters of Horace Wells, Discoverer of Anesthesia.* Journal American College of Dentists, Vol. 11, No. 2, June, 1944; and Vol. 12, No. 2, June, 1945.

Beecher, H. K., and Ford, C., *Some New Letters of Horace Wells Concerning an Historic Partnership.* Journal of the History of Medicine and Allied Sciences, Vol. 9, No. 1, January, 1954.

Beecher, H. K., and Ford, C., *Nathan P. Rice's "Trials of a Public Benefactor."* Journal of the History of Medicine and Allied Sciences, Vol. 15, No. 2, April, 1960.

Boland, Frank, *The First Anesthesia.* Athens, Georgia, University of Georgia Press, 1950.

Camac, C. N. B., *Epoch-making Contributions to Medicine, Surgery, and the Allied Sciences.* Philadelphia, W. B. Saunders Co., 1909.

Cartwright, F. F., *The English Pioneers of Anaesthesia.* Bristol, John Wright & Sons, Ltd., 1952.

Fifty Years of Pharmacy in Nova Scotia. Halifax, 1925.

Flexner, James T., *Doctors on Horseback.* New York, The Viking Press, 1937.

Ford, William W., *William Thomas Green Morton.* More Books, Vol. 21, No. 8, October, 1946, Boston Public Library.

Fuller, R. C., *The First Authentic Record of the Use of Chloroform on This Side of the Atlantic.* Canadian Pharmaceutical Journal, Vol. 58, 118, October, 1924.

Hurwitz, Alfred, and Degenshein, George A., *Milestones in Modern Surgery.* New York, Hoeber-Harper, 1958.

Keys, Thomas E., *The History of Surgical Anesthesia.* New York, Schuman's, 1945.

Redman, Kenneth, *Some Memorials on Crawford W. Long, The First Performer of an Ether Anesthesia.* The South Dakota Journal of Medicine and Pharmacy, Vol. 11, No. 2, February, 1959.

Robinson, Victor, *Victory Over Pain.* New York, Henry Schuman, 1946.

Taylor, Frances Long, *Crawford W. Long and the Discovery of Ether Anesthesia.* New York, Paul B. Hoeber, Inc., 1928.

Thorwald, Jurgen, *The Century of a Surgeon.* New York, Pantheon Books, 1956.

Wilson, R. C., *Drugs and Pharmacy in the Life of Georgia.* Athens, Georgia, University of Georgia Press, 1959.

Semmelweis: Defender of Motherhood

Camac, C. N. B., *Epoch-making Contributions to Medicine, Surgery, and the Allied Sciences.* Philadelphia, W. B. Saunders Co., 1909.

Edgar, I. I., *Ignatz Philipp Semmelweis, Outline for a Biography.* Annals of Medical History, Third Series, Vol. 1, No. 1, 74-96, January, 1939.

Kelly, E. C., *Medical Classics*, Vol. 5, p. 338. Williams & Wilkins, 1905.

Robinson, Victor, *Pathfinders in Medicine.* New York, Medical Review of Reviews, 1912.

Sinclair, Sir William J., *Semmelweis, His Life and His Doctrine.* Manchester, University Press, 1909.

Slaughter, Frank G., *Immortal Magyar.* New York, Henry Schuman, 1950.

Thompson, Morton, *The Cry and the Covenant.* New York, Doubleday & Co., 1954.

Founding of The American Medical Association

Davis, N. S., *History of the American Medical Association from its Organization up to January, 1855.* Philadelphia, Lippincott, Grambo & Co., 1855.

Fishbein, Morris, *A History of the American Medical Association.* Philadelphia, W. B. Saunders, 1947.

Virchow and Cellular Pathology

Ackerknecht, E. H., *Rudolf Virchow, Doctor, Statesman, Anthropologist.* Madison, University of Wisconsin Press, 1953.

Edgar, I. I., *Pathology and Rudolf Virchow.* Journal of the Michigan State Medical Society, Vol. 59, 626-631, April, 1960.

Sigerist, H. E., *The Great Doctors.* New York, W. W. Norton & Co., 1933.

Helmholtz: Physicist-Physician

Arrington, George E., Jr., *A History of Ophthalmology.* New York, MD Publications, 1959.

Friedenwald, H., *The History of the Invention and of the Development of the Ophthalmoscope.* The Journal of the American Medical Association, Vol. 38, No. 9, March 1, 1902.

Goodspeed, A. W., *Contributions of Helmholtz to Physical Science.* The Journal of the American Medical Association, Vol. 38, No. 9, March 1, 1902.

Hall, W. S., *The Contributions of Helmholtz to Physiology and Psychology.* The Journal of the American Medical Association, Vol. 38, No. 9, March 1, 1902.

Knapp, H., *A Few Personal Recollections of Helmholtz.* The Journal of the American Medical Association, Vol. 38, No. 9, March 1, 1902.

Koenigsberger, L., *Hermann von Helmholtz,* 3 vols. Braunschweig, 1902.

McKendrick, J. G., *Hermann Ludwig Ferdinand von Helmholtz.* London, T. Fisher Unwin, 1899.

Randall, B. A., *The Debt of Otology to Helmholtz.* The Journal of the American Medical Association, Vol. 38, No. 9, March 1, 1902.

Sigerist, H. E., *The Great Doctors.* New York, W. W. Norton & Co., 1933.

Wood, C. A., *Hermann von Helmholtz, The Inventor of the Ophthalmoscope.* The Journal of the American Medical Association, Vol. 38, No. 9, March 1, 1902.

J. Marion Sims: Gynecologic Surgeon

Ackerknecht, E. H., *American Gynecology Around 1850.* Reprint from the Wisconsin Medical Journal, March, 1952.

A Century of Service. The Times—News of The Woman's Hospital, Division of St. Luke's Hospital, New York, Vol. 7, No. 2, May, 1955.

Harris, Seale, *Woman's Surgeon.* New York, Macmillan Company, 1950.

Heaton, Claude E., *The Influence of J. Marion Sims on Gynecology.* Reprint from the Bulletin of the New York Academy of Medicine, Second series, Vol. 32, No. 9, September, 1956.

Marr, James Pratt, *James Marion Sims.* New York, 1949.

Marr, James Pratt, *Pioneer Surgeons of the Woman's Hospital.* Philadelphia, F. A. Davis Company, 1957.

Sims, J. Marion, *The Story of My Life.* New York, D. Appleton & Co., 1889.

Claude Bernard: Explorer of Physiologic Frontiers

Bernard, Claude, *An Introduction to the Study of Experimental Medicine.* New York, Macmillan Co., 1927; also, Dover Publications, Inc., 1957.

Bernard, Claude, *The Origin of Sugar in the Animal Body.* Source Book of Medical History, Logan Clendening. New York, Dover Publications, Inc., 1960.

Binet, Léon, *An Alleged Skeptic: Claude Bernard.* Médecins, Biologistes et Chirurgiens, Paris, Segep, 1954.

Foster, Michael, *Claude Bernard.* New York, Longmans, Green & Co., 1899.

Olmsted, J.M.D., *Claude Bernard, Physiologist*. New York, Harper & Brothers, 1938.

Robinson, Victor, *Pathfinders in Medicine*. New York, Medical Life Press, 1929.

Sigerist, Henry E., *The Great Doctors*. New York, W. W. Norton & Co., 1933.

Virtanen, Reino, *Claude Bernard and His Place in the History of Ideas*. Lincoln, University of Nebraska Press, 1960.

Pasteur:
The Chemist Who Transformed Medicine

Binet, Léon, *Louis Pasteur*. Médecins, Biologistes et Chirurgiens, Paris, Segep, 1954.

Clendening, Logan, *Source Book of Medical History*. New York, Dover Publications, Inc., 1960.

Dubos, René J., *Louis Pasteur, Free Lance of Science*. Boston, Little, Brown & Co., 1950.

Langumier, René, *L'Institut Pasteur*. La Documentation Française Illustrée, No. 149, July, 1959.

Longstreth, Morris, *Against the Germ Theory of Disease*. The Therapeutic Gazette, 3rd series, Vol. 2, 1886.

Paget, Stephen, *Pasteur and After Pasteur*. London, Adam and Charles Black, 1914.

Robinson, Victor, *Pathfinders in Medicine*. New York, Medical Life Press, 1929.

Sigerist, Henry E., *The Great Doctors*. New York, W. W. Norton & Co., 1933.

Vallery-Radot, Pasteur, *Images de la Vie et de L'oeuvre de Pasteur*. Paris, Flammarion, 1956.

Vallery-Radot, Pasteur, *Louis Pasteur*. New York, Alfred A. Knopf, 1958.

Vallery-Radot, René, *The Life of Pasteur*. Translated by Mrs. R. L. Devonshire. New York, Doubleday, Page & Co., 1926; and Dover Publications, Inc., 1960.

Lister Introduces Antisepsis

Camac, C.N.B., *Epoch-Making Contributions to Medicine, Surgery, and the Allied Sciences*. Philadelphia, W. B. Saunders Co., 1909.

Clendening, Logan, *Source Book of Medical History*. New York, Dover Publications, Inc., 1960.

Edgar, Irving I., *Modern Surgery and Lord Lister*. Journal of the History of Medicine and Allied Sciences, Vol. 16, No. 2, April, 1961.

Frowde, Henry, *The Collected Papers of Joseph, Baron Lister*. London, Oxford University Press.

Godlee, Sir Rickman John, *Lord Lister*. London, Macmillan & Co., Ltd., 1918.

Guthrie, Douglas, *Lord Lister, His Life and Doctrine*. Edinburgh, E. & S. Livingstone, Ltd., 1949.

Lister, Joseph, *On a New Method of Treating Compound Fracture, Abscess, etc., With Observations On the Conditions of Suppuration*. London, The Lancet, 1867, Vol. 1, pp. 326-329; 357-359; 387-389; and 507-509.

Paget, Stephen, *Pasteur and After Pasteur*. London, Adam and Charles Black, 1914.

Patrick, John, *A Short History of the Glasgow Royal Infirmary*. Glasgow, David J. Clark, Ltd., 1940.

Sigerist, Henry E., *The Great Doctors*. New York, W. W. Norton & Co., 1933.

Vallery-Radot, René, *The Life of Pasteur*. Translated by Mrs. R. L. Devonshire. New York, Doubleday, Page & Co., 1926; and Dover Publications, Inc., 1960.

Wrench, G. T., *Lord Lister, His Life and Work*. New York, Frederick A. Stokes Co., 1913.

Charcot: Master of Neurology

Garrison, Fielding H., *Charcot*. International Clinics, (35S) 4:244-272, Dec., 1925.

Guillain, Georges, *J.-M. Charcot, His Life—His Work*. Translated by Pearce Bailey. New York, Paul B. Hoeber, Inc., 1959.

Schneck, Jerome M., *Jean-Martin Charcot and the History of Experimental Hypnosis*. Journal of the History of Medicine and Allied Sciences, Vol. 16, No. 3, July, 1961.

Wechsler, I. S., *Jean-Martin Charcot*. In Haymaker, W., The Founders of Neurology. Springfield, Illinois, Charles C Thomas, 1953.

The Hopkins:
A Revolution in Medical Education

America's Medical Schools. Chicago, American Medical Association, and Association of American Medical Colleges, 1961.

Bernheim, Bertram M., *The Story of the Johns Hopkins*. New York, McGraw-Hill Book Co., 1948.

Changing Concepts in Medical Education. Therapeutic Notes, Vol. 69, No. 1, January, 1962.

Chesney, Alan M., *The Johns Hopkins Hospital and The Johns Hopkins University School of Medicine*, Vols. 1 and 2. Baltimore, The Johns Hopkins Press, 1943, and 1958.

Chesney, Alan M., *John Shaw Billings and The Johns Hopkins Medical School*. Bulletin of the Institute of the History of Medicine, Vol. 6, No. 4, April, 1938.

Chesney, Alan M., *The Johns Hopkins Hospital, 1889-1939*. Fiftieth Anniversary celebration folder.

Chesney, Alan M., *The Johns Hopkins University School of Medicine, 1893-1943*. Fiftieth Anniversary commemorative folder.

408

Cushing, Harvey, *The Life of Sir William Osler.* Oxford, Clarendon Press, 1926.

Flexner, Abraham, *I Remember.* New York, Simon and Schuster, 1940.

Flexner, Simon, and Flexner, James T., *William Henry Welch and the Heroic Age of American Medicine.* New York, The Viking Press, 1941.

Johns Hopkins Medical School Catalogue. Baltimore, The Johns Hopkins Press, 1893.

Minutes of the Advisory Board of the Johns Hopkins Medical Faculty. 1884, handwritten, unpublished.

Parker, Franklin, *Influences on the Founder of the Johns Hopkins University and the Johns Hopkins Hospital.* Bulletin of the History of Medicine, Vol. 34, No. 2, March-April, 1960.

Randers-Pehrson, Justine, *The Surgeon's Glove.* Springfield, Illinois, Charles C Thomas, 1960.

Shryock, Richard H., *The Unique Influence of the Johns Hopkins University on American Medicine.* Copenhagen, Ejnar Munksgaard, Ltd., 1953.

Röntgen:
Invisible Rays That Save Lives

Bleich, A. R., *The Story of X-Rays from Röntgen to Isotopes.* New York, Dover Publications, 1960.

Burry, James, *A Preliminary Report on the Röntgen or X-Rays.* Journal of the American Medical Association, Vol. 26, No. 9, Feb. 29, 1896.

Fletcher, Gilbert H., *Recent Advances in Radiotherapy.* The New Physician, Vol. 10, No. 12, December, 1961.

Glasser, Otto, *Dr. W. C. Röntgen.* Springfield, Illinois, Charles C Thomas, 1958.

Illuminated Tissues. Medical Record, Vol. 49, p. 71, Jan. 11, 1896.

Leucutia, Traian, *Roentgen Therapy of Skin Cancer.* The New Physician, Vol. 10, No. 12, December, 1961.

The Conquest of Yellow Fever

Burnet, F. M., *Viruses and Man.* London, Penguin Books Ltd., 1955.

Kelly, Howard A., *Walter Reed and Yellow Fever.* New York, McClure, Phillips & Co., 1906.

Peller, Sigismund, *Walter Reed, C. Finlay, and Their Predecessors Around 1800.* Bulletin of the History of Medicine, Vol. 33, No. 3, May-June, 1959.

Reed, Walter; Carroll, James; Agramonte, Aristides; and Lazear, Jesse W., *The Etiology of Yellow Fever, A Preliminary Note.* Philadelphia Medical Journal, Vol. 6, No. 17, Oct. 27, 1900.

Reed, Walter; Carroll, James; and Agramonte, Aristides, *The Etiology of Yellow Fever, an Additional Note.* Journal of The American Medical Association, Vol. 36, No. 7, Feb. 16, 1901.

Reed, Walter, *The Propagation of Yellow Fever; Observations Based On Recent Researches.* Medical Record, Vol. 60, No. 6, Aug. 10, 1901.

Reed, Walter, and Carroll, James, *The Etiology of Yellow Fever, A Supplemental Note.* American Medicine, Vol. 3, No. 8, Feb. 22, 1902.

Ross, Ronald, *Malaria and Mosquitoes.* Nature, Vol. 61, No. 1587, March 29, 1900.

Ruiz de Zarate, Serafin, *Dr. Carlos J. Finlay and the Hall of Fame of New York.* Havana, Ministry of Health and Hospital's Assistance, 1959.

Rush, Benjamin, *An Account of the Yellow Fever as It Appeared in Philadelphia in 1797.* Philadelphia, Thomas Dobson, 1798.

Theiler, Max, *Yellow Fever.* In Rivers, Thomas M., and Harsfall, Frank L., Jr., *Viral and Rickettsial Infections of Man.* Philadelphia, J. B. Lippincott Co., 1959.

Williams, Greer, *Virus Hunters.* New York, Alfred A. Knopf, 1959.

Yellow Fever. A Symposium in Commemoration of Carlos Juan Finlay. The Jefferson Medical College of Philadelphia, 1955.

Walter B. Cannon:
Physiologic Investigator

Alvarez, W. C., *Dr. Walter B. Cannon Passes.* Gastroenterology, Vol. 5, No. 5, Nov., 1945.

Cannon, Walter B., *The Mechanical Factors of Digestion.* London, Edward Arnold, 1911.

Cannon, Walter B., *Bodily Changes in Pain, Hunger, Fear and Rage.* New York, D. Appleton & Co., 1915.

Cannon, Walter B., *The Way of an Investigator.* New York, W. W. Norton & Co., 1945.

Cannon, Walter Bradford, A Memorial Exercise. Harvard Medical School, 1945.

Dale, Sir Henry H., *Prof. W. B. Cannon.* Nature, Vol. 158, No. 4003, July 20, 1946.

Spillman, Ramsay, *Walter Bradford Cannon.* The American Journal of Roentgenology and Radium Therapy, Vol. 55, No. 1, Jan., 1946.

Ehrlich:
Chemotherapy Is Launched

Ackerknecht, E. H., *Aspects of the History of Therapeutics.* Bulletin of the History of Medicine, Vol. 36, No. 5, Sept.-Oct., 1962.

Bender, George A., *The Development of Chemotherapy*. A History of Pharmacy In Pictures, Detroit, Parke, Davis & Company, 1960.

Bulloch, William, *The History of Bacteriology*. London, Oxford University Press, 1938.

Cowen, David L., *Ehrlich, the Man, the Scientist*. American Journal of Pharmaceutical Education, Vol. 26, No. 1, Winter, 1962.

Marquardt, Martha, *Paul Ehrlich*. New York, Henry Schuman, 1951.

Sigerist, Henry E., *The Great Doctors*. New York, Doubleday & Co., 1958.

Sonnedecker, Glenn, *Paul Ehrlich and Chemotherapy*. American Journal of Hospital Pharmacy, Vol. 17, No. 9, Sept., 1960.

Stevenson, Lloyd G., *Nobel Prize Winners in Medicine and Physiology, 1901-1950*. New York, Henry Schuman, 1953.

Urdang, George, *Two Centenaries*. The Pharmaceutical Journal (London), March 13, 1954.

Ramón y Cajal: Charting The Nervous System

Cannon, Dorothy F., *Explorer of the Human Brain*. New York, Henry Schuman, 1949.

Garrison, F. H., *Ramón y Cajal*. Bulletin of the New York Academy of Medicine, Vol. 5, No. 6, June, 1929, pp. 483-508.

Jelliffe, S. E., *Santiago Ramón y Cajal, M.D.* Transactions of the American Neurological Association, 60th Annual Meeting, 1934, pp. 234-236.

Obituary. The British Medical Journal, Vol. 2, 1934.

Obituary. The Lancet, Vol. 2, 1934, p. 959.

Penfield, Wilder, *The Career of Ramón y Cajal*. Archives of Neurology and Psychiatry, Vol. 16, 1926, pp. 213-220.

Penfield, Wilder, *Santiago Ramón y Cajal*. Archives of Neurology and Psychiatry, Vol. 33, No. 1, Jan., 1935, pp. 172-173.

Ramón y Cajal, S., *Recollections of My Life*. 2 Vols. Translated by E. Horne Craigie. Philadelphia, American Historical Society, 1937.

Schuck, H., *et al.*, *Nobel, The Man and His Prizes*. Norman, University of Oklahoma Press, 1951.

Sherrington, C. S., *Obituary*. Nature, Vol. 134, 1934, pp. 871-872.

Sprong, Wilbur, *Santiago Ramón y Cajal*. Archives of Neurology and Psychiatry, Vol. 33, No. 1, Jan., 1935, pp. 156-162.

Stevenson, Lloyd G., *Nobel Prize Winners in Medicine and Physiology, 1901-1950*. New York, Henry Schuman, 1953.

Harvey Cushing and Neurosurgery

Evans, Joseph P., *Harvey Cushing, Surgeon and Teacher*. Reprint from Surgery, Vol. 49, No. 4, April, 1961.

Fulton, John F., *Harvey Cushing*. Springfield, Illinois, Charles C Thomas, 1946.

Thomson, Elizabeth H., *Harvey Cushing, Surgeon, Author, Artist*. New York, Henry Schuman, 1950.

Goldberger: Dietary Deficiency and Disease

Ackerknecht, E. H., unpublished monograph.

Bicknell, F., and Prescott, F., *The Vitamins in Medicine*, third edition. London, William Heinemann, Ltd., 1953.

Kagan, Solomon R., *Joseph Goldberger*. Medical Record, Vol. 146, 1937, pp. 473-476.

Goldberger, Joseph, *The Etiology of Pellagra*. Public Health Reports, Vol. 29, No. 26, Part 1, June 26, 1914.

Goldberger, Joseph; Waring, C.H., and Willets, D.G., *The Prevention of Pellagra*. Public Health Reports, Vol. 30, No. 43, Part 2, October 22, 1915.

Goldberger, Joseph, and Wheeler, G.A., *Experimental Pellagra in the Human Subject Brought About by a Restricted Diet*. Public Health Reports, Vol. 30, No. 46, Part 2, Nov. 12, 1915.

Goldberger, Joseph, and Wheeler, G.A., *The Experimental Production of Pellagra in Human Subjects by Means of Diet*. U. S. Public Health Hygienic Laboratory Bulletin No. 120, February, 1920.

Goldberger, Mary Farrar, *Dr. Joseph Goldberger, His Wife's Recollections*. Journal of the American Dietetic Association, Vol. 32, 724-727, August, 1956.

Nelson, E.M., and Sebrell, W.H., in *The Vitamins*. Chicago, The American Medical Association, 1939.

Parsons, R.P., *The Adventurous Goldberger*. Annals of Medical History, New Series, Vol. 3, 1931.

Parsons, R.P., *Trail to Light*. Indianapolis, Bobbs-Merrill, 1943.

Paterson, G.R., *The Romantic History of a Vitamin*. Canadian Pharmaceutical Journal, June, 1960.

Vitamins and Nutrients. Remington's Practice of Pharmacy, 12th Edition. Easton, Pa., Mack Publishing Co., 1961.

Banting, Best, and Diabetes

Banting, F. G., and Best, C. H., *The Internal Secretion of the Pancreas*. Journal of Laboratory and Clinical Medicine, Vol. 7, 1922.

Banting, F. G., Best, C. H., and Macleod, J. J. R., *The Internal Secretion of the Pancreas*. American Journal of Physiology, Vol. 59, 1922.

410

Best, C. H., *A Canadian Trail of Medical Research*. Journal of Endocrinology, Vol. 19, 1959.

Best, C. H., *Selected Papers of Charles H. Best*. Toronto, Canada, University of Toronto Press, 1963.

Dale, Sir Henry H., *Opening Address*. Diabetes, Vol. 3, No. 1, 1954.

Dolger, H., and Seeman, B., *How to Live With Diabetes*. New York, W. W. Norton & Co., 1958.

Feasby, W. R., *The Discovery of Insulin*. Journal of the History of Medicine and Allied Sciences, Vol. 13, No. 1, 1958.

Feasby, W. R., *The Discovery of Insulin*. Bulletin of the Medical Library Association, Vol. 48, No. 1, 1960.

Harris, Seale, *Banting's Miracle*. Philadelphia, J. B. Lippincott Co., 1946.

Lentz, John, *Sir Frederick Grant Banting*, in *Sixteen American Health Heroes*. New York, Metropolitan Life Insurance Co., 1955.

McFarlane, Leslie, *The Seekers*. (Manuscript for a screenplay, unpublished.)

Stevenson, Lloyd, G., *Sir Frederick Banting*. Toronto, Ryerson Press, 1946.

Wrenshall, G. A., Hetenyi, G., and Feasby, W. R., *The Story of Insulin*. London, The Bodley Head, 1962.

The Era of Antibiotics

Antibacterial Dynamite. Therapeutic Notes, Vol. 51, No. 1, Jan., 1944.

Bender, George A., *The Era of Antibiotics*. Modern Pharmacy, Vol. 43, No. 3, 1958.

Brunel, Jules, *Antibiosis from Pasteur to Fleming*. Journal of the History of Medicine and Allied Sciences, Vol. 6, No. 3, 1951.

Chain, Ernst B., *Academic and Industrial Contributions to Drug Research*. Nature, Vol. 200, No. 4905, Nov., 1963.

Chain, E., Florey, H. W., *et al.*, *Penicillin as a Chemotherapeutic Agent*. The Lancet, 2:226-28, 1940.

Clarke, H. T., Johnson, J. R., and Robinson, Sir Robert, *The Chemistry of Penicillin*. Princeton, N. J., Princeton University Press, 1949.

Duggar, B. M., *Aureomycin: a Product of the Continuing Search for New Antibiotics*. Annals of the New York Academy of Science, 51: 177-181, 1948.

Ehrlich, J., Bartz, Q. R., Smith, R. M., Joslyn, D. A., and Burkholder, P. R., *Chloromycetin, a New Antibiotic from a Soil Actinomycete*. Science, 106:417, Oct. 31, 1947.

English, J. P., *The Chemotherapy of Infectious Disease, 1909-1959*. Journal of Chemical Education, Vol. 37, No. 4, April, 1960.

Fleming, Alexander, *On the Antibacterial Action of Cultures of a Penicillium, with Special Reference to Their Use in the Isolation of B. Influenzae*.

British Journal of Experimental Pathology, 10:226-236, 1929.

Florey, H. W., Chain, E., Heatley, N. G., Jennings, M. A., Sanders, A. G., Abraham, E. P., and Florey, M. E., *Antibiotics*, 2 vol. London, Oxford University Press, 1949.

Florey, H. W., and Abraham, E. P., *The Work on Penicillin at Oxford*. Journal of the History of Medicine and Allied Sciences, Vol. 6, No. 3, 1951.

Fulton, John F., *Introduction* (to Antibiotics number). Journal of the History of Medicine and Allied Sciences, Vol. 6, No. 3, 1951.

Harrell, W. E., *Penicillin and Other Antibiotic Agents*. Philadelphia, W. B. Saunders Co., 1945.

Hobby, Gladys L., *Microbiology in Relation to Antibiotics*. Journal of the History of Medicine and Allied Sciences, Vol. 6, No. 3, 1951.

Lister, Joseph, *Commonplace Books*. Annals of the Royal College of Surgeons, Vol. 6, 140-141, February, 1950.

Maurois, André, *The Life of Sir Alexander Fleming*. London, Jonathan Cape, 1959.

Stevenson, Lloyd G., *Nobel Prize Winners in Medicine and Physiology, 1901-1950*. New York, Henry Schuman, 1953.

Urdang, George, *The Antibiotics and Pharmacy*. Journal of the History of Medicine and Allied Sciences, Vol. 6, No. 3, 1951.

Waksman, Selman A., *Streptomycin, Isoltaion, Properties, and Utilization*. Journal of the History of Medicine and Allied Sciences, Vol. 6, No. 3, 1951.

Woodward, T. E., Smadel, J. E., Ley, H. L., Jr., Green, R., and Mankikar, D. S., *Preliminary Report on the Beneficial Effect of Chloromycetin in the Treatment of Typhoid Fever*. Annals of Internal Medicine, Vol. 29, No. 1, July, 1948.

Woodward, T. E., Smadel, J. E., and Ley, H. L., Jr., *Chloramphenicol and Other Antibiotics in the Treatment of Typhoid Fever and Typhoid Carriers*. The Journal of Clinical Investigation, Vol. 29, No. 1:87-89, 1950.

Medicine Today and Tomorrow

Chain, Ernst B., *Academic and Industrial Contributions to Drug Research*. Nature, Vol. 200, No. 4905, Nov., 1963.

English, J. P., *The Chemotherapy of Infectious Disease, 1909-1959*. Journal of Chemical Education, Vol. 37, No. 4, 1960.

Leake, Chauncey D., *The Scientific Status of Pharmacology*. Science, Vol. 134, No. 3496, 1961.

Major, Ralph H., *A History of Medicine*. Springfield, Illinois, Charles C Thomas, 1954.

INDEX

References in bold face indicate the text pages upon which the person's biography or the medical subject is covered in detail.

412

413

415

417

Société de Biologie, 251, 252
Société de l'Ecole, 181
Socrates, 37, 52
Sodium glucosulfone, 389
Sophocles, 37, 52
Sorbonne, 250, 253, 258, 261, 263, 264, 267, 276, 280, 322
Soubeiran, Eugéne, 189
Southern Medical and Surgical Journal, 191
Spallanzani, Lazaro, 260
Spanish-American War, 309, 310, 338
Spanish Military Hospital, 176
Speculum, Sims, 241
Spermatozoa, 112
Spigelius, A. van der, 134
Spine, injury, 66
Spirochetes, 112
Spleen, 55
Splenectomy, 344
"Spongia somnifera," 187
Spontaneous generation, 224, 259-262
Squibb, E. R. & Sons, 380
Stain
    chrome silver, 336
    gold sublimate, 337
    Golgi's, 337
    silver carbonate, 338
Staphylococcus, 375, 377, 378
Stargazing, 17, 28
State Institute for Serum Research and Testing, Steglitz, 327
"Steel," 38
Stegomyia fasciata, 313
Sterility, 38
Sternberg, George Miller, 309
Steroids, 389
Stethoscope, **176-183,** 211, 393
Stevens, Alexander H., 214-216
Stewart, F. Campbell, 214
Stillé, Alfred, 213-215
Stockton, Richard, 156
Stokes, Adrian, 314
Stone Age, 26
Streptococcus, 375, 378
Streptomyces griseus, 382
Streptomycin, 382, 383
Strophanthin, 28
Stuart, Henri Luther, 242
Studies on Beer, 264
Sugar, 250
Sulfa drugs, 374, 376, 389
Sulfanilamide, 374, 388
Sulfur, 18
Sulfuric acid, 82, 187
Sulfuric ether, 192, 194
Surgeon's Corporation, 147;
    see also Corporation of Surgeons
Surgery, 11, 12, 16, 20-25, 43, 45, 46, 54, 79, 83, 90, **92-98,** 144-151, 184, 236, 239, 268-277, 342, 388, 390
    eye, 197
    see also Neurosurgery
Susruta, **40-49,** 187
Susruta-samhita, 43-45, 48
Sutures, 274, 275
"Sweet vitriol," 187
"Sweet whiskey," 189, 195
Sydenham, Thomas, **116-122,** 160
Sydenham, William, 118

Sylvius. *See* du Bois
Syme, James, 271, 275
Sympathin, 320
Syphilis, 81, 82, 92, 136, 149, 267, 324, 329, 330, 388
Syringe, hypodermic, 196

Taboos, 26, 28, 29
Tabulae Anatomicae Sex, 88
Talbott, John H., 218
Talleyrand, 143
Tamarinds, 128
Tannic acid, 11
Taylor, Isaac E., 196
Telesphorus, 36
Tello y Munzo, J. F., 337
Terramycin, 382
Tetanus, 12, 48, 53, 55, 240, 268, 391
Tetracyclines, 382, 384
Texture of The Nervous System of Man and of the Other Vertebrates, 338
Theiler, Max, 306, 314, 315
Theophrastus, 187
Theory
    of evolution, 225
    germ, 83, 114, 256, 259-261, 264, 393
    humoral, 50, 55, 59, 132, 220
    phlogiston, 141
Therapeutic Gazette, The, 262
Theriac, 95
Thermometer, clinical, 282
Thessalus, 52
Thiamin, 357
Thom, Charles, 379
Thom, Robert A., 3, 4, 7
Thomas, Miss M. Cary, 292
Thompson, John, 148
Thompson, Leonard, 367
Thomson, Elizabeth, 340
Thornton, Matthew, 156
Thyroid extract, 388
Tin, 82
Tintoretto, 86
Titian, 86, 88
Today's Health, 218, 219
Tooth-brushing, 49
Toronto Academy of Medicine, 366
Toronto General Hospital, 367
Toronto Hospital for Sick Children, 362
Tourniquet, 105
Townsend, Solomon D., 193
Toxoids, 324
Traité Elémentaire de Chimie, 141
Traité médico-philosophique sur la manie, 167
Tranquilizers, 160, 389, 390
Treatise on the Diseases of the Chest and on Mediate Auscultation, A, 182
Treatise on the Natural History of the Human Teeth, 148
Treatise on the Scurvy, A, 129
Tréfouël, J., 374
Tréfouël, Mme. J., 374
Trephining, **20-25,** 54
Treponema pallidum, 329
Trichinosis, 224, 310
Trismus nascentium, 240
Trotter, 130
Trusses, 98
Trypanosomes, 328, 329
Trypan-red, 328
Tubercle bacillus, 326

Tuberculosis, 38, 48, 55, 136, 178, 179, 182, 225, 310, 382, 391
Tuke, William, 164
Tumors, 24, 136, 224, 389
    brain, 338, 342, 346, 347
Turpentine, 11, 96
Twort, Frederick William, 375
Typhoid fever, 178, 309, 344, 384, 391
Typhus, 130, 179, 353, 383, 384
Tyrocidine, 376
Tyrothricin, 376

Ulcer, 45, 46
Underwood, E. A., 173
Unicorn, 98
United States Army Medical School, 309
United States Dispensatory, 190
United States Pharmacopoeial Convention, 208
United States Public Health Service, 219, 348, 351
University
    of Barcelona, 335
    Basel, 80, 81
    of Berlin, 233, 326
    of Bologna, 64, 90, 134
    of Bonn, 232
    of Buffalo, 218
    Cambridge, 102, 103, 120, 337
    of Chicago, 353
    Clark, 338
    College, London, 270
    of Cologne, 78
    Columbia, 208
    of Edinburgh, 127, 128, 155, 271, 275, 281
    Erfurt, 78
    Ferrara, 78
    Freiburg, 78
    of Georgia, 190
    of Giessen, 302
    Glasgow, 272
    Harvard, 211; *see also* Harvard Medical School
    Heidelberg, 78, 232
    Johns Hopkins, The, **286-297,** 340; *see also* Johns Hopkins School of Medicine
    Kaiser-Wilhelm's, 301
    of Leipzig, 326
    of London, 270, 369
    of Louvain, 86, 87, 113
    Ludwig-Maximilian's, 304
    of Madrid, 334, 337, 339
    of Minnesota, 362
    of Montpellier, 64, 119, 164
    Oxford, 106, 119, 291, 372
    of Padua, 87, 88, 102, 103, 132, 134, 135
    of Paris, 86, 263, 280
    of Pennsylvania, 156, 157, 190, 208, 291, 343
    of Pest, 200, 204
    of Pisa, 90
    Princeton, 154
    Rutgers, 382
    of Strasbourg, 259
    of Toronto, 360-370
    of Tuebingen, 78, 202
    of Utrecht, 301
    of Vienna, 78, 200